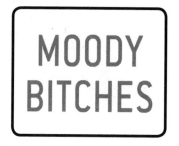

ALSO BY JULIE HOLLAND

Weekends at Bellevue

PENGUIN PRESS | NEW YORK | 2015

MOODY BITCHES

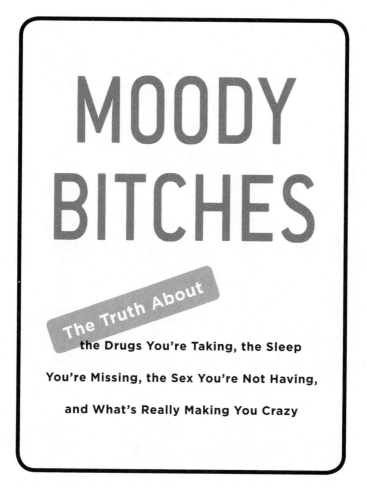

The Truth About the Drugs You're Taking, the Sleep You're Missing, the Sex You're Not Having, and What's Really Making You Crazy

JULIE HOLLAND, M.D.

PENGUIN PRESS
Published by the Penguin Group
Penguin Group (USA) LLC
375 Hudson Street
New York, New York 10014

USA · Canada · UK · Ireland · Australia
New Zealand · India · South Africa · China

penguin.com
A Penguin Random House Company

First published by Penguin Press, a member of Penguin Group (USA) LLC, 2015

ISBN 978-1-59420-580-4

Printed in the United States of America
1   3   5   7   9   10   8   6   4   2

DESIGNED BY AMANDA DEWEY

Neither the publisher nor the author is engaged in rendering professional advice or
services to the individual reader. The ideas, procedures, and suggestions contained
in this book are not intended as a substitute for consulting with your physician.
All matters regarding your health require medical supervision. Neither the
author nor the publisher shall be liable or responsible for any loss or damage
allegedly arising from any information or suggestion in this book.

For Sara Starr Wolff,
teacher, therapist, and gardener,
who wanted what she had, and said what she meant.
And for her son, Jeremy,
whose shining love and acceptance
allow me to blossom.

CONTENTS

Introduction   1

PART ONE   MOODY BY NATURE

One Own Your Moods   *13*

Two Bitchy Like Clockwork   *35*

PART TWO   MATING, MILFS, MONOGAMY, AND MENOPAUSE

Three This Is Your Brain on Love   *59*

Four Marriage and Its Discontents   *75*

Five Motherhead   *95*

Six Perimenopause: The Storm Before the Calm   *117*

PART THREE   THE MOODY BITCHES SURVIVAL GUIDE

Seven Inflammation: The Key to Everything   *147*

Eight Food: A Drug We Can't Resist   *165*

Nine So Tired We're Wired   *195*

Ten A Sex Guide That Actually Works   *215*

Eleven Your Body: Love It or Leave It   *245*

Twelve You. Need. Downtime.   *267*

Conclusion: Staying Sane in an Insane World   *289*

Acknowledgments   *297*

Appendix: Naming Names: A Guide to Selected Drugs   *301*

Glossary   *343*

Notes   *349*

Index   *407*

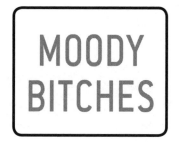

Introduction

W omen today are overworked and exhausted. We are anxious and frazzled, yet depressed and burned out. Our moods and libidos are at a rock-bottom low, our vital energies drained as we struggle to keep up with work, family, and hundreds of "friends" online. We blame ourselves for how bad we feel, thinking we should be able to handle it all. We dream of being perfect; we even try to make it look effortless, but we were never meant to be so static. We are designed by nature to be dynamic, cyclical, and, yes, moody. We are moody bitches, and that is a strength—not a weakness.

We evolved that way for good reasons; our hormonal oscillations are the basis for a sensitivity that allows us to be responsive to our environment. Our dynamism imparts flexibility and adaptability. Being fixed and rigid does not lend itself to survival. In nature, you adapt or you die. There is tremendous wisdom and peace available to us if we learn how our brains and bodies are supposed to work. Moodiness—being sensitive, caring deeply, and occasionally being acutely dissatisfied—is our natural source of power.

Yet we have been told just the opposite. From a young age, we are taught that moodiness, and all that comes with it, is a bad thing. We learn to apologize for our tears, to suppress our anger, and to fear being called hysterical. Over the course of women's lives, the stresses and expectations of the modern world interfere with our health and hormones in ways big and small, and the result is the malaise so many women feel. There simply is a better way.

Moody Bitches opens the playbook on how we can take hold of our moods and, in so doing, take hold of our lives. By integrating timeless wisdom with today's science, we can master our moods. If we can understand our own bodies, our naturally cycling hormones, and how modern medicines derange our exquisitely calibrated machines, then we can make informed choices about how to live better.

Women's hormones are constantly in flux. They ebb and flow over a month-long cycle and they wax and wane throughout decades of fertility, vacillating with particular volatility during adolescence and perimenopause, the spring and autumn of the reproductive years. Compare this to men's stable hormone levels throughout most of their lives. Our hormonal variations allow us to be empathic and intuitive—to our environment, to our children's needs, and to our partners' intentions. Women's emotionality is normal. It is a sign of health, not disease, and it is our single biggest asset. Yet one in four American women are choosing to medicate away their emotionality with psychiatric medications, and the effects are more far-reaching than most women realize.

Whether it's food, alcohol, drugs, cell phones, or shopping, we all rely on something in order to numb ourselves during difficult times. Whatever the chosen substance, it offers a welcome promise: that things will be different and better once it is consumed. But you can never get enough of something that *almost* works, and because our solutions are usually synthetic, not natural, we come up short. We are uncomfortable in our own skin, with our own desires; we are not at ease in our homes and offices, in our roles as parents or caretakers of our parents. Plowing forward, we think we can outrun the angst if we just stay "insanely busy."

In my psychiatric practice, my patients, like most women, are starved for information about the drugs they're taking and how they can change how they're feeling. *Moody Bitches* is an answer to both problems. I name names (which medicines I love, and the ones I avoid) and discuss the real side effects I've observed—weight gain, libido loss, becoming blasé—and what you can do about them. I share straight talk about enhancing your sex life, the direct link between food and mood, sticking to exercise or sleep schedules, and perhaps the most important piece: tuning in to your body to realign with your natural, primal self.

When I started my practice twenty years ago, women came to me confused by their symptoms and unsure of what to do. They complained of difficulty getting back to sleep or agitation or tearfulness, but they didn't quite know what was wrong. I helped them put a name to their symptoms and explained that there were medicines that could help. I needed to do more teaching about drug therapy back then, and a lot more hand-holding. I would set aside the last ten or fifteen minutes of the hour-long initial consultation in order to quell the fears of people who were wary of taking something that would alter their brain chemistry.

These days, new patients come to me sure that they need medicine for their nerves or their moods, like most of the other women they know. They want me only to help them figure out which one. The confusion used to be: "I can't understand why I keep waking up at four in the morning"; "It's so hard to get out of bed and I don't really care about anything"; "I'm angry all the time, and I don't know why." But over the years, the conversation has morphed, so that now it usually begins with something like this: "Can you tell me the difference between Wellbutrin and Effexor?"; "I can't figure out if I have ADD or OCD"; "Do you know that ad with the woman riding the horse on the beach?"; "Is that new butterfly sleeping pill better than Ambien?" And the one I hear more than you can imagine from my established patients: "Is there anything *new* I can try?"

The drug companies started direct-to-consumer advertising in the 1980s. Soon after I started my private practice in the mid-1990s, it became less heavily regulated. Ads started springing up on television and in magazines, trumpeting the latest antidepressants and sleeping pills. I went along for the ride as America's use of all prescription psychiatric medications tripled during the nineties, as a direct result of this powerful marketing. By 2006 the antidepressant Zoloft had made more money than Tide detergent, and it became clear to me that something new was happening. Drug companies are spending billions of dollars to turn normal human experiences like fear or sadness into medical diseases. They aren't developing cures; they're creating customers. The problem is not our emotionality; the problem is that we are being persuaded to medicate it away.

The latest news is particularly terrifying. Abilify, a medicine originally formulated to treat people with schizophrenia, expanded into the depression market and is now our nation's top-selling medication, and not just of psych meds. America's number one moneymaking medicine is an antipsychotic. As a psychiatrist, I must tell you, this is insane. There is an ancient Greek word, *pharmakon,* which held disparate meanings— sacrament, medicine, and poison. It is a common saying in medicine that sometimes the treatment is worse than the disease. There are many medications (chemotherapy is a good example) that are helpful or curative at lower doses but dangerously toxic in higher amounts. It is also true that there are powerful medicines that are appropriately used for one diagnosis but are complete overkill for another. Prescribing antipsychotics to treat depression seems particularly out of balance, especially given the risks of irreversible side effects like diabetes or movement disorders inherent in this class of medicine.

We represent 5 percent of the global population, yet we take 50 percent of the world's pills. (We also take 80 percent of the world's painkillers.) Meanwhile, the percentage of people labeled with psychiatric diagnoses is continually growing. Is it possible there really is an epidemic of mental illness and disability happening in our lifetime, or are physicians too quick to reach for their prescription pads instead of offering harder solutions to their patients' complaints? Medical journals are full of only one kind of ad: pages of information on the newest drugs and exactly how to prescribe them. Four out of five prescriptions for antidepressants are not even written by psychiatrists but rather by general practitioners, and more often than not they're prescribed for patients without an actual diagnosis of depression. Particularly troubling: surveys of primary care doctors show they routinely overestimate what the antidepressants can do. They've been hoodwinked by the ads, like the rest of America.

Just as offering your toddler the choice between the red dress and the blue dress moves the conversation forward, beyond "you need to wear a dress," the barrage of antidepressant advertising advances the question from *Should I take an antidepressant?* to *Which one should I take?* Don't let pharma-con change the way you manage your moodiness. I'm here to tell you that there are healthier ways to treat depression, anxiety, and irritability that don't include pills.

It is not solely the right cocktail of neurotransmitters that dictates mood; more than anything, it is how we live our lives. We can improve how we feel by changing behaviors around food, sex, exercise, addictions, and work/family balance. The problem with taking your happy pills and puttering along as before is that it's no better than sweeping dirt under the carpet. I want you to take that rug out back and beat the hell out of it.

But this is not drudgery. It begins with awareness, with the natural process of reconnecting with yourself and your body. Understanding the meaning and utility of your moods is empowering. Reclaiming your authentic, natural self is liberating. It is wholesome and it is healing. Not just for you, but also for your partner, your family, and your community.

This book begins with information about our complex inner workings, revealing the science behind why, as caregivers and nurturers, women have evolved to think and feel differently from men. I explain the wisdom of feeling deeply, and the dangers of cutting ourselves off from that depth. I look closely at why the twenty-eight-day cycle brings on tears and insatiable hunger (and what you can do about it), and how oral contraceptives and antidepressants can disrupt natural phases of desire and connection, potentially leading you to choose "Mr. Wrong," or even to opt out of any mate choice entirely.

The second section delves into relationships and family, with a particular focus on how women's moods mirror critical transition points in our lives. From menarche (the very first menstrual cycle) to mating, from motherhood to menopause, our ever-fluctuating hormones not only dictate but also respond to our behaviors. Testosterone may make you horny to go out and find a guy, but, more likely, seeing a hot new guy will make your testosterone levels rise. We tend to think of love and sex as distinct, but falling head over heels is a physical experience as powerful as any mind-altering drug, and orgasmic sex can trigger hormones that change how attached you are to your partner, complicating your casual hookups. The early stages of a relationship are difficult enough to navigate, but long-term commitment poses its own complications. *Moody Bitches* tells the truth about monogamy and desire, and why it is that your SSRI (antidepressants like Paxil or Zoloft) is likely not doing you any favors in the bedroom. I also explain the physical and emotional consequences of pregnancy and child rearing; becoming a mother changes not just your body but your brain.

Change is the constant in women's lives, and never more so than in perimenopause, the transitional period before fertility ends that recalls the turmoil of pubescence. *Moody Bitches* unpacks the biology behind the "cougar" stereotype, describes the herbs and supplements that can combat hot flashes, and paves the way for the peace and freedom that await on the other side.

The third section, the Moody Bitches Survival Guide, is an instruction manual for well-being at any age. We begin with a comprehensive introduction to inflammation, the basis of nearly every medical disease, including depression. Stress and inflammation are inextricably linked, and the key to combating both lies in a system you've probably never heard of, the endocannabinoid system. When stress nearly knocks you overboard, your internal cannabinoid system helps to right the ship. Even if you've never smoked a joint, your brain and body use cannabis-like molecules to make you resilient to stress, similar to the way your endorphin system provides you with natural pain relief. These cannabinoids tamp down inflammation and reactivity in the body, maintaining metabolism, immune functioning, learning, and growing. The endocannabinoid system is mentioned throughout *Moody Bitches*, because it is involved in nearly everything we do, like eating, sleeping, exercising, having sex, giving birth, and nursing.

The practices detailed in the survival guide are critical tools for establishing and preserving mental and physical health; they are designed to reduce stress and inflammation and augment the body's own spectacular capacity for producing pleasure. You'll learn about natural nutrition, so you can stop dieting and start eating for health, and normal sleep, so you can prioritize the hours your body needs. In fact, better sleep, nutrition, and regular cardio in the sunshine may just replace your SSRI. The survival guide also includes practical advice on sex that actually works and addresses the main obstacles women face in reaching orgasm. Getting into and enjoying your body, whether through sex, exercise, or that dreaded word *mindfulness,* will help you achieve the balance and harmony we're all clamoring for.

Moody Bitches is a rallying cry for a new way of living. Our lives are out of sync with nature. I fear that the further away we get from what's natural for us, the sicker we're going to get. Our disconnection is our pathology. We need to get back in tune with our bodies and with the natural world around us. In our digital distraction we've lost a basic truth: fresh air, sunlight, and movement make us feel better. Daily cycles of light and dark will do more for our sleep than any pill, being sedentary is our biggest health hazard, and we miss a lot when our relationships become virtual.

Moody Bitches is grounded in research and informed by my experiences in working with my patients. Health begins with understanding, and my aim is to demystify women's inner lives to enable change. I'm speaking as a psychiatrist, a wife, and a working mother of two children; the prescriptions I share here are what have worked for me, and for my patients.

Our bodies are wiser than we ever imagined, and so much of what plagues them is interrelated. Overmedication has robbed us of our sense of control, and modern life has separated us from the restorative rhythms of nature. It is understandable to respond to the man-made madness of this world with tears and frustration; those feelings of distress are a pathway toward health and wholeness. We need to tune in to our discomfort, not turn it down. Being sensitive, being irritated, and being vocal about our needs and frustrations will improve our lives.

Once we begin to listen to our bodies and align with our moodiness, we can take action. That action might be to try a natural remedy when you had relied on a prescription. It might be to reappraise all that you ask of yourself in your many roles as a woman. The answer for each of us will be unique. But all of us need to stop and listen when we get bitchy. Embracing our moods will, in the end, make us happier.

We need to begin anew, to realign with our bodies and learn how to treat them right. It's time to embody the wisdom inherent in nature, and in our natural animal selves. *Moody Bitches* will show you the way, giving you the tools you need to take care of yourself.

PART ONE

MOODY BY NATURE

One

Own Your Moods

While I spend most of my workday having one-on-one sessions with my patients, I've made several television appearances as a psychiatric expert over the years. One afternoon not long ago I sat down across from a newswoman in the studio. We were chatting before we rolled tape. She seemed pert, energetic, and emotionally connected. We hit it off immediately and were enjoying the hushed banter that ensues before taping; then I noticed her fingernails were bitten down quite a bit. When I asked her about it, she told me her therapist had consistently recommended she take medication to "calm her nerves," but she was resistant to the idea.

"I bet your anxiety helps you in your work," I offered. "You have to be hyperaware to know what's a good story to cover, and perceptive about when and how to push certain questions during an interview. Also, I would guess you have some obsessive traits that help you stay organized and productive, leaving no stone unturned."

She looked at me like I truly understood her. "Yes." She stared at me, dumbfounded. "Yes!" she repeated. "It's also just who I am: I am nervous, jumpy. I've always been like this. Why would I want to medicate away my own basic personality?"

Why indeed?

More women than ever before are taking psychiatric medications, creating a new normal that isn't normal at all. It is at odds with our biology. Our brains are wired differently from men's brains, and our hormones do make us more moody.

Women feel more, and for good reasons. By evolutionary design, women's brains have developed to encourage empathy, intuition, emotionality, and sensitivity. We are the caretakers and the life givers; our ability to recognize and respond to the needs and moods of others is key to their and our survival, the basis of family, community, and connection. We need to intuit when our children are in danger or in need, or when the men around us might have malevolent intent. We will subordinate when that's safest, but we will also aggressively protect those in our charge, whether family or friends.

Women have always been asked to do difficult work, and our bodies have powerful coping mechanisms to meet these challenges. But living with mechanisms like moodiness and acute sensitivity can be a trying experience on a daily basis. If that weren't enough, like the newswoman I met on set, we are all under constant pressure to restrain our emotional lives and our natural strengths.

THE ALTERED STATES OF AMERICA: ONE NATION, FEELING LIKE CRAP

It's not just that our hormones make us more moody. It's also that the pharmaceutical industry has exploited this biological attribute through advertising. Antidepressants are overwhelmingly marketed to women, stigmatizing depression as a feminine illness, making men less likely to seek treatment, and giving women the go-ahead to take their daily dose so they can cook for their families and dote on their children. Ads for antidepressants (and antipsychotics used to treat depression) are commonplace in women's magazines like *Good Housekeeping* and *Better Homes and Gardens,* and on daytime talk shows. They typically feature pictures of women with sad faces, staring out the window, unable to play with their neglected, frowning children or text their friends. (I wish I were kidding about this last one. The "after" picture for one antidepressant shows a woman now on meds, happily texting someone on her phone.) Many ads now encourage a woman to ask her doctor to consider adding an antipsychotic into the mix after a mere six-week trial of her antidepressant has "failed."

While the number of Americans on antidepressants has skyrocketed year after year, two big bumps are seen historically. The first was when direct-to-consumer advertising broadened in 1997, completely orchestrated by the Big Pharma lobbies. The other jump in sales came after 9/11, when pharmaceutical marketing homed in on women even more. That September, the women I saw in my office were acutely anxious, fearful for the safety of their Wall Street husbands or their children who were in downtown elementary schools near the attack. They were tense, twitchy, and unable to sleep. Coincidentally, the makers of Paxil came out with a print ad of a woman on a crowded city street, clutching her bag, jaw clenched, surrounded by words like "sleep problems" and "worry," with the tagline "Millions could be helped by Paxil." Drug makers had found 9/11 to be a marketing opportunity. Glaxo doubled its advertising to $16 million in October 2011, compared with the previous October's $8 million. That's just one month of advertising dollars to hook all the women who had a natural, fearful response to a terrorist act. And it paid off big. They got on their meds and stayed on them.

All of this direct-to-consumer advertising has given many of us, especially people who came of age in the 1990s, an inflated sense that we are lay psychopharmacologists. We've seen enough ads to know which medicines have lower incidences of sexual side effects (Wellbutrin, an antidepressant that does not raise serotonin levels) and which ones report an increased risk of sudden death (Abilify, an antipsychotic prescribed for depression, when used in elderly dementia patients). My mother often said, "A little bit of knowledge is a dangerous thing." Gen Xers are quick to stock up on pharmaceuticals garnered from friends, the Internet, and physicians, and dole them out to friends and family. As the *New York Times* explained, "they choose to rely on their own research and each other's experience in treating problems like depression . . . a medical degree, in their view, is useful but not essential."

At this point, everybody and their cat are on antidepressants. Seriously—one of my patients has an underweight cat that was recently prescribed Remeron, an antidepressant that can cause increased appetite. In today's insurance-driven health-care system, handing over a prescription is the easiest, quickest way for doctors to get someone out of their office so they can see their next patient. It also keeps the patients coming back for easy, efficient refills. Unfortunately, shorter doctors' visits, now the norm, mean more time spent alleviating symptoms with pills and less spent digging down to really fix the problem. There is simply no talking about the harder but healthier ways to treat the symptoms. Cholesterol-lowering medicines called statins are a good example. A doctor can spend twenty minutes trying to educate a patient about dietary changes and exercise that could lower cholesterol levels, or can hand over a prescription for a pill being pushed by every drug rep who comes to the office bearing a tray of cheese Danish.

Women are particularly vulnerable to overprescribing. Numerous medical chart reviews consistently show that doctors are more likely to give women psychiatric medications than men, especially women between the ages of thirty-five and sixty-four, who often present with complaints of nervousness, difficulty sleeping, sexual dysfunction, or low energy. A patient recently asked me if he should take Risperdal, an anti-psychotic, for his nervousness, because his female colleague told him it had been helping her with anxious thoughts. Risperdal was originally formulated for use in schizophrenia, but people with schizophrenia make up only 1 percent of the world's population. It's obviously better business to target 50 percent of the population: women. This is pharma-con in action.

I'm not suggesting that all use of psychiatric medicines is counter-productive. People who don't really need these meds are taking them, while people who are genuinely psychiatrically ill remain undiagnosed and untreated, often due to socioeconomic factors. Clearly there are times when we need to pull out the big guns. Vegetative depressions that last for weeks, when you can't get out of bed, bathe, or feed yourself, are not going to resolve themselves through soul-searching. Manic episodes where there is no sleep to be had for many days in a row will require mood stabilizers. But we've gotten ourselves into a situation in America now where more women are taking antidepressants and antianxiety medications for years on end, and it's lowering the bar for all of us, creat-ing a new normal in terms of invulnerable posturing and emotional blunting, and, more important, it is changing the tipping point for when other women will seek chemical assistance.

Cosmetic psychopharmacology is not unlike cosmetic surgery. As more women get breast implants, the rest of us feel flat chested. And so it is with more women taking antidepressants and antianxiety medica-tions. Suddenly, you're the odd one out if you aren't like your friends, tak-ing something to "take the edge off" or give you a little lift to withstand the slings and arrows on your journey. More women are feeling lousy and finding themselves on psychiatric medications, and staying on them far longer than they were ever meant to be used. And we're not necessarily getting any better.

MADE TO BE MOODY

As women, our interior lives are complex and ever changing. Our neurotransmitters and our hormones—estrogen in particular—are intricately linked. When estrogen levels drop, as in PMS, postpartum, or perimenopause, it's common for moods to plummet as well. Waxing and waning levels of estrogen help us to be more emotional, allow us to cry more easily and even to break down when we're overwhelmed. There are estrogen receptors throughout the brain that affect our mood and behavior, and there are complex back-and-forth interactions in the brain between estrogen and serotonin, the main neurotransmitter implicated in anxiety and depression. Although it's more complicated than I'm making it out to be, it's helpful to think of serotonin and estrogen as yoked. When one is up, the other is likely to be as well. So it is not your imagination. Where you are in your reproductive cycle, monthly and over your lifetime, is an enormous factor in determining what you are feeling.

Think of serotonin as the "it's all good" brain chemical. Too high and you don't care much about anything; too low and everything seems like a problem to be fixed. When serotonin levels are lower, as is seen in PMS, emotional sensitivity is heightened. We're less insulated and end up more cranky, irritable, and dissatisfied. The most common antidepressants, also used to treat anxiety, are serotonin reuptake inhibitors (SSRIs). These are medicines (such as Prozac, Zoloft, Paxil, Celexa, and Lexapro) that block the brain's natural recycling of the serotonin back into the nerve cell, so more can get across to the next neuron. If your serotonin levels are constantly, artificially high, you're at risk of losing the emotional sensitivity that makes you *you*. You may be less likely to cry in the office or bite your nails to the quick, but you're also going to have a harder time reacting emotionally and connecting fully with others, especially sexually.

SSRIs not only affect behavior, they alter perception of the environment. If the "it's all good" chemical is bathing your brain, will you really try very hard to fix anything? At higher doses, SSRIs sometimes promote apathy and indifference. Patients report having less motivation overall. When one of my patients becomes blasé about things, making the big *W* sign for "whatever" about life, it's a sign to me that she might be overmedicated, and it's time to taper down the happy pills. Being more complacent and apathetic can have disastrous effects on your life, both at home and at work.

Sometimes, if I see a patient with crippling depression or anxiety, then prescribing an SSRI is the right call, but even if it is the best initial treatment, it might not be the forever cure. Feeling deeply may, at times, be difficult to navigate, but it's also a powerful tool, in the workplace and at home, and it's essential for growth. We are built to be highly attuned and reactive, and embracing that truth is the first step in gaining mastery of our inner lives and our health.

HARDWIRED TO FEEL

Women's brains develop differently from men's, and the distinctions make for profound differences in how we process and communicate emotions. All brains develop along the same pathway in the womb, but things change for boys at eight weeks, once the testes become functional. With testosterone in the mix, a surge in the male sex hormone kills off many cells in the communication centers and grows more neurons slated for action, aggression, and sexual drive. In men, these brain areas take up two and a half times the space they do in women.

Even more brain changes occur after gestation, during adolescence, when sex hormones surge, further differentiating the sexes. As the female brain develops, more space and more brain cells are reserved for language, hearing, and memory. Our memory center, the hippocampus, is larger than men's, perhaps reflecting an evolutionary advantage of remembering details of emotional events and the crucial behaviors of our potential mates, especially what they said they'd do versus what actually happened. Our memories have an influence on our emotions. The hippocampus can calm the hair-trigger responses of the amygdala, the area of the brain devoted to fear, aggression, and anger. The amygdalae are larger in men and have receptors for testosterone.

Ever wonder why you can lose it and then calm down, but those feelings continue to echo for your husband? Women's larger hippocampi and smaller amygdalae may add up to our having better control over our emotional outbursts than men, particularly when it comes to actions involving fear or aggression. We might react emotionally, but then we pull it together, thanks to the hippocampus.

We are not living in a world that is kind to this sort of behavioral response, though. When under acute stress, the amygdala gains in functionality and the hippocampus loses, one reason you panic and can't remember as well when pushed. The biggest problems come with chronic stress, where the hippocampus loses not just functionality but brain cells. It becomes atrophied, can no longer quiet the raging amygdala, and then all responses to stressors are amplified. This is what is seen in post-traumatic stress disorder, and it may well be seen in anyone undergoing chronic stress.

Intuiting the motives and feelings of others is an essential social skill that is employed unconsciously and automatically and has been characterized as quintessentially feminine. The better we are at sensing our body's signs of arousal (feeling our own heartbeat, for example), the better we are at judging emotions in ourselves and others. The insula, thought to be the seat of self-awareness, empathy, and interpersonal experience, helps us to understand others and is noticeably bigger in women. The insula not only helps us process "gut feelings," to figure out what we and others are feeling emotionally, but also enables us to experience and recognize body sensations. What has often been labeled "female intuition" has served women well in their traditional roles as caregivers and nurturers. The ability to intuit the emotions and desires of others has helped women better predict whether a man may become violent or abandon the children, or whether our nonverbal babies are hungry or in pain.

Men aren't built to be as sensitive as women are. Women have more brain circuitry not only for expressing language and emotion but also for detecting emotional nuance and anticipating what others are feeling. Given that there is such a gender discrepancy with this empathic system, it's likely not your imagination that your boyfriend has no idea what he's feeling half the time (called alexithymia) and has even less facility at communicating it. Testosterone impairs empathy and the ability to intuit others' emotions by reading their eyes. Being aware of or oblivious to others' needs is bound to affect how giving a person is, one reason you might think of him as selfish.

We register conflict more deeply than men, and get more stressed out about it as well. No doubt some of this is learned behavior, as girls are often encouraged to keep the peace more than boys, but there is a strong biological component. When men are threatened, their bodies go into "fight or flight" mode, with adrenaline surging to provide energy to muscles. When stress levels are high in women, "tend and befriend" behavior often predominates. Women are more likely to band together in the face of adversity, creating strength in numbers, huddling together to save the children and one another. Oxytocin, the hormone released in women after orgasm and during cuddling or nursing, encourages prosocial, trusting behavior, while testosterone tends to fuel aggressive, competitive behavior. In both men and women, high testosterone levels blunt oxytocin levels, and vice versa, so there is give-and-take between aggression and bonding. Oxytocin's release affects women more powerfully than men, helping us to be more generous and connected. It also helps us to figure out who is in and who is out of our circle of contacts, our tribe. In hostile environments, or with unsupportive contacts, oxytocin may actually enhance the stress responses, even playing out as aggression toward strangers. Protective mothers' maternal aggression has been linked to oxytocin, for example.

Girls flock together and keep social harmony, often through language. Staying connected via gossip and verbal intimacy leads to a rush of dopamine, one of the brain's pleasure chemicals, and oxytocin. Estrogen triggers dopamine and oxytocin production in pubescent girls. Midcycle, these hormones peak, as do verbal output and desire for intimacy. Whereas women tend to discuss troublesome issues with peers, men tend to process their troubles alone, nonverbally. This may reflect the balance of oxytocin versus testosterone. Testosterone inhibits talking and the drive to socialize. For boys, self-esteem comes from being independent, not interconnected. Boys aren't as communicative, and they aren't nearly as derailed by conflict and competition. It's part of who they are, and, perhaps equally important, who they're expected to be.

The connections between the areas of the brain that process emotion are more active and extensive in women. Women have nine areas devoted to this function, compared with only two in men. Women also have more bilateral processing of emotions in their brains, going left to right, right to left, connecting the analytic and emotional areas, whereas men tend to stay more within each hemisphere. So we could say that women are using their whole brains while men are often using only half of theirs at a time. Women do seem to be better at multitasking than men. Men not only have more difficulty juggling multiple priorities but they are also slower and less organized than women when switching between them.

Men's brains have more linkages with their cerebellum, the control center for movement, so for men, there may be less time between seeing and doing than there is for women. Men tend to outperform women on motor and spatial cognitive tasks, while women are faster in tasks of emotional identification and nonverbal reasoning. We also outperform men on a "lost key" challenge; maybe this is why our families ask us where everything is, and, more important, why we know the answer. Because men were primarily the hunters and we the foragers, it was crucial that we remembered where we last found the good food.

Obviously, we must be cautious in discussing differences between the sexes because there is a large variation within each gender, and nurture and culture factor in nearly as much as nature does. There is interplay between our natural abilities and how we are molded to behave that is impossible to fully tease apart. Case studies of children with ambiguous genitalia who are raised to be male or female even though they possess the opposite genetic material are rare, but they do help to teach us one thing: the influence of biology cannot be underestimated. Often, our own balance of testosterone and estrogen levels dictates how aggressive we'll be in a pickup game of basketball (or if we'd ever be caught dead in a pickup game of basketball) more than anything our parents ever taught us.

THE DOWNSIDE TO FEELING DEEPLY

While biology may provide women with a set of attributes, from brain structures to hormones, that are advantageous in our traditional roles of nurturing and caregiving, there is a downside. These same attributes may also make us more inclined to suffer from depression and anxiety. In childhood, no difference exists in the prevalence of depressive disorders between girls and boys. In adulthood, women are twice as likely as men to experience depression and two to four times more likely to be diagnosed with an anxiety disorder like panic attacks or generalized anxiety.

The increased risk begins early in adolescence as puberty strikes. It ends by age sixty, when hormonal cycling ceases. Although some of the increased incidence of depression in women may result from societal factors like body image pressures, or their greater tendency to seek help for mental health issues, or diagnostic bias among doctors, there is strong evidence that much of the gender difference in mood disorders is linked to hormones.

Some women are more susceptible to hormonal fluctuations than others. There is a subgroup of women who seem to be at risk for what's called reproductive depression, that is, mood changes caused by variations in hormone levels, like those seen prior to menstruation or after delivery. If you're the PMS type, you're also more likely to have postpartum depression or perimenopausal mood instability. Certain women have a specific sensitivity to these hormonal changes while some lucky ones don't, possibly dictated by genes governed by changing estrogen levels. The good news is, when your hormones aren't fluctuating, like when you're postmenopausal, the risk for depression isn't elevated. After menopause, the risks even out, especially two years after the final menstrual period, when the dust has settled. There is truth to the idea that the years after menopause are a real prime time of life for many women, both professionally and personally.

Again, there are likely evolutionary reasons for mood variability being tied to hormonal fluctuations. There is a positive mood state (called euthymia) in the first half of the menstrual cycle, leading up to ovulation, that encourages a woman to connect with mates and conceive. The more depressed, progesterone-heavy state in the second half of the cycle helps to ensure the safety of the product of conception by keeping the woman passive, cautious, and out of danger. Progesterone rises during the second half of the menstrual cycle and surges even higher if an egg is fertilized. It is the main hormone that maintains pregnancy. Progesterone is implicated in premenstrual syndrome, postpartum depression, and dysthymia, a chronic low-grade depression. The increased incidences of depression and anxiety during pregnancy (particularly in the first trimester) and the immediate postpartum period come during crucial periods for the baby, when more cautious and isolative maternal behavior can help ensure the baby's survival. If women develop these behaviors, whether conserving precious energy or avoiding dangerous situations, then these traits will be passed on. Viva Darwin.

Anxious and depressed behaviors have survived in our gene pool for millennia because they are adaptive. They confer an advantage to our survival and that of our offspring. An anxious, obsessive forager will not only find more food, but will also return home safely. She is also more likely to keep her children out of harm's way. Likewise, a depressed woman will more quickly withdraw from wasted enterprises, whether pursuing food or a mate, and conserve her energy. This may be the basis for seasonal affective disorder, which causes lower energy and motivation when food supplies are most scarce.

When women feel under threat, estrogen helps us to "maintain," to be resilient and bounce back. In this way, estrogen is really acting as a stress hormone. One of the ways estrogen builds resilience is by enhancing serotonin levels, which help to keep us fortified, calmer, more rational, and less emotional. Serotonin activity is greater during higher estrogen levels. When estrogen surges, it causes more serotonin to be made, and it also causes serotonin receptors to be made. But, as with most things in the body, what goes up must come down. The natural process of stress triggering surging estrogen levels has a built-in stop mechanism, which then normalizes our serotonin levels.

SSRIs are the most common treatment for depression and anxiety, but if you're on SSRIs, with steady serotonin levels, you miss out on this natural ebb and flow of serotonin in response to estrogen. You stay more rational and less emotional. Estrogen fluctuations help to keep us sensitive. SSRIs deaden our sensitivities.

More women than men get depressed, and estrogen may have a lot to do with this. Estrogen affects how serotonin functions in the brain. Women are more vulnerable to changes in serotonin levels and more responsive to drugs and medicines that affect serotonin. This is one reason that women may be more affected by sexual side effects of SSRIs than men. So where you are in your menstrual cycle or your perimenopausal staging will have effects on your mood, like how irritable, sensitive, or impulsive you are, as these behaviors are affected by serotonin. As you'll see in the next chapter, it's normal to have times in your cycle when your estrogen is lower, which means your serotonin will follow suit and you'll feel lousy. It's temporary and it's natural. You don't necessarily need daily antidepressants to mask these moods.

SSRIs can do many wonderful things for people with serious depression, and I have to admit that my patients love the way they make them feel, at least at first, but they can also take many sensations away. SSRIs tend to blunt negative feelings more than they boost the positive ones. On SSRIs, you probably won't be skipping around gaily with a grin plastered on your face; it's just that you're less likely to feel tearful, irritable, and hopeless. People on SSRIs report less of many other human traits: an ability to cry, irritation, care about others' feelings, sadness, erotic dreaming, creativity, surprise, anger, expression of their feelings, and worry.

One of my best friends from college told me a story of when she was first prescribed Prozac. "It really scaled back my empathy. Since I was a young girl, I've always felt bad if someone else felt bad. It's a big part of who I am. I would let the other kids find the Easter eggs during the hunt, because they seemed to want them more than I did. When I first went on Prozac, I remember seeing another woman crying and thinking, *Looks like you have a personal problem. Sucks to be you.* This is what it must feel like to be a dude." SSRIs affect emotional processing and turn down the empathy response. This can have devastating effects on the ability to parent or to maintain relationships.

IT'S ALL RIGHT TO CRY AND GET ANGRY

Antidepressants can be utilized as a starting point for benefiting from psychotherapy or creating lifestyle changes, but once those behaviors are firmly in place, the medications often can and should be tapered off. If you break your leg, you don't keep the cast and crutches forever. Before you commit to a lifelong SSRI prescription, consider the dynamic emotional range you might be giving up.

My patients on SSRIs will report, "I knew the situation was upsetting. I was supposed to be feeling sad, but I couldn't cry." Crying isn't just about sadness. When we are frustrated, when we are angry, when we see injustice, when we are deeply touched by the poignancy of humanity, we cry. And some women cry more easily than others. It's normal. It's how we're designed, and it doesn't mean we're weak or out of control.

Crying allows us to deeply feel what we're feeling and then move on. It is a crescendo that naturally leads to a denouement of intensity. For most women, this depth of feeling is a birthright, but if you really can't stand crying, or get frustrated because you can't speak when your throat tightens, here are two tricks that work well instead of meds. Simply think up lists of rhyming words, or subtract sevens from one hundred. Shunting blood away from the emotional centers and over to the rational verbal or calculating areas will mollify most people. (You just have to remember to do it, which means relying on your hippocampus to tamp down your amygdala.)

There are times when it's inconvenient, to say the least, to cry, but there are other times when it's to your advantage. Letting yourself cry can be important in communicating with your partner. A clear, visible sign that we're upset may be just what men need. Women pick up subtle signs of sadness in others 90 percent of the time. Men are better able to discern anger and aggression; when trying to decide whether their female partner is sad, men are right only 40 percent of the time. That's less than if they flipped a coin to help them answer. This is also a reason to express your feelings verbally and not expect your male partner to know how you're feeling by how you look or act. They're simply not constructed for intuiting emotion the way we are. As for families, sometimes it's a good idea to let your kids see you cry, especially if they've scared you with reckless behavior or frustrated you with thoughtlessness. Tears can underscore lessons in how their behavior affects others.

But we clearly have issues around our tears. Have you ever noticed how often women apologize for crying? In part it's because men are uncomfortable with expressed emotion, and so they, and we, have been socialized to shut it down. Another part is that emotion interferes with the forward-momentum agenda so prevalent in our society. The problem with shutting it down is that we're stifling a piece that we need, that our partners and families need, and that the world needs.

Being sad can help us make clear-eyed assessments of our lives. Depressed people are no longer in denial about unpleasant or hurtful truths. SSRIs can create complacency in times when action is needed, perhaps to leave an abusive spouse or a dead-end job. Medication can make a bad situation tolerable and mask the need for change. In one study of medicated women, "these patients continued to lead dysfunctional lives, and their motivation for major lifestyle changes seemed to decrease as depressive symptoms improved." In such situations, the symptoms of depression, unpleasant though they may be, can be the clarion call to action.

Another issue to consider: stuffing down your feelings is going to make you miserable. The suppression of anger in particular is a crucial factor in depression. People who've experienced depression are more likely to hold in their anger and fear expressing it, believing they must hide their feelings to preserve their relationships. Depressed patients have higher levels of anger than control subjects; the more anger, the more severe the depression.

In my office, I see evidence of this link frequently. Many of my female patients have no idea how to express their anger in healthy ways, and their suppressed anger contributes to their depression and, I believe, other medical symptoms as well. They weren't taught as young girls that it was okay to be angry, and they weren't schooled in how to handle this kind of emotion. Sugar and spice don't make space for anything that's not nice. When we don't even know we're angry, we can't converse with the person responsible or otherwise tackle the problem. We cry; we eat; we soothe ourselves a thousand different ways. Instead, we need to fully feel our feelings of anger, figure out where they are coming from, pull ourselves together, and then head out the door for a face-to-face conversation. I had a patient who called me from her office in tears, saying she needed to go up on her SSRI because she couldn't be seen crying at work. After dissecting why she was upset (her boss had humiliated and betrayed her in front of her staff), we decided that what was needed was calm confrontation, not more medication.

In an examination of women's employment reviews, certain words show up repeatedly, like *bossy, abrasive, strident,* and *aggressive.* This is when they lead; words like *emotional* and *irrational* are used when they object. Men are exhorted to be more aggressive in the workplace, but not so with women. What's interesting is that SSRIs reduce aggression, poor

impulse control, and irritability while increasing cooperation and affiliative behaviors. Primate research shows that SSRIs augment social dominance behaviors, elevating an animal's status in the hierarchy. So they
may well help women get along, and even get ahead, in the workplace,
but at what cost?

I notice in my female patients a certain self-consciousness about
being assertive. "I think, maybe" is the way a woman begins her sentence
even when she knows damn well that she's right. We hem and haw to
seem as if we're unsure, even though we should trust our gut and speak
firmly and bravely. Growing up, I was taught, directly and indirectly,
how to couch my ideas so they'd be taken as suggestions or opinions and
not as statements of facts. I will not teach my daughter to tone down her
self-confidence when she speaks. Little girls need every ounce of self-
esteem they can get. It's much easier to soften the edges later in life than
it is to build up a foundation of self-worth. And girls who hold on to their
assertiveness and self-esteem are less likely to grow up to be depressed
women.

THE H WORD

In the nineteenth century, hysteria was a uniquely female diagnosis that
became a catchall for many women's complaints that couldn't be immediately remedied. Nearly all physicians were men in the 1800s, and they
lumped a number of physical and emotional symptoms reported by
women under one heading, derived from the Greek word for uterus, *hys-
tera*. Criteria for hysteria included malaise, headaches, irritability, nervousness, insomnia, fatigue, low libido, high libido, water retention, and,
eventually, any behavior undesirable to society, such as organizing the
right for women to vote. One treatment for hysteria involved bringing the
patient to orgasm, while another, clitoridectomy, involved surgical re-

moval of the clitoris, and was performed throughout the 1880s and into the 1920s.

These days, hysteria has a more specific meaning: excessive expression of emotion, especially vulnerabilities such as despair or panic. If a woman behaves in a way that a man finds uncontrollable or inconvenient, she will be accused of being hysterical, basically being told she doesn't have a right to feel or act that way because it isn't in line with how a man would feel or act. Keep in mind, many a boy grows up at the mercy of his mother's emotions, and so men fear the emotionality of women. This may be one reason that some male doctors are quick to squelch any expression of emotion in their female patients, most easily by reaching for a prescription pad.

While the term *hysteria* is no longer officially used in medicine, there is the increasingly common diagnosis of the "women's disease" fibromyalgia. Symptoms include mysterious muscle aches, joint pain, and exhaustion. Coincidentally, the current treatment for fibromyalgia is antidepressants. Epidemiological studies show a female-to-male preponderance of three-to-one for chronic pain diagnoses like fibromyalgia. Men are less apt to receive a diagnosis of fibromyalgia than women, even if they have the same symptoms.

In my office, I often hear stories of misdiagnosis from my female patients. They offer lists of physical complaints to their male doctors, who are quick to dismiss them as hysterical, though they never utter that word if they're smart. "You're just stressed" is a popular conclusion offered instead, or else they're saddled with the diagnosis of fibromyalgia and treated, conveniently, with the same medicine they'd get if they were "just stressed"—antidepressants. Over the years, I've had multiple patients misdiagnosed with fibromyalgia when in fact they had Lyme disease, lupus, hypothyroidism, rheumatoid arthritis, or, in one case, ovarian cancer.

Women's sensitivities extend to the physical; our bodies feel more pain than men's do. There is overwhelming laboratory evidence that women have lower thresholds for pain, experience greater pain intensity, and have a lower tolerance for experimentally induced pain. Women are also more apt to notice aches and pains in their bodies, due to their neurologic underpinnings, particularly their more active insulae. We have more serotonin receptors to process pain, and our hormones estrogen and progesterone affect endorphin transmission and opiate receptors, leading to higher perceptions of pain.

It is important to note that where we are in our menstrual cycle also affects our pain sensitivity. We are more sensitive not just to social slights before our periods but to physical pain as well. Add to this the fact that many of us do somaticize, that is, focus on how our body feels and convey that to others. Again, this may be the insula in action. Some of our awareness and discussion of our physical pain may be caused by our experiencing, but not giving a voice to, the psychic pain of feeling put-upon or burdened. Our psyches are silently screaming for attention and relief, but we translate that psychic pain into bodily pain, which is easier to attempt to eradicate with medications and the attention of (often male) physicians.

The study of pain specific to women is in its infancy. In the journal *Pain*, nearly 80 percent of the studies included male subjects only, with only 8 percent studying females only. Medicine is not keeping pace with the pain so many women suffer. Men presenting with the same symptoms as women are taken more seriously and given a more thorough diagnostic workup. You see this in reports of chest pain, in lung cancer, and in general complaints and diagnostic workups. Without a doubt, you see it the most in psychiatric complaints.

Women are still, very simply, second-class citizens in the world of medicine. Until recently, surgeons knew much less about female pelvic anatomy and nerve-sparing surgery for women than for men. This ignorance has translated into thousands of hysterectomies (our country performs this operation more than any other) with avoidable complications, like diminished or absent orgasms or urinary incontinence.

Nearly all medical research, and in particular drug research, is still performed on male subjects, whether animal or human. Later, when the drugs come to market, problems specific to women may surface only after the drug has been in use for many years. Eight of ten drugs withdrawn from the market between 1997 and 2001 posed greater health risks for women than for men. After twenty years on the market, the sleeping pill Ambien finally has a separate recommended dose for women, half the strength of the usual dose, because it turns out that women metabolize the drug differently, having higher levels in their blood from the same dose. People are finally talking about the fact that women are unrepresented in clinical studies, but until the medical community better recognizes the complexity of the female brain and body—and how they differ from men's—we will be at a disadvantage.

We are not men. We are women. We feel more deeply, express our emotions more frequently, and get moody monthly. It's normal. It's nature's way. And we don't necessarily have to medicate away the essence of who we are to make others more comfortable. In fact, once we better understand our bodies and our own moods, we will realize that as women we have many natural tools for tackling all of the challenges of our busy, complex lives.

Two

Bitchy
Like Clockwork

S ome days you feel like a rock star. Some days you feel like a rock. This has a lot to do with where you are in your monthly cycle. Your mood is likely at its best during the first half of your menstrual cycle, called the follicular phase, where the ovary nurtures a developing egg. This is when estrogen levels climb and dominate progesterone levels. Estrogen helps you feel alluring, nurturing, and forgiving— all qualities that help you attract and entrance a mate, as your egg matures and becomes ready for ovulation. Because estrogen acts as a stress hormone, little difficulties slip away like water off a duck's back. Who wouldn't want to be with you? You're so easy to be with!

The second half of the cycle, the luteal phase, is the two weeks between when the egg is released from the follicle and when your period starts. This is where mood complaints will occur, when progesterone dominates estrogen. Progesterone can make you feel sluggish and cranky, and it peaks at day twenty-one. Right before your period, estrogen levels drop hard and fast, and so does your goodwill toward others. If you get a little bitchy like clockwork every month, blame low estrogen and high progesterone. Welcome to PMS, premenstrual syndrome.

PMS is natural. Not fun, but normal. But in the "bible" that psychiatrists use to diagnose illness, the *Diagnostic and Statistical Manual of Mental Disorders,* premenstrual dysphoric disorder (PMDD), an extreme form of PMS, is listed as a pathological state, implying that it requires psychiatric treatment. Somewhere between 3 and 8 percent of women of reproductive age meet the criteria for PMDD. About 15 to 20 percent of women have horrendous PMS or none at all; the rest of us fall somewhere in between, and where we lie can shift from month to month and, more important, from menarche (the beginning of monthly periods in adolescence) to perimenopause, the two phases of our lives where PMS tends to worsen due to more erratic hormone fluctuations.

Crying at the drop of a hat, having a short fuse, feeling overwhelmed and underappreciated, craving chocolate, and not being able to get off the couch are all fair game during the days leading up to your period. Lower estrogen levels cause serotonin levels to drop precipitously a few days before menstruation, which may be the biological basis of many PMS symptoms. Low levels of serotonin are implicated in depression, panic disorder, and obsessive-compulsive disorder (OCD), so don't be surprised if you feel a bit like a psych patient (or three) before your period starts. Less serotonin is like less insulation available to protect you from the outside world. You're even more physically sensitive to pain than usual, and more emotionally sensitive to criticism. You're less resilient in the face of stresses and feel sadder, hungrier, and more scared, tearful, and angsty. When you stack up PMS symptoms against those of a major depressive episode, there is a massive overlap. The big difference is that PMS goes away once your period starts. Major depression persists for weeks or months.

Typically PMS arises in the three or four days before your period starts, but a handful of my patients report their PMS symptoms starting a day or two after ovulation. They become terribly depressed, hopeless, and despairing. They get into fights more easily with family members and coworkers. They have trouble getting to sleep or staying asleep and feel bloated and crabby. A few of my patients assure me their PMS is mild, but pretty much everyone notices that "the period before their period" does bring some significant and noticeable changes in mood. Because it is perfectly normal to have mood fluctuations throughout your monthly cycles, you don't necessarily need to medicate PMS away, but you do need to educate yourself about it. I also strongly recommend that you keep track of your cycle, jotting down when your period starts and when you ovulate. If you keep track of when certain mood symptoms occur, not only will it help you to plan your monthly calendar but it might help to keep certain family members, and maybe even coworkers, in the loop on what to expect.

Besides getting a good sense of when you're fertile, keeping track of your cycle will give you a heads-up about when you're going to be more emotionally sensitive and reactive. You can plan to take on more challenging assignments at the beginning of your cycle right after your period, when your resilience is higher. The peak estrogen levels seen toward the middle of your cycle mean improvement of verbal and fine motor skills, so plan your business presentations and sewing projects for that time of the month. You should definitely leave the tasks best suited to someone with OCD, like cleaning out your closets, for during the PMS part of your cycle. Also, your pain tolerance is at its lowest point during PMS. Not a great time to go to the dentist or get waxed. Schedule those appointments during the first half of your cycle.

Commonly my patients tell me that it's easier for them to cry during the few days before their period. There is a phenomenon called rejection sensitivity that is often seen in clinically depressed patients. When your serotonin levels are bottomed out in depression, you're more sensitive to everything, and it takes less of an insult or slight from someone for your feelings to be hurt. It's no different in the days leading up to your period. Hurtful comments are going to hit you harder. Women cry more easily during PMS, and it's not just the mean things that others say. There is an increased sensitivity to schmaltzy television commercials and corny country songs on the radio. If I get a lump in my throat when I see anything poignant on the streets of New York—a homeless schizophrenic rooting through the garbage, a businessman stopping to help tourists fumbling with a map—I know just where I am in my cycle.

Our emotional lives revolve around our own internal clockwork, and understanding that schedule requires attention. Keep track of when you're horny, when you're bitchy, when you're flirty, and when you want to kick ass and take names. Becoming intimate with your rhythms will allow you to use natural fluctuations to your advantage, and establishing a baseline is the only way to accurately identify changes. This becomes especially important when starting or stopping a medication, especially those—such as oral contraceptives or SSRIs—that provide an unnatural stability. Their potential impact on mood, libido, and more is real, and you may find that that they're taking more than they're giving.

LEARNING FROM PMS

Being a crybaby is one thing, and maybe you could say that it is an endearing exacerbation of womanly empathy and vulnerability, but it hardly ends there. This increased sensitivity, especially to criticism, can cause explosive reactivity. My patients with PMS notice that they get snappy and easily irritated by things they would typically let slide the rest of the month. They become more unpredictable in their responses, and they can let loose with utterances or actions that are not in their repertoire the other three weeks of their cycle. This has to do with the frontal lobes inhibiting the emotional centers, which require solid doses of serotonin. Closer to PMS means lower serotonin levels, so for some of us, the closer we get to our periods, the more likely it is that the "bitch switch" is on. But it's not that we're getting upset over nothing.

We are getting upset over real things, it's just that we usually hide our sadness and anger better. Thanks to high estrogen levels, we are usually more resilient. Breezy, even. We allow for others' needs better and can remain detached more convincingly. Natural cycles of caring less and more correlate with our menses. A good way to think of estrogen is as the "whatever you want, honey" hormone. Estrogen creates a veil of accommodation. Designed to encourage grooming and attracting a mate, and then nurturing and nourishing our family members, estrogen is all about giving to others: keeping our kids happy and our mates satisfied. When estrogen levels drop before our periods, that veil is lifted. We are no longer alluring and fertile; we are no longer so invested in the potential daddy sticking around. It's time to clean house. During the rest of the month you put up with all kinds of bull that you won't tolerate the week before your period.

I say, let it be a lesson to you. Perhaps you should be putting up with less all month long. The dissatisfaction that comes on a monthly schedule is a gift to you, a chance to make some much-needed changes in how you're living your life and how much you're giving, bending, and stretching to meet everyone else's expectations. What I stress with my patients is this: the thoughts and feelings that come up during this phase of your cycle are real; they are genuine. If you're feeling overwhelmed or underappreciated, that you're taking on more than your partner, or that things are out of balance, chances are it's all true.

Remember that our animal imperative is to reproduce. Every cycle is a chance to propagate the species. Just as your hormones allow your uterus to fluff up and prepare for a new embryo, they also push you to "nest." When a woman is in the later months of her pregnancy and progesterone levels are at their highest, there is a frenzy that overtakes her to clean the house and prepare for the arrival of her baby. Every month, when your body prepares for a possible embryo implantation, progesterone levels are building and causing a smaller form of nesting. Toward the end of the cycle, a woman might become dissatisfied with her environment and obsessive about making changes in order to make sure the setting is appropriate next month for the burrowing of the embryo into the uterine lining. PMS is a time of psychological inventory, to take stock and make sure you are where you want to be in your life. Every cycle is an opportunity for a fresh start, to make your life over the way you want it. Pay attention to that critical eye, to those judgmental thoughts. They are probably more valid than you'd like to believe, and I bet they're actionable, too.

Women's empathic skills can be a great source of useful information and strength, and there is some evidence that they are highest during our premenstrual days. PMS is a great time to tune in to intuition. Because of lower serotonin levels, we are more "raw" and less emotionally blanketed before we menstruate. It is a time to rest and reflect and to honor deep feelings. Sensitivity is dismissed in our culture, but it really does have its advantages. PMS is an opportunity to listen to your body and to honor your feelings. Trust your PMS bitchiness. And put it to good use the rest of the month. Harness the knowledge you garner when you're more critical, write it down, and put it into action when you're more genteel and diplomatic, as soon as your period ends. Try this for a month or two and see if you don't have some "new month's resolutions" of your own.

CHOCOLATE AND OTHER TREATMENT OPTIONS

In both depression and PMS, food cravings, typically for carbohydrates, are common. The usual suspects are comfort foods like breads, pastas, and desserts, particularly those of the chocolate persuasion. I'm not typically a dessert person, but if I find myself scrambling through the cabinets for leftover Halloween candy, I know my period is exactly two days away. There are studies that claim that craving chocolate during PMS is specifically American and therefore a learned cultural phenomenon and not related to anything physiological. The theory is that we have been taught that it's okay to eat chocolate during PMS and we're taking advantage of that accepted behavior by indulging when it's our time of the month. I don't buy that for a minute. First, your body requires more calories when you're premenstrual, and sweets and carbs can provide them quickly. Second, your magnesium levels are low (premenstrual migraines are a reflection of this), and chocolate can boost magnesium levels.

The most important piece of the puzzle is again serotonin. In depression and in PMS, when serotonin drops, your body tries to fix that imbalance. It begins to want carbs, specifically sugar, and particularly chocolate. Eating carbs is known to boost serotonin levels, but try to stick with complex carbs like whole grains instead of sugary concoctions to avoid the insulin surge and crash of blood sugar levels that follow. Tryptophan is the amino acid your body uses to create serotonin, so it makes sense to eat foods high in tryptophan specifically, instead of carbs in general. One thing I tell my patients about chocolate cravings is that they can sometimes be satisfied by eating bananas, which are high in tryptophan. Milk, lentils, and turkey are also high in tryptophan, especially the dark meat, so the truth is, you'd be better off pulling a

King Henry and munching on a turkey leg than scarfing down all those Oreos.

Here's an even lower-calorie way to boost serotonin levels: the amino acid supplements L-tryptophan and 5-hydroxytryptophan (5HTP), the building blocks for making your own serotonin, are available in any health food store. Nutritional supplements, vitamins, minerals, and amino acids can offer significant symptom relief, but you'll need to do more legwork to educate yourself about what's recommended and how to take it. Because of aggressive lobbying, these supplements are not regulated by the FDA to the same extent that prescription medicines are; there can be tremendous variability among brands and even within brands. Enlisting the assistance of an herbalist or naturopath would be wise in many situations.

Vitamin B_6 is also helpful for PMS, as it is a cofactor for serotonin synthesis. Adding a magnesium supplement, which can lower anxiety and prevent insomnia, is also a good idea in the days leading up to your period. Magnesium is a diuretic, so it'll also help with your swollen boobs and bloated pelvis. Calcium can also lessen irritability and help with insomnia, so a calcium-magnesium supplement would work nicely. Sometimes caffeine (or pineapple or asparagus, natural diuretics) can help to get rid of some degree of the bloating and fatigue. Omega-3 fatty acids found in oily fish or fish oil supplements may also help cut down on reactivity and irritability.

Here's the biggest tip I can give regarding PMS: regular exercise. Cardio, in particular, can help to reduce many symptoms of PMS and moodiness in general. It has been shown to be as effective as antidepressants in improving mood and energy level and reducing feelings of malaise. In many situations, daily cardiovascular exercise can do as much for you as SSRIs, without the weight gain and deadened libido.

Your diet also matters. Estrogen dominance can lead to heavier periods. Hormones in processed meat and certain chemicals in plastics, soaps, and pesticides can mimic estrogen, as can soy, which is added to many processed foods. If you do eat meat and poultry, make sure it's organic, or at least labeled "hormone-free," as the hormones used in the meat industry can potentially cause heavier periods. My patients who have switched to a vegetarian or vegan diet are enjoying lighter, less crampy periods. Also, keeping your weight at an optimal level can make a big difference in your monthly symptoms. The more body fat you have, the more estrogen your body is going to make, so aim for a leaner frame if you have significant PMS symptoms or especially heavy periods.

Timing is everything. When you do and don't have sex can affect a slew of things. For instance, when you started having sex, and how often you have it, can affect fertility. If you started earlier and engage in it weekly, your cycles are more likely to be regular. Weekly sex, with its regular dose of pheromone exposure, also means you're less likely to have heavier, painful periods, your fertility will more likely stay on track, and your menopause may even arrive later. One more important timing tip: abstaining from intercourse and from orgasm may be just what your uterus needs during menstruation. In a group of women with heavy periods, 83 percent reported sex during menses, compared with 10 percent in the group with lighter periods.

For severe PMS that affects functioning (missing work or school, being unable to perform household chores, having huge, regular blowups with everyone around you), there are prescription medication options. Psychiatrists will commonly prescribe SSRIs or SNRIs (serotonin and norepinephrine reuptake inhibitors like Effexor, Pristiq, and Cymbalta; see the appendix for details). You can take these pills all month long or just during the week before your period. The shorter-half-life medicines, like Paxil and Effexor, are not good choices here, as coming off them tends to be uncomfortable; you don't need to deal with antidepressant withdrawal every month. I prefer to use Lexapro, which starts working quickly and is easier to taper. I have quite a few patients who used to take antidepressants every day but now take only 5 milligrams of Lexa-pro for the four to seven days before their period every month, and this can be perfectly effective.

Another treatment option is to go on oral contraceptives, which create steady hormone levels. For many women, PMS is markedly re-duced, as are cramping and heavy bleeding. Often, the longer you're on the Pill, the lighter your periods are. There is also the option of taking oral contraceptives continually, where you stop the hormones only three or four times a year to have withdrawal bleeding. More gynecologists are recommending continual use of the Pill, especially in patients with endo-metriosis (a condition that causes extremely painful menses). Just how often you need to come off the hormones in order to shed the uterine lining is a subject of some debate, but the FDA has approved the use of Seasonale and Seasonique, which allow only four periods a year. And I certainly have patients who are enjoying fewer than that.

However, I have a few complaints and caveats about oral contracep-tives, so I'd prefer that you don't rush to use them to treat PMS until you read on.

THE PILL'S DIRTY LITTLE SECRETS

Using oral contraceptives to manage PMS is not an option for everyone. Flatlined hormone levels have the potential to throw things off dramati-cally; it's not what's natural for us. It is extremely hard to predict who is going to do well on the Pill versus who won't. I have some patients who are typically very moody and erratic, seemingly tossed about on a stormy sea of hormones throughout the month. Those patients often do better on the Pill, having fewer mood swings and minimal PMS once they get past the first few months of taking oral contraceptives. For them, the Pill ends up being stabilizing, providing steady levels of the same hormones day in and day out, which is what they need to manage their moods and minimize PMS.

But many of my patients find that they cannot tolerate how emotional the Pill makes them, and after trying several different brands over the years, they abandon the idea of using oral contraception for birth control. For these patients, the Pill is destabilizing. I have heard this sentence countless times when first meeting a patient and asking about contraception: "The Pill made me crazy." Those exact words. It's not clear why so many women in my office are reporting this phenomenon, except that many are coming to me for complaints of depression, not just PMS. In one study of women who started oral contraceptives, 16 percent noted that their moods had worsened, while 12 percent noted improvement in their moods and 71 percent had no change in their moods. Women who had PMS prior to the Pill reported significant improvement in their PMS on the Pill, while those with a history of depression, not just PMS, had worsening moods.

Some women are simply more sensitive to hormones affecting their moods than others are. The Pill works by presenting just enough estrogen and progesterone to the pituitary that it thinks ovulation has already occurred and so won't trigger the follicle to release an egg. Estrogen and serotonin regulate each other in a complicated dance, like so many things in the brain and body. Anything that affects estrogen is going to have an impact on serotonin. One possible reason the Pill may make some women a bit bonkers: estrogen causes the manufacture of a serotonin receptor called 5HT2A. This is the receptor that mediates the effects of hallucinogens like LSD and is the target of some antipsychotic medications. About a third of women have variations on this receptor that may cause problems when estrogen levels are higher.

But the bigger culprit is likely the progesterone. Synthetic progestin is horrible for your mood, and about 10 percent of women really can't tolerate it at all. The oral contraceptives Yaz and Yasmin are preferable when it comes to mood effects, perhaps due to one component, drospirenone, which is more similar to natural progesterone than other synthetics are, or due to the fact that it acts more like a diuretic, lessening water retention during the premenstrual phase. (Being bloated does bad things to your brain.)

Another reason oral contraceptives may worsen mood is that synthetic hormones seem to interfere with tryptophan metabolism and vitamin B_6 levels, both of which are necessary to make serotonin. If you're on the Pill, you should supplement with B_6.

You could say that the Pill basically tricks your body into thinking it's pregnant already, so that no egg gets released. Also, the cervix becomes plugged up with thick mucus, the way it does in pregnancy. Because there is no thinner cervical mucus flowing, the Pill can make your vagina drier, and sex may become painful. If you're not on the Pill, your cervical mucus is an easy way for you to track your cycle and fertility. Midcycle, the mucus is runny like egg whites. When you're fertile, nature ensures you'll be naturally more lubricated when you need it. On the Pill, you're not fertile, so there is less mucus and you're not well lubricated.

For many women, the Pill makes their skin clearer; estrogen does help give you that peaches-and-cream complexion. Your breasts tend to get a bit larger on the Pill, just as they do in pregnancy, likely due to the steady progesterone levels the Pill provides. So lighter periods, less acne, and lovely boobs sound great, I know, but there are some downsides to being on the Pill. First, there is the issue of weight gain, but, more accurately, a change in weight distribution. Estrogen dictates where fat gets placed in the body. It makes you put on weight in your hips and thighs, and also in the backs of your arms. There is a logical reason for this. Women of childbearing potential need a different center of gravity. If you're going to carry a baby in your belly, you need ballast in your back-side; estrogen tends to make your stomach flatter because that's not where fat distribution is needed. (FYI, when you're perimenopausal, your belly starts to store fat because your estrogen levels are waning. Beware the menopot.)

Second, oral contraceptives can really cut into your sexual desire. I tell my patients this is the "dirty little secret" of the Pill. For some women, being liberated from the fear of unwanted pregnancy may allow them to relax and experience sexual pleasure more, but a slew of other women are unhappy to discover that their desire for sex and their ability to achieve orgasm are muted by being on the Pill. There are two factors at work here. The first is, the longer you're on the Pill, the lower your testosterone levels become, and the less horny you are over time. Taking extra estrogen orally increases levels of something called sex hormone binding globulin (SHBG), a protein in the blood that binds up testosterone, so you end up with lower circulating levels of "free" testosterone, one-tenth to one-twentieth of normal. If the hormone is bound up, it doesn't hit the receptor, so it's useless to your brain. It gets worse: a research study showed that women who'd been off the Pill for four months still had SHBG levels four times that of normal. When I spoke with one of the investigators, he told me it never returns to normal. Another gynecologist told me, "It should be a warning on the box," but instead it's something no one seems to talk about.

Testosterone, while twenty times more prevalent in men, is also present in women, and it is the primary hormone responsible for sexual drive and desire. Part of every woman's monthly cycle includes testosterone levels that rise and fall, peaking just as fertility peaks, midcycle. Normal testosterone levels not only vary throughout the cycle but also go up and down throughout the day (higher in the morning in most women) and in response to various circumstances and behaviors (rising after vigorous exercise, success at work, and having regular sex). Women's testosterone levels tend to be highest in their early twenties and fall after menopause, after all the other hormones have declined. So not only is there a peak in testosterone midcycle but there may also be one during a brief, magical time right around age forty, a woman's "sexual peak," where testosterone levels are relatively higher than those of the other hormones. When you're on the Pill, you miss out on all of that.

OVULATION AND PHEROMONES: CHOOSING A CAD OR A DAD

Many women have significant shifts not just in their hormones but in their horniness all month long. It wasn't until my forties that I became aware of how much my libido, and, more important, my feelings about my husband, varied from week to week. When I read about this in a book called *Sexy Mamas,* I felt validated: "My husband knows that my monthly cycle provides me with about a week of feeling romantic, a week of lust, a week of slowing down, and a week of no desire. We work around that."

Fertility increases gradually up to ovulation and rapidly decreases afterward. Your desire to have sex naturally follows that pattern. While most primates have a period of "heat," it is generally assumed that the human female doesn't have such a cordoned-off time frame and is sexually available all month long, called "extended sexuality." As you may have experienced, there are a few days in your cycle when you're more up for sex than at other times, and, logically, Mother Nature has been smart about when that is. Women are more likely to be horny midcycle, during peak fertility, in the day or two leading up to the egg being released, when their testosterone levels are at their highest. The perfect storm of ovulation, optimum fertility, and peaking testosterone levels creates one red-hot mama (to be).

The baboon's backside turns bright red when she is in heat (called estrus), signaling to nearby males that she's ready for love. Humans are not quite so overt, though our midcycle high estrogen levels do cause a subtle dilation of blood vessels in our cheeks, enhancing our natural blush. Studies show that men are more sexually attracted to women wearing red than other colors. Also, men are more likely to assume that a woman is sexually active and receptive if she is wearing red. This may be partly cultural and partly biological. Perhaps unconsciously, women know this, as we are more likely to choose to wear red when expecting to meet and chat up an attractive man.

Ovulation is the only time every month when you're pretty much guaranteed to be horny. Your desire is easier to arouse, and your sexual response is heightened. Greater feelings of attractiveness also peak during this time. All kinds of important things happen midcycle, when you ovulate. Oxytocin peaks, which means increased rates of orgasm and wanting to bond with others. Also, testosterone and estrogen levels are higher, which puts you in an ultrareceptive and horny place. Your pupils even dilate more in response to seeing your sex partner when you're midcycle, but not if you're on the Pill.

We have a repertoire of not-so-covert behavior that makes it clear we're fertile. Women who are ovulating are more likely to feel sexually attractive and to choose provocative, clingy clothing. They dress more fetchingly, wear more jewelry and perfume, and go out more when they're midcycle and fertile. They're also more likely to casually hook up, and less likely to use condoms. Women feel more attractive around ovulation, and men are able to tell which women are closer to ovulation and trying to look more attractive by examining their photos. In studies, men pay strippers who are ovulating more money than those who aren't, and they rate the voices of women who are ovulating as sexier than the voices of those who aren't.

For that day or two when you have a viable egg, your body is being told by your hormones (especially testosterone) to go out and find a sperm donor. And not just any sperm donor. Our evolution dictates that we find the finest, fittest mate to donate his genetic material to our lineage. Introducing the alpha male—the best hunter, but not necessarily a good sharer. Women are also more likely to choose "bad boys" when they're ovulating—the kind of guy with a five o'clock shadow and a motorcycle, who'd most likely arouse you but maybe won't stick around and help you raise your kids. This dual sexuality is called conceptive and not conceptive. Some sex researchers call this dilemma "cad versus dad." We want cads when we're fertile, and dads when we're not.

In my office, the younger gals tend to go for men who excite and intrigue them, who have an edge and are hard to pin down. Women prefer men with a lower voice (more testosterone and likely more infidelity prone) for short-term mating but not for long-term relationship building. I've had countless heart-to-hearts with these patients about their choices in men. Often, as they mature, I remind them that the criteria need to change; they are shopping for a husband now, not a boyfriend.

When women are ovulating, their mate selection focuses on masculine traits that signal good genetic material, the alpha-male DNA. When not fertile, women still seek out men, but are more attracted to "nongenetic material and assistance"—those with resources who'll stick around to help with child rearing. Women, regardless of their own wealth, may still seek out men with adequate resources and social status. I know you have a job and a good credit rating and you don't need a man for anything, but your brain is still more like a cavewoman's than you'd like to admit. There have been no major changes to our genetics since we were hunter-gatherers. We're naturally attracted to men who not only have money, power, and social rank but also have shown they will share it. Just not all month long.

Women find classically masculine faces more attractive around the time they ovulate, choosing less chiseled-looking guys when not fertile. Fertile women are also more attracted to men acting in dominant, competitive ways. When we're fertile, it's all about genetic material, not social graces, which means if you're in a relationship with a dad, you may still end up flirting with a cad midcycle. Like men, it's natural for us to seek out the best genetic donor for our offspring. And also like men, even with a bird in the hand, we still go poking around the bush. Partnered women are more likely to choose the scent from a dominant man, while single women respond to the scent of men who are nurturing and willing to commit. It may be that even when a woman is partnered with a good provider (a dad), she can't help but still be attracted to a man midcycle who could lend his exceptional genes to her next offspring (a cad).

So what happens with women who are on oral contraceptives and never have a fertile phase? Just what you'd expect with static hormones. There's no midcycle peak in oxytocin to push bonding and orgasms, and no surge in estrogen or testosterone stoking desire. As far as the brain is concerned, the deed is already done. If there's a bun in the oven, there's no need to attract a baker, and so the midcycle preference for the chiseled cad is gone. Women on the Pill act like women who are already pregnant, where the focus is to attract someone with other things to offer and share besides their manly genetic virtues. Pill users show weaker or no preferences for facial and vocal masculinity.

The biological drives for food, drink, and sex ensure first our own survival and then the survival of our progeny. Clearly, women and men go about this differently, focusing on separate attributes we deem important. When searching for the best possible genetic donors, men follow their eyes and women follow their noses. Men are actually more likely to fall in love at first sight, and neuroimaging of men in the early stages of romantic love show increased brain activity in the visual centers. Men are swayed by facial symmetry, glowing skin, and a particular waist-to-hip ratio. These help to signal that a woman is healthy and able to bear children.

When it comes to mating, women are influenced by scent. The sense

of smell is the oldest and least mediated sense in our brains and processes information more quickly than the other sensory systems. Because
the brain cells for smell are only one synapse away from the amygdala,
our emotion center, we have no real control over liking or being repulsed
by an odor. Women have a more sensitive sense of smell, and more brain
space devoted to processing smells and pheromones, thanks to estrogen.
Estrogen helps us to detect pheromones, the signature scent of a potential mate, more adroitly than men do, especially during ovulation, when
estrogen levels are highest. For optimal mating, we need someone who's
in the Goldilocks zone of different but not too foreign: genetically similar and compatible, but not family. Pheromones from the male sweat
glands allow us to make this determination. Women prefer the smell of a
stranger's armpit over that of family members, which is an ageless signal
to prevent inbreeding.

When it comes to mate selection, so much happens unconsciously
that we don't really have much control over. Pheremones are a good example. When a patient tells me she has a new boyfriend, I usually ask her
if she likes the way he smells. I don't mean his cologne or deodorant, and
I definitely don't mean his stink when he walks off the basketball court,
but rather his scent, his natural odor. "If you stuck your nose in his armpit, would you be happy?" You'd be surprised how often this question is
met with a resounding yes. When I hear "I could live there!" then I know
they're a good match. How someone smells to you matters tremendously.
This is one of the reasons I'm not a huge fan of online dating. Pheromones help us to pick ideal mates for ourselves, and this process is based
primarily on genetics, not on Photoshopped selfies.

In 1995, Swiss researcher Claus Wedekind performed a study that
has come to be known as the sweaty T-shirt experiment. He asked
women to sniff T-shirts that men had been donning for three days without showering or using cologne. Wedekind found, and further research

has confirmed, that most of the women were attracted to the scent of men whose major histocompatibility complex (MHC) was markedly different from their own. The MHC indicates a range of immunity to various disease-causing agents. When you're mating, you want someone with different immunities than you have, so that your offspring can benefit from the variety. Optimally, children will have more disease-fighting capacity than either of their parents. Too-similar immune systems of potential parents can lead to complications in fertility and pregnancy. Also, if a woman partners with a man whose genetic makeup is too similar to hers, she's more likely to cheat on him. The more genes they share, the more likely she'll be attracted to other men.

Pheromones are typically processed unconsciously, but lately this issue has come to the fore, and there have been more sweaty T-shirt parties going on around the country, a riff on the Wedekind experiment. Male invitees are told to bring a T-shirt they've worn for twenty-four hours (including overnight). They are assigned a number and the shirt is placed in a Ziploc bag. Women smell the shirts, choose the one they like the best, and find their lucky date through his number. "Pheromone party" organizers say they have created lasting pairs in this way. Follow your nose to marital bliss. Being attracted to someone's pheromones can help carry you through some significant bumps in the relationship. Taking in another's scent helps with bonding. Primates are prosocial, and they solidify bonds in their community by grooming, which involves sitting close to each other and breathing in each other's scent, never mind picking and eating bugs off each other's fur. The next time you're mad at him, smell your man's armpits or T-shirts, and see if that doesn't help you feel a bit better about who he is and what you have together. If and when you have them, smell your kids, too. There's research on mother-infant bonding via pheromones as well.

Men rate not just a woman's visible sexual attractiveness as highest when she's midcycle; they like her scent more then, too. If she's on the Pill and not ovulating, she doesn't have the same "cyclical attractiveness of odors" that naturally cycling women do. A much bigger deal: being on the Pill affects the way women process pheromones in terms of these important genetic compatibility issues. Women on the Pill don't seem to show the same responsiveness to male scent cues. They tend to pick mates who are more similar to them, and less "other." Scottish researcher Tony Little found that women's assessment of men as potential husband material shifted drastically if they were on oral contraceptives. In a replay of the sweaty T-shirt experiment, women who were using birth control pills chose men's T-shirts randomly or, even worse, showed a preference for men with similar immunity to their own. One study remarked that a woman on the Pill might go off it only to realize she is with someone who is more like a brother than a lover.

The good news is that she will probably pick a dad and not a cad. Women on the Pill favor less masculine men, which could mean he will stick around for child rearing. But do you want him? Women who were on oral contraceptives when they chose their mates scored lower on measures of sexual satisfaction and partner attraction. If there was a separation in their relationship, they were more likely to have initiated it than the men were, and more likely to complain of increasing sexual dissatisfaction. But they were also happier with how their partners provided for them, and often ended up having longer relationships.

These days, I actually recommend to my patients who are on oral contraceptives that they go off them for three or four cycles to make sure the man they met when they were on the Pill is still the man they want to bed down year after year and create a family with when they're off it. Once you're already in a relationship, it gets mighty complicated to stop your birth control to reassess the man you've already chosen. Better to do your mate selecting while not under the influence of any other hormones besides your own, which means finding a nonhormonal form of birth control—such as condoms, an IUD, a diaphragm, or a cervical cap—while you're on the lookout for the man of your dreams. I also recommend spending some time in his armpit to make sure he's the one. I'm not kidding. The body, undisrupted, is powerfully intuitive and worth listening to.

PART TWO

MATING, MILFS, MONOGAMY, AND MENOPAUSE

Three

This Is Your Brain
on Love

The way we're wired, neurologically and hormonally, has a lot to do with how we think and feel—and when we think and feel it. But relationships exert their own powerful effects on the body and the mind. The first few months of attraction create a heady mix of neurotransmitters that no drug can adequately mimic. As a psychiatrist, I will say this: falling in love turns women into manic, obsessive, delusional junkies. At its most unromantic, falling in love is the neural mechanism of mate selection, evolved to ensure that we pine for, obsess over, and pursue the one person we believe will provide us with not only the fittest offspring but also the support to nurture that child through infancy. Falling in love with someone is an elaborate dance in the brain and body that motivates and focuses us on mating with this preferred partner. And in the early stages, the difference between falling in lust and falling in love can be difficult to distinguish. The progression from attraction to attachment is a physical process as much as it's an emotional one. (Attachment, the phase that comes after attraction, has its own brain chemistry, which I'll get to in the next chapter.)

Dopamine is the key chemical element of attraction, underlying the experiences of paying attention, sensing pleasure, and seeking reward. Dopamine tells us two things: "Notice this important thing" (called salience) and "This feels good; do it again." The reward circuitry runs on dopamine, the molecular cornerstone of addiction. Drugs that enhance dopamine levels, like cocaine and speed, are more likely to be addictive than other drugs; many researchers believe a drug can't be addictive without at least secondarily increasing dopamine transmission.

When you fall in love, dopamine makes you crave and need your newfound crush. The object of your affection is specific, partly because dopamine has tagged him or her as salient. Experiments with prairie voles, typically monogamous, showed that higher levels of dopamine were responsible for preferring a particular partner, and blocking dopamine decreased that partner preference. In anthropologist Helen Fisher's brain scans of people who fell deeply in love, their dopaminergic reward systems were kicked into high gear, reminiscent of brain scans of people high on cocaine. Increased blood flow was seen in the caudate nucleus, an area fed by dopamine neurons. Sometimes referred to as the "motor of the mind," the caudate directs your body to approach the target, motivating you to go after the reward. Dopamine ensures that this is a pleasurable process, making the behavior reinforcing, meaning you'll gladly do it repeatedly.

Addiction is characterized by three things: sensitization, tolerance, and withdrawal. Over time, smaller triggers will induce a craving, more substance is required to induce pleasure, and going on the wagon feels terrible. You see the same increase in wanting, in appetite and desire, whether for a drug or for a crush. And if the object of your desires breaks it off, your brain chemicals nosedive into abrupt withdrawal. Expect a bad crash. Crying, sleeping, and bingeing on food and alcohol are common in my jilted patients. If you reunite, some portion of the feel-good chemistry reappears, convincing you that you were meant to be together. But don't be fooled by your pharmacological homecoming party—junkies feel good when they relapse, too, at first. It doesn't necessarily mean he's the one, but it should help to explain the particular pleasure of makeup sex. You fight; you feel ultraterrible because you're in withdrawal from your lover and a whole lot better, and higher, once you are reunited.

The dopamine reward circuitry underlies not just pleasure but the anticipation of more pleasure and the motivation to get it. This may be the biological logic underlying the age-old advice to play hard to get and the dating advice book *The Rules*. Studies show that getting the reward too early in the game reduces the intensity and the duration of the brain's dopamine activity. A delay in the win gives the most pleasure, potentially benefiting both of you.

But dopamine alone is not responsible for that blissful feeling of finding Mr. Right. Falling in love stimulates the release of norepinephrine, a chemical cousin of adrenaline, which keeps you excited and energized, with sweaty palms and a rapid heartbeat. Norepinephrine revs up all five senses, the better to heighten awareness and remember every detail of your love object and his or her effect on you. Your brain and body are on high alert, primed for action and reaction. Sleep is optional. So is food, for that matter.

Norepinephrine also contributes to the release of estrogen, which stimulates courting behavior. Increased levels of these two chemicals are seen in laboratory animals striking a sexually inviting pose known as lordosis. Arching the back and sticking the butt up in the air makes it easier for rear-entry penetration. There may be a human equivalent of lordosis, seen in the posture created by high heels, or, more obviously, in Miley Cyrus's twerking.

Add to the cocainelike mix of dopamine and norepinephrine a healthy shot of endorphins, our naturally circulating opiates, nature's painkillers and stress relievers. So falling in love is pharmacologically a bit like a speedball, the combination of cocaine and heroin. But there's more, because experiencing intense infatuation, and especially love at first sight, is like taking a psychedelic drug, too. Phenylethylamine (PEA), sometimes dubbed the "molecule of attraction," floods the brain when the initial magnetism occurs. PEA is responsible for some of the dreaminess and giddiness when first falling in love. It may underlie love at first sight, and it's likely present in your brain during that all-important first kiss. Phenylethylamines naturally occur in your brain, but they're also found in a group of drugs that includes ecstasy (MDMA) and some hallucinogens. PEA also kills appetite and can work as a short-term antidepressant. It is present in good chocolates, and it may also spike during orgasm, causing that trippy, out-of-body feeling that some women are lucky enough to experience.

With all of these stimulating chemicals bathing the brain, it's no wonder many women who fall in love find it easier to lose weight and exercise and harder to fall asleep at night. One thing I've noticed repeatedly: when my patients fall in love, they can more easily go off their antidepressants and quit me. I can't devise a medication cocktail that can compete with what your brain will concoct in the early glow of a relationship. In fact, there are those who so enjoy the brain chemistry of the infatuation phase that they become serial attraction junkies. They fall in love, stay high for three to six months, and when the magic fades they move on.

There are other chemical players on the team during the initial attraction phase. The levels of the sex hormones testosterone and estrogen are higher when falling in love. They enhance sexual desire and receptivity, respectively. Estrogen and progesterone both enhance the love/trust circuits, so as long as you're not in PMS land, you may be more open to loving and nurturing behavior. But in terms of being horny, it's all about testosterone. Men and women with higher levels of circulating testosterone engage in more frequent sex and have more orgasms. Men who inject testosterone (for performance enhancement on the athletic field or on Wall Street) experience more sexual thoughts and more morning erections and have more sex. But they don't necessarily fall in love.

When women fall in love, increased dopamine levels can enhance testosterone levels. Also, inhaling male pheromones can trigger testosterone release in a receptive woman. Just thinking about your new guy can raise your levels. Interestingly, men who are falling in love have slightly lower levels of testosterone than usual, perhaps so they don't scare off their new mate with how horny they typically are the rest of the time! So while we fall in love, women's testosterone levels bump while men's dip, which may give us a chemically unifying feeling that we're in this experience together, and we are evenly matched in terms of libido.

How all of this works when gay men or lesbians form lasting unions is hard to fully address, mostly because there's a lot less research in this area. Obviously, same-sex couples can and do create healthy, loving unions and families. Their brains give them the same pleasurable, heady mixes when they become infatuated, fall in love, and form binding attachments, proof that what brings us together is about more than just procreating.

HUGS, NOT DRUGS

Oxytocin makes you feel great. Do you know that ultrarelaxed feeling you get when you hold your baby? How about the bliss after you've just had orgasmic sex and are being held closely? That's oxytocin, the hormone of bonding and of trust. A twenty-second hug will trigger oxytocin release, as will exchanges of friendly signals, like being smiled at and returning the grin. Think of oxy as superglue for your relationship. It cements a nursing mother and her child, and it bonds lovers from the first time their eyes lock across a crowded room. Holding hands, kissing, and sex will all get your oxy levels zooming. Smiling babies and hugs with boyfriends activate not only oxytocin release but also dopamine-associated brain reward circuits, encouraging us to keep doing it. In that way, you could say that oxytocin makes you crave even more physical contact. Oxytocin helps to protect us against stress and promote relaxation. There are even some studies showing it can help to speed healing. So hugging, cuddling, and orgasmic sex are good for not just your heart and soul but your body as well.

Women have more oxytocin receptors in their brains, and oxytocin works better in an environment rich with estrogen. So you may be more likely to connect and fall in love during the first half of your cycle, before estrogen levels drop. Oxytocin, in both men and women, creates feelings of trust, connection, and contentment around the preferred partner. Oxytocin reduces heart rate and blood pressure, enabling social bonding and trusting behaviors. A sense of calm and security quiets the typical fear of strangers, allowing more generosity. In experiments, people given oxytocin are more willing to trust a stranger or give them money. That may be the reason why people who are touched while spoken to are more likely to honor a request or keep a promise. It also may be why falling in love can be dangerous for some. I had a patient who lent way too much money to a new boyfriend who later disappeared.

Infatuation overrides rational thought. At higher levels of oxytocin, you may become forgetful, and your ability to think clearly may be diminished. Falling in love squelches anxiety and skepticism. Oxy, in particular, seems to be crucial for inhibiting fear and anxiety, allowing bonding and sex to occur. When people fall in love, their fear circuitry gets turned way down, so the critical thinking system (anterior cingulate cortex) and the fear center (amygdala) are less active. The brain's Miracle-Gro fertilizer, a nerve growth factor called brain-derived neurotrophic factor (BDNF), which helps to foster new connections between nerve cells, is elevated in people who've fallen in love, triggering a massive neuronal reorganization. (Remember BDNF, because you're going to be learning about it again. Neuroplasticity is involved in pregnancy, perimenopause, and exercise, and it's important.) Tons of brain cells have to be "obliterated and replaced with new ones. This is one reason falling in love feels... like a loss of identity." Is all of this dangerous? Probably not, but it's good to keep your wits about you when falling in love. You're not in your typically critical "right mind." You're not even yourself!

YOU'RE MY OBSESSION

Ask my husband about how we met and he'll say he's never been pursued by anyone more aggressively in his life. Ask me, and I'll tell you about love at first sight. I remember every moment of that party where I set my eyes on him. I had to lock myself in the bathroom to calm down my breathing and pounding heartbeat (norepinephrine in action). In the days that followed, I would check countless times to see if he'd contacted me. All day long, I could think of nothing but him, Him, HIM.

It's normal, it's nature's way, and it's likely that lower than normal serotonin levels were underlying my obsessive thoughts and activities. When serotonin levels are high, there is a sense of satiety; you want for nothing. When levels are lower, you become obsessive and angsty. Blood serotonin levels in those newly in love resemble levels in people with OCD. They're abnormally low for both, about 40 percent of the normal controls.

Dopamine and serotonin tend to act like they're on opposite sides of a seesaw. When one is up, the other is often down. Infatuation and initial attraction are characterized by higher dopamine and lower serotonin levels. Higher serotonergic states make it harder to climax, as anyone on Zoloft can tell you. So this low serotonergic state helps explain not only why it's easier for you to climax with your new lover but also your tremendous feelings of angsty need and obsessive ruminations about your newfound love.

One thing I'd like to stress: women on SSRIs likely won't experience some of the chemical cocktail of attraction and infatuation. SSRIs create artificially high serotonin levels, decreasing impulsive and compulsive behavior. You have more behavioral control, and you don't obsess as much about anything, even if you just fell in love, which you may not even do on an SSRI. SSRIs interfere with mating in a few crucial ways. As serotonin and dopamine often balance each other out, if serotonin is too high, dopamine levels will be low. Emotional blunting and apathy result. It's hard to go out and chase down a guy when your "Go get 'em, tiger!" neurochemical is lacking. Also, there's less chance of your getting obsessive and fixated on one preferred partner when you are taking a medicine meant to treat OCD. If high dopamine and low serotonin drive the rewarding and obsessive nature of falling in love, being on an SSRI, with its resultant low dopamine and high serotonin levels, won't drive the behavior. Female rats treated chronically with SSRIs reduce the amount of time they spend near males. Sex researchers are currently conducting studies showing that women on SSRIs rate men as less attractive and spend less time poring over images of their faces than women who aren't on SSRIs, being "less likely to find those of their chosen sex physically attractive or desirable as a potential romantic or sexual partner." Just as I recommend my patients get off oral contraceptives when mate shopping, there are reasons to slowly taper off antidepressants as well. If being on SSRIs means you already feel satiated and don't even look twice at a guy, it's going to be hard to move forward from attraction and infatuation to attachment.

Falling in love and choosing a mate rely on sexual attraction and sexual energy. If libido is lowered and sexual response is muted by an SSRI, it seems obvious that this will have a negative impact on the entire process. The neural systems associated with attachment and pair bonding also rely on orgasm and its resulting surge of oxytocin. Because SSRIs make orgasm much more difficult, they jeopardize this major trigger. One way that a woman can judge a potential partner is by how much time and attention he's putting toward her pleasure. "Scientists think the fickle female orgasm may have evolved to help women distinguish Mr. Right from Mr. Wrong." A man who can pay extra time and attention to a woman's needs may also be a better father and more willing to share what he has (a dad and not a cad). Perhaps unconsciously, a woman may use her ability to climax with a certain partner to help her decide whether he is the one for her and her future children, or not so much. If it's nearly impossible for her to be aroused all the way to orgasm because of her SSRI, then she can't make use of this measuring device.

LUST

From an evolutionary perspective, you could say lust is practice for love. Learning to flirt to attract a mate, and practicing what to do when you find a potential partner, need to be finessed repeatedly over time. The chemistry of lust and attraction are similar, but not the same. Testosterone makes us horny, dopamine keeps us moving forward, and oxytocin frees us up from the fear of strangers so we can shed our clothes and get close. But with lust, a biological drive for sexual gratification, it's more about testosterone and less about oxytocin.

Estrogen may make us more receptive to sex, taking the brakes off and helping us to be uninhibited, but testosterone is the gas pedal. Even flirting seems to have some basis in testosterone. While romantic love is reserved for one preferred partner, the target of lust isn't the perfect man, but rather "almost any semi-appropriate partner"; it's not Mr. Right so much as Mr. Right Now. Also, the neural mechanism of attraction won't allow you to fall in love with two different people at once, but you can lust after more than one person at a time. Another key difference is that the fires of lust are quickly doused once the sex is over; with attraction, repeated sex just adds to the buildup of good feelings.

In women, testosterone is made in the adrenal glands and ovaries, spurring our competitive drive, our assertiveness, and our lust. In adolescence, a girl's level of testosterone rises five times above normal, but it is in the context of her estrogen increasing ten to twenty times above normal, so it's balanced out to a large extent. Adolescent boys have a twenty-five-fold increase in their testosterone, unabated by other mitigating hormonal factors, which means they have much higher sex drives than the girls. Also, in boys these levels are static, whereas girls have cyclical variation. Boys' behavior ends up being much more consistent, basically a constant stream of horny. Boys have more frequent sexual thoughts and more masturbation, which is not to say girls aren't doing it, too, just not as much. Interestingly, surging testosterone levels in an adolescent girl can signal the time of first intercourse.

Women have different standards for hookups versus getting hitched. In the past few years, numerous articles have been written about how today's women, whether in college or out in the world soon after, are so focused on getting their careers off the ground that they prefer more casual sex over complicated long-term relationships. They'd rather get their gratification on their own terms and not muck it up with messy feelings like love. Since "women's lib" and oral contraceptives have become commonplace, women have had growing freedom in this arena. Having sex has become uncoupled from committed relationships and the responsibilities of motherhood. This is a relatively new phenomenon, and I totally get it. But one warning about one-night stands, just so you aren't fooling yourself. Lust and sex can trigger feelings of attraction and even love. Rising testosterone levels can enhance dopamine and norepinephrine transmission and lower serotonin, matching the brain chemistry of someone who's falling in love. And sex can definitely trigger attachment and bonding, due to oxytocin. Testosterone can trigger oxytocin release, and an orgasm will definitely trigger oxytocin release. If you orgasm or cuddle after sex, the bonding hormones may sneak up on you, though you intended your sex to be casual. Thanks to oxytocin, you may find yourself with loving, attached feelings for your Mr. Right Now.

There is a strong desire in women to be held and cuddled. Many of us will use sex as a means to an end, hoping to have some afterglow and snuggling, willing to trade sex for that experience. Men, too, are eager to be held. A common complaint among men in sex therapy is that they don't receive enough nonsexual touching. But getting naked and cuddling is going to trigger oxytocin, the bonding hormone. So you may find that it's hard for you to keep your "friend with benefits" in that same category for long.

THE CHEMISTRY OF SEX

Your brain on sex is like a series of loops. Hormones may trigger behaviors, but just as often, behaviors trigger hormones. Sexual activity stimulates testosterone release, which further revs up desire and triggers dopamine release. This dopamine-laden euphoria and arousal further trigger testosterone release. Sensitivity to touch is enhanced by dopamine and particularly by oxytocin. The more skin-to-skin contact, cuddling, kissing, eye gazing, and nipple stimulation, the more oxytocin gets released, which triggers testosterone, then dopamine.

Oxytocin and endorphins not only stoke arousal and pleasure but also help produce feelings of closeness and relaxation. As a woman becomes aroused by stimulation of her nipples, oxytocin gets released, just as it is when suckling a newborn. Further attention to her vagina, clitoris, or cervix creates more oxytocin and estrogen release, resulting in an acute drive to become penetrated, and an expansion of the vaginal muscles in case that's what will happen. Estrogen is involved in every phase of sex, making women more sexually receptive and lubricated and triggering oxytocin release. As sex progresses, oxy increases, culminating in an orgasmic burst. Estrogen and testosterone put the brain on high alert, so that dopamine and norepinephrine, our two "stand up and take notice" chemical friends, can get involved. Dopamine, of course, makes us pay attention to a potentially rewarding stimulus like sex. It gives us pleasure, enhances sensory input, and triggers the reward circuitry that motivates us to keep going, driving us toward orgasm.

You have two competing systems in your body: sympathetic and parasympathetic. The sympathetic is the fight-or-flight system, while the parasympathetic is the rest-and-digest system. Norepinephrine jump-starts the sympathetic nervous system, increasing heart rate, raising blood pressure, and causing heavy breathing. Balancing this out, the parasympathetic system also gets in on the act, directing blood flow to the genitals. Sex is a delicate balance of sympathetic and parasympathetic stimulation, toggling back and forth. Too much adrenaline-like arousal early on, and plateau or orgasm may be difficult, if not impossible, as is seen with stimulants like cocaine and speed. (There are those people, though, who need a short burst of adrenaline in order to get over the finish line.)

For the finale, endorphins take center stage, helping us to feel great and make sex something we'll want to do repeatedly. Endorphins also raise our pain threshold. Response to pain is just half of normal during the peak of sexual arousal. Does that help explain nipple clamps? Not only do they hurt less when you're extremely aroused and high on your brain's own heroin, but there is some overlap in the brain when it comes to sexual pleasure and pain, as their circuitry is closely linked. If you're also curious about anal sex or toe sucking, anal sensations travel some of the same routes as genital sensations, and the area in the brain that maps out physical sensations from the genitals is right next to the one for the toes. Stimulate either area enough and you get some carryover into the genital sensation part of the brain. And breast and genital neural circuitry overlap as well, which may explain why some women can orgasm from nipple stimulation alone. Isn't the brain marvelous? Also, there is mounting evidence that sexual pleasure triggers the endocannabinoid system as well, your body's internal cannabis molecules.

THE CHEMISTRY OF ORGASM

Orgasms are good for you. They reduce mortality, are good for your heart and cardiovascular system, help to prevent endometriosis, and when the time is right, they help you to conceive and carry a pregnancy to term.

The beginning of sexual pleasure is dopamine mediated, while the second act is primarily endorphins, which crescendo with orgasm. Oxytocin and dopamine are the big players leading up to orgasm, but the climax itself owes its mind-bending effects to the triple threat of oxy, endorphins, and PEA, the hallucinogen-like brain chemical, which just might make you feel like you really were "way out there" when you climaxed. Trippy, out-of-body experiences, or laughing, crying, and switching between the two, are all possible and normal during an orgasm.

Oxytocin keeps you feeling connected to your lover. It also permits relaxation, helping you feel calm, secure, and trusting enough to climax. Peaking at orgasm, oxytocin causes uterine contractions, which help to "suck up" semen into the cervix. It also can engender tremendous feelings of openness, trust, and bonding. The oxy afterglow lasts between one and five minutes postorgasm in women.

After orgasm, serotonin peaks, creating one happy, relaxed, sexually satisfied, and satiated sensation. In some women after orgasm, a negative feedback loop is triggered, with prolactin secretion making them

sleepy, dopey, and, often, significantly less horny. Still other women respond to the heightened pleasure with one thought in mind: I wanna go
again. Sometimes all that dopamine, norepinephrine, and testosterone
continue to trigger sexual desire. Also, the oxytocin creates more touch
sensitivity and a desire for more skin-to-skin cuddling, which can trigger
another round of testosterone surge.

> ## BRAIN BLOOD FLOW IN ORGASM—
> ## ALL THE WONKY DETAILS

Barry Komisaruk's lab at Rutgers University in northern New Jersey is
the world's largest orgasm research laboratory. Here, men and women
are slid into an MRI chamber, where they must lie completely still, their
heads held immobile in a mesh cage. Their brain blood flow is then measured while they give themselves, or receive, orgasms. Over the years,
this lab has studied just what it takes to climax, including looking at
women who can orgasm through fantasy alone and others who've had
their spinal cords severed, to see if they can climax. (They can, as long as
their vagus nerve, which innervates the genitalia, is intact.)

The lab's more recent studies are delineating the difference between
self-stimulation and partner stimulation. Most of us would be quick to
agree that these two orgasms are qualitatively different, especially in the
emotional realm. The question is: are they physiologically different?
Early results suggest they are.

During orgasm, fresh oxygen- and nutrient-rich blood floods the
brain. Leading up to orgasm, a series of brain blood flow changes occur.
First is activation of the somatosensory cortex, the part of the brain that
maps out bodily sensations. Next seen is decreased blood flow to the
frontal cortex. You want less frontal flow because you need your foot off
the brakes to move a car forward. Frontal inhibition will put the kibosh

on the entire sequence. Soon after, the secondary somatosensory cortex, which adds the emotional piece to your physical sensations, is activated. Then increased blood flow is seen in the amygdala, your emotional center, and then in the part of the hypothalamus that is responsible for the release of oxytocin.

The last piece of the puzzle is the dopamine circuitry that underlies reward seeking, pleasure, and euphoria. The final push into orgasmic bliss is the job of this brain area. Dopamine not only helps you pay attention, focus, and keep your eyes on the prize, but it also marks an event as salient. So don't be surprised if the guy you were only moderately into suddenly becomes more important in your eyes after he's given you the big O. Dopamine surges also decrease sensory thresholds for more sensation, priming the brain for more pleasure. Multiple orgasms, anyone? (For more on sexual pleasure, please enjoy the sex chapter.)

Four

Marriage and Its Discontents

The chemistry of attraction changes over time, ebbing over six to eighteen months, being slowly supplanted by the chemistry of attachment. Committed love is calmer, with none of the sweaty palms and churning stomach, thanks to less circulating dopamine, norepinephrine, and phenylethylamine (PEA). Because of that seesaw effect, lower dopamine means higher serotonin. The reward circuitry isn't firing, and the frontal lobes are fully online, so rational thought wins out over emotional upheaval, due to normalized serotonin levels. The study comparing the serotonin levels of patients with OCD to those who were infatuated showed that the levels do finally normalize during the attachment phase, as your lover becomes less of an obsessive fixation. Less dopamine also means less testosterone, for both of you, so the lust factor has died down considerably. Men's testosterone levels are lower after they've been partnered for more than a year compared to those in the first six months of a committed relationship.

Recall the dads-versus-cads issue. In men, higher levels of testosterone (cad) can reduce the attachment drive. A manly guy may be great pickings for a one-night stand and may provide top-shelf genetic material, but it may not be in his nature to stick around to change diapers. Birds that are given an extra dose of testosterone abandon their nests. A man with lower testosterone may be a great father and less likely to stray, but he may not have the most chiseled chin. One plus: typically, during the parenting phase, lower testosterone levels help ensure that fathers will focus on their newborn and not stray. So parenthood could potentially help turn a cad into a dad. Not only are men with lower testosterone levels more responsive to infants' cues but "paternal effort" can lower a man's testosterone levels.

Longer-term, attached love is sometimes called companionate love. This familiarity and companionship creates feelings of comfort, well-being, a sense of calm, and even decreased perceptions of pain, courtesy of oxytocin and endorphins that are still on board.

While the neurochemistry of committed love may lack the intensity of the early attraction phase, the effect of a long-term relationship on your well-being can hardly be underestimated. But once the chemical dependence of the early days fades away, couples who choose to stay together have to work harder to remain connected. Monogamy can complicate libido in particular and may affect women more than men.

Emotional connectedness is all about oxytocin (and estrogen, which enhances oxy's functioning) in women and a hormone called vasopressin in men. These are the molecules of attachment and bonding. Vasopressin, in particular, is considered the molecule of monogamy and exclusivity. Vasopressin not only enhances a man's commitment to a woman but also underlies male bonding (the "bromance"). In the same way that oxytocin and testosterone compete with each other, vasopressin and testosterone are often at odds as well. Vasopressin diminishes the impact of testosterone on competition and aggression, encouraging the defense and protection of progeny and, importantly, preventing promiscuity and infidelity. In monogamous prairie voles given a vasopressin blocker, their testosterone takes the lead; they screw one female and then abandon her for another.

Studies of the vasopressin receptor gene (dubbed the "monogamy gene" in *The Female Brain*) show two versions, long and short. The longer version of the gene is associated with improved bonding and mating behaviors and more appropriate social behaviors. This version is present in our primate cousins the bonobos, who are quick to hug, kiss, and even have sex to keep the peace. The shorter gene variant is seen in the more aggressive chimp population. Also, interestingly, the shorter gene is seen in autism in humans, where there are some deficits in social and bonding behaviors.

Vasopressin also facilitates clear thinking, attention, memory, and emotional control. In Helen Fisher's brain-imaging studies, people in longer love relationships show increased activity in the anterior cingulate cortex (where attention, emotion, and memory interact) and the insular cortex, which processes emotions. So the brain is formulating and filing emotional memories. The early phases of attraction are fiery and passionate. Attachment is calmer, more relaxed, and solidified. Oxytocin is the common chemical in both phases, pulling two people together, lowering their defenses that are suspicious of trusting and connecting, and then keeping them bonded. Eye contact, the "anchoring gaze," is a powerful way to connect with women, creating intimacy and, often, sexual longing. Looking away, turning away, or doing anything that threatens bonding can trigger stress hormones that get in the way of oxytocin and endorphins.

We are wired to connect and to need other people. In more than ninety countries surveyed worldwide, more than 90 percent of us are married at least once by the time we're forty-nine. In the United States,

we marry, divorce, and remarry at higher rates than in any other country, but half of American adult women over the age of eighteen are
unmarried. Since 2000 that number has risen from 45 million to 56 million. First-time marriages end in divorce four out of ten times. The lowest rate, among upper-middle-class couples with college degrees, is one
in three. That's as good as it gets in America.

The Maslow hierarchy of human needs starts with the basics of food
and shelter and then moves onward and upward, through safety and
security to love and belonging and self-esteem, finally peaking at self-
actualization. And so it's been with the evolution of marriage, from
institutional, where marriage started out as protection from violence,
assuring that food and shelter were maintained, to companionate, focusing on love and sex, and finally to the self-expressive marriage. Now
more than ever, we're looking for our partnership to foster personal
growth and self-discovery. The quality of a marriage helps to predict personal well-being; marital distress is associated with depression and other
psychiatric complaints, while the positive effects of a strong union help
to keep us healthy and strengthen over time.

YOU COMPLETE ME. I HATE YOU.

We naturally mate with someone whose immunity is different from our
own because it expands the repertoire of defenses in our children. Just as
with the MHC complex and immune status, what is healthiest for our
children comes from a union of two opposites. My kids like knowing that
they should go to Dad for certain things and to Mom for others. We each
bring opposite talents and skills to the table, and that helps to create not
only a stronger, more complete team but also healthy hybrids when we
procreate.

In relationships, we often want our partner to be the things that we are not. Certain behaviors in others echo long ago, deeply repressed parts of ourselves. As children, we were molded by our parents' reactions toward us. We put away bothersome behaviors, suppressed our emotional intensity, and hid our needs in order to make their jobs easier. Down the line, we miss those abandoned facets of who we were. We would love to be reunited with our discarded selves to make an imagined whole. That's where the magic comes in, when two people come together, igniting a spark that shines light on where those repressed parts have been hidden. You complete me. You're everything I'm not, and we make something bigger and better than either of us alone could create.

In the early stages of love, words of endearment like *sweetie* and *baby* remind us of our very first successful love relationship, as a babe in arms. As in early childhood, our need to be securely attached to someone who loves us and cares for us is being met, and all is well. After the magic comes the power struggle, where annoying tics and habits begin to irk us. The very things that drew us to someone are the ones that now drive us crazy. We realize the person we married or otherwise committed to is nothing like us and needs to change or we're going to need to be committed. As in mental hospital.

The former answer to our prayers becomes a living nightmare as we struggle to continue to get those early childhood needs of love and attachment fulfilled. We maneuver and manipulate, withdraw and intimidate, cry and criticize, but our partner comes up short in meeting our demands. We alternate between screaming matches and dry accountings on an emotional ledger of tit for tat. You won't do this for me, so I'm not going to do that for you. Eventually, you both realize you can't change the other or make the other love you the way that you need. At that point, it's often time for an affair, or a divorce, or a détente of a sexless marriage (very common in my office population), or, hopefully, couples therapy.

Understanding why this phase happens is a crucial weapon in the armory of trying to make love work. Like magnets flipped around, attraction can turn to repulsion. We are repelled by those who remind us of what we are not. Because we were taught to detest those things that we'd hidden away at our parents' insistence, we end up rejecting those parts of ourselves. So when someone is really getting on your nerves and you're incensed by some of their behaviors, turn it around and look at your own. Chances are good there's projected self-hatred fueling that burning rage.

Something else to keep in mind: we re-create our childhood environment as we project our hurts, insecurities, fears, angers, and anything else from our traumatic pasts onto our partners. If our parents were reliable and warm, we'll be drawn to that type of relationship in adult life. If they were disengaged, neglectful, inconsistent, or self-involved, that's the type of person we'll pick for our mate.

The brain isn't very good at discerning past from present social pain. Partners often unwittingly trigger each other by re-creating early scenes that were tagged as emotionally salient in the past. No matter how idyllic your childhood was, you had psychological trauma. At some point your needs weren't met and it left you devastated. Any reminder of an early attachment failure will set off alarm bells in the stress network of the brain and body. The memory centers of the hippocampus will grade how emotional an experience is with help from the amygdala, the fear center. Frontal input gives the final yes or no on what gets expressed. This is why the more mindful and present you are, the less emotionally reactive you'll be. Mindfulness strengthens that final frontal inhibition, the "don't do it or you'll be sorry" part of the brain. Higher cognitive functions are shut down by intense emotions. Cultivating mindfulness can help maintain an emotional balance within you and between you and your partner. Enhancing awareness can help to strengthen the "top-down" control, enhancing rationality and dampening emotional reactivity. Here we have the conscious marriage, using mindfulness to keep your attachment strong.

In yoga, the postures that you hate performing are the ones your body likely needs the most. That's why they're the hardest. They reveal your weakest, most inflexible parts. In life, the people whom you find the most challenging inevitably are the ones who have the most to teach you. Unlike codependent couples who enable unhealthy behavior, conscious couples enable positive, healthy aspects of each other's behavior, and in the process they heal each other's childhood wounds. The goal is for each of you to stretch toward the middle, widening your shared repertoire of behavior. As opposites, you each have the blueprint for the other's personal growth. Individuals need to harmonize their own feminine and masculine qualities; so do couples. Balancing the yin and yang qualities that each of you brings to the table will benefit both of you.

To my patient who's always complaining about her husband, I said something like this: "Stop fixating on how he isn't like you. Nobody is, and you wouldn't want to be yoked to your carbon copy anyway. The fact that he's so many things you're not, and vice versa, is exactly what makes your partnership work. Opposites attract for a reason. The two of you make something bigger than each of you alone ever could. An effective team."

DIVISION OF LABOR: SEX AND POWER

Interesting news: we're becoming the men we wanted to marry. The number of women who are their family's sole or primary breadwinner has soared, to 40 percent today from 11 percent in 1960. Things are switching around from where they were in the fifties, when women were warned, "If you sink into his arms, you'll find your arms in his sink." Back then, men had career goals, and women wanted those men. These days, women are bringing home the bacon, and one out of five married moms has a higher income than her husband. A recent business school survey showed more women defining success through work, while men chose personal growth as a priority. A common configuration in New

York City is the alpha woman working at an executive-level position married to a guy who works at home on his computer, if he works at all. He picks the kids up from school and might do some household chores while Mommy has meetings and travels for work. Powerful woman, slacker husband. See, opposites really do attract.

Because nearly two-thirds of families have two working parents, it's a toss-up to see who's going to be doing which chores. My thinking is, some people are more or less meticulous about particular things, so you divide the chores accordingly. Fess up to each other about the housework you don't mind doing. Owning up to your traits is one way to be more authentic in your relationship. Sharing earnings and household chores decreases the likelihood of divorce, unless the wife earns more than her husband—then they're more likely to report marital troubles and consider separating. The best odds arise if the wife earns around 40 percent of the household income and the husband does about 40 percent of the housework.

Even though the egalitarian marriage creates higher emotional satisfaction and promotes longevity of a relationship, there is a casualty. Sex. On one hand, women surveyed made clear that marrying a man who was willing to help out with the child care and household chores mattered more than his level of income or his religious beliefs. We want to marry a housewife as much as they do. The problem is, we don't want to have sex with the maid. It turns out that sexism is sexy. We want the men to do the manly chores, like taking out the garbage and maintaining the car. When our husbands are doing dishes and laundry, we're less likely to have sex with them.

I can't tell you how many of my patients are in sexless marriages, but it's more than I ever would have thought. These are perfectly peaceful partnerships where the division of labor seems adequate, and there's love and comfort there, just no sex for very long stretches—months or years. There's a spark missing, a frisson between partners that's required for animal coupling. One requirement for sexual energy is gender differentiation. You're manly and I'm womanly and those opposites attract. In households with stay-at-home dads, it may be that he feels less confident without his "day job," and his harried, working wife may start to lose some respect for his position. Men who take care of the children and the house may seem a little less manly to us when we finally plop into bed at night, even though we tell them how happy we are with the division of labor during the day. What's the problem? Equality and "consensual everything" just isn't sexy.

For many of us, part of what makes sex hot is shifts in power. Being controlled, dominated, or "taken" is a common factor in arousal. As much as we're for women's liberation, some habits die very hard, especially in the bedroom. There is often a direct correlation between being powerful outside the home, in the boardroom, and then wanting to be submissive in the bedroom. It may be that when a man spends his days loading the dishwasher according to his wife's tutorial, or folding laundry just so, he's got no more mojo for doing his wife to her specifications.

Then there's resentment. So unsexy, and so common. Wives in my office regularly voice their complaints about how hard they work, how they don't get the help and support they desire and deserve, and it's impossible to ignore these discrepancies at the end of the day when they finally turn in. Sometimes the bedroom is the only place where we can say no and have it be a complete sentence.

THE SEVEN-YEAR ITCH IS REAL

As might be expected, the longer a couple stays together, the more likely sexual infidelity will eventually happen, with a spike in the numbers around seven years of marriage. When gender is teased out, the timing differs. Women are more likely to cheat in their twenties and less likely in their fifties, while men are most likely to cheat in their thirties. The likelihood of an affair peaks in the seventh year of marriage for women and then ebbs from there. For men, the likelihood of an affair decreases over time, until the eighteenth year of marriage; then it increases. High-risk times for men straying tend to cluster around pregnancy and the months following the birth of a child. This may be psychological more than biological as men's testosterone levels naturally recede a bit when they're new dads. But if their needs for sex and attention aren't being attended to, they may look elsewhere. For women, it's all about fertility. Women may be more likely to cheat on their husbands when they're ovulating, thanks to the surge in testosterone, the hormone of novelty.

MONOGAMY IN NATURE? NOT SO MUCH

Very few animals are actually sexually monogamous: 3 percent of mammals, and only one in ten thousand invertebrates. Pair-bonding is rare among mammals; only 3 percent rear their young in this way. "But what about penguins and swans?" you ask. Well, sorry to burst your bubble, but they don't have sex with one partner forever. Penguins are monogamous only until their eggs hatch; the next year they choose new mates. Over his lifetime the "monogamous" penguin may have created two dozen families. And though they do pair-bond to raise their young, swan nests were found to have young from multiple fathers. In fact, when you look at the offspring of the few "monogamous" birds and mammals, infidelity is present in 100 percent of species examined. This is why I think of monogamy as unnatural. Not undesirable, not unattainable, but certainly not natural.

So let's look at our own family tree, where the primates are. First of all, we didn't descend from apes; we *are* apes. We are part of the same family, the great apes (Hominoidea) containing gorillas, orangutans, chimpanzees, bonobos, and humans. Chimps and bonobos (formerly called pygmy chimps) are our closest primate relatives. Female bonobos and chimps mate multiple times with multiple males in a row, raising children fathered by different males. Humans and bonobos, but not chimps, have missionary sex, face to face. We both kiss deeply and look into each other's eyes when mating. We also both carry the genetic codes for oxytocin release, which helps to bond lovers. Chimps stick to rear entry; the female's vulva faces back, not forward, as in bonobos and humans.

In bonobo troops, the female status matters more than the male status, with older females outranking the youngsters. Bonobos are significantly less aggressive than chimps. Sex is used to keep social order, and genital rubbing between female bonobos is common, used to solidify female bonding. It should be noted here that the bonobo clitoris is three times bigger than ours, taking up two-thirds of the vulva, and positioned optimally for ventral stimulation, so all that rubbing has a big payoff. Suffice to say, none of this matriarchy or genital rubbing to keep the peace is seen in chimps. Also, only humans and bonobos have a significant percentage of homosexual sex and, most important, have sex outside of ovulation, a rarity in the animal kingdom. Pair-bonded monogamous animals have infrequent sex and only for reproduction. Sex to keep the peace or solidify the relationship is not practiced.

Among all the social, group-living primates, monogamy is not the norm. The one ape that is monogamous lives in treetops and is solitary, part of the lesser ape family, the gibbon. As humans are the most social of all the primates, except for perhaps the bonobos, it is unwise to assume we'd naturally be monogamous. Body dimorphism (different sizes for different genders) is correlated with male competition for mates. If men and women were monogamous, we'd be the same size, as the gibbons are. If we were completely polygynous (men taking multiple female partners), men would be twice the size of women, as male gorillas and orangutans are. Chimps, bonobos, and human males are all around 10 to 20 percent larger and heavier than females, which implies we have similar rates of promiscuity.

THE BIOLOGY OF FIDELITY—VASOPRESSIN AND PRAIRIE VOLES

The well-studied monogamous prairie voles maintain a single pair bond while raising several litters. As in humans, sex triggers oxytocin release in the females and vasopressin release in the males. The meadow voles, on the other hand, are solitary, asocial, and promiscuous. The vasopressin receptor is quite different in this species. When genes from the monogamous male prairie voles were injected into the brains of the promiscuous male meadow voles, more vasopressin receptors were formed, and the animals started to fixate on and mate with one female vole only.

Vasopressin in the males peaks during sexual arousal. It not only triggers partner preference but is also involved in male parental care. I know what you're thinking: *Can I inject vasopressin into my husband?* No, and some guys have more vasopressin than others. There are different genes that code for vasopressin, and some men have certain genes that others don't have. Men who have a gene variant called 334 score lower on feelings of attachment for their spouses and are more likely to have experienced a marital crisis during the past year or to be in a relationship without being married.

Testosterone levels not only affect sex drive and sexual response but also have a lot to do with fidelity and parenting impulses. Married men and fathers have lower testosterone levels than single and childless men. Right after his child is born, a man's testosterone levels might fall as much as 30 percent. Men who maintain multiple female partners (polygyny) have higher testosterone levels than monogamously married men. Not surprisingly, married men with higher testosterone levels have sex more frequently than those with lower levels, and men who cheat have higher testosterone levels than those who don't. Unconsciously, women may know this. In one study, women rated men with lower voices (more testosterone) as being more likely to be unfaithful and were more likely to select more masculine men with lower voices as short-term, rather than long-term, partners.

THE COOLIDGE EFFECT

Named for Silent Cal, the story goes that he and the missus were separately being shown around a farm. Upon hearing that the rooster mated dozens of times a day, Mrs. Coolidge said to the guide, "Tell that to my husband." Later, when he heard his wife's remark, the president asked, "With the same hen?" "Nope. It's a different hen every time." "Tell that to my wife."

The Coolidge effect, that varying the sex partner invigorates the libido, has been documented in many male mammals, including humans. But it turns out that female primates are aroused by novelty as well. Unfamiliar males are more attractive than the known quantity. "The search for the unfamiliar is documented as a female preference more often than is any other characteristic." Nature has bred philandering into our genes, enhancing the mating strategy of more copulations in order to increase the likelihood of passing those genes on. If guys who are players make more babies, there will be more players in the gene pool.

Ever wonder why men who seem to have it all—fame, fortune, and a loving family—throw it all away for a bit of strange? It's nature, trumping both reason and willpower. Novelty is the strongest attractor. Many of us are "novelty seeking." We enjoy new restaurants, new music, new friends, and new hobbies. Research suggests that people who cheat are not only novelty seekers but also more likely to be extroverts than their partners are. They're also simply more easily bored.

THE SPACE BETWEEN

Couples who spend all their time together may end up being too close. Like a fire deprived of oxygen, sexual energy sputters when there's no room to breathe. You each need to bring something separate and "other" to the partnership, which means you have to go out there and have your own experiences. Girls' night out is good for both of you. Don't confuse love with merging. Eroticism requires separateness; there must be a synapse to cross.

Typically one partner will be clingier while the other will be squirming away. Some people comfort themselves in a dyad, while others soothe themselves solo. Compromise is key here, as we all have our sweet spot regarding intimacy. Some of us want to share everything and be bound at the hip, while others of us would like a little elbow room, please.

Part of the problem is that we've been fed this idea that our spouse should be able to provide everything we need: love, security, companionship, and hot sex. But the intimacy and comfort of a committed relationship carry a completely different energy (not to mention brain chemistry) than eroticism and lust do. Some of the hottest sex you've ever had probably occurred with someone you didn't know all that well, right? The excitement of two people coming together rests on the uncertainty of where it's going and whether it will last. Once you're committed to each other, that spark is history. The trick is to balance the need for unpredictability and novelty with the need for consistency and reliability. And it's no easy trick.

Our sex may be less hot unless we each "get a life," but there's a competing theory about spending time together for the good of the partnership. Couples who spend weekly time talking or being active together are more likely to be happy than couples who take less time to bond. Spouses who share friends spend more time together and have better marriages. Since the 1970s, we're spending less time with our partners (from thirty-five to twenty-six hours a week) and more time doing other things outside the home, mostly work. For couples with kids, the number of hours spent together has gone from thirteen to nine.

Our emotional needs may be clamoring for more time together, while our animal, lusting selves may require time apart for a sense of novelty. Balancing our needs for intimacy and isolation is challenging and a frequent source of stress in our relationships. The first step is to honestly appraise what your needs and desires are and then to lovingly communicate them to your partner. You can't negotiate what isn't on the table, so you're going to have to show your hand in order to win. There is one-way autoregulation, which is "I can do this for myself" or "You can do this for me." Then there's two-way mutual regulation: "We do this for each other." If two people heal the relationship actively, the relationship will heal the two people. Pour your attention into the space between and it will nurture you in return.

SURVIVING AN AFFAIR

Nearly a third of marriages survive an infidelity. Sometimes the discovery of an affair can lead to positive outcomes in the relationship. There may be a willingness to work through problems or improve communication or the quality of the partnership. It is an opportunity to rewrite the rules of your marriage and to become aware of unconscious behaviors that threaten to put anything before your relationship. One of you went outside the safe space of your "couple bubble" to get your needs met. This is crucial information to help make your conscious marriage stronger.

Typically, the man who has an affair will realize that the wife he left is better suited to his needs and caretaking than the woman he left her for. Unfortunately, many women are schooled to reject a repentant cheater because he'll likely do it again. Serial monogamy—falling in lust, becoming attached and committed, only to eventually fall for another partner all over again—is our way of trying to grapple with two competing masters, biology and society.

REWRITING THE RULES

Some couples opt for honesty over fidelity. They accept that their partners are occasionally going to be interested in other lovers and don't want to forfeit the entire relationship. I have a few trailblazing patients who are consensually nonmonogamous. That is, they both know what's going on with the other. Some are swingers, others are in open marriages, and a few call themselves polyamorous. The bottom line with all three is consciousness, and dare I say conscientiousness. Rules are clearly conveyed and adherence is monitored and discussed. Everything is out in the open, which allows both partners to go through the process as one. Their trust is based on truth.

Sometimes people have sex outside their primary relationship for reasons not involving their partner's or the relationship's inadequacy. For example, what if one member of the dyad is bisexual? In Esther Perel's book *Mating in Captivity,* she describes "couples who negotiate sexual boundaries" as "no less committed than those who keep the gates closed. It is their desire to make the relationship stronger that leads them to explore other models of long-term love."

It's normal and natural for both sexes to have a wandering eye and a thirst for novelty in the form of new partners. To pretend otherwise is delusional. How we respond to those desires is up to us. We should at least begin with open communication about our wants and needs with our partner. Candid talk may reveal some surprises; for instance, some men are aroused by the thought of their wives with other men. Talk about your fantasies and share your experiences out in the world when you get home. Hiding and lying will bring only shame, stress, and their eventual discovery. Don't wait until things have progressed before you reveal the details to your partner. Maintaining a secure attachment will assist both of you in navigating these waters together, helping to make your relationship watertight.

MAKING LOVE LAST: THE TEMPTATION OF MONOGAMY

Many committed partnerships feel the fizzle at about three to four years, a common spike in when divorces occur. Anthropologists reckon that this is biological more than anything else. Attachment, trust, security— all of these vasopressin- and oxytocin-powered devices evolved so partners would stay together at least long enough to raise a child. Pairs mate and rear an infant through toddlerhood, and when the heavy lifting of parenting has passed, there is a biological drive to move on and partner with another, always searching for the best genetic material for their lineage. Hence, serial monogamy, sequential committed relationships.

Because we're living longer, couples are spending many more years together than was the case in generations past. So the question is, how do you keep love alive and make it last over these many bumps in the road? Have fun, have sex, and give each other space. Fun, in this case, needs to be about novelty and adrenaline. Novel experiences increase dopamine levels as the brain turns on the gas to pay attention and enjoy. Dopamine can trigger testosterone release, so new activities that require focused attention can help create desire. Dopamine injected into the male rat's bloodstream stimulates copulating behavior, and horny rats that copulate frequently have higher circulating dopamine levels. If you can find a way to inject a sense of danger into your activities, go for it. Norepinephrine, the brain's version of adrenaline, can also stimulate the production and release of testosterone, which will rev sexual desire. So anything that's moderately stressful, threatening, transgressive, or mildly painful can potentially be sexually arousing as well. In sex research, this is known as excitation transfer. You may simply know it as "kinky."

Having sex can trigger the hormones you need to make you horny. I often encourage my patients who report low desire to just go ahead and start the process of sex. Once you get going, some of the desirable brain changes will start to kick in, and before you know it, you'll actually be enjoying yourself. "Use it or lose it" definitely applies to sex. Having orgasms regularly keeps all your sex hormones in play; the more sex you're having, the more sex you'll have. Regular exposure to male pheromones keeps hormone levels healthier, so keep smelling your man. Also, the chemistry that results from orgasm triggers closeness and bonding and possibly even monogamy, all of which might lead to more sex. But this is where it gets complicated.

The warm waters of attachment have been known to douse the fires of lust. Oxytocin can interfere with dopamine and norepinephrine, lessening their impact. And we all know about familiarity breeding contempt. Am I right, married ladies? For many of us, and certainly for laboratory animals, proximity dampens desire. The sex researchers who run primate labs say they have to give the females new males every three years or so. (Jealous?)

We have a natural drive toward novelty in our sexual partners. Biologically speaking, as mammals, "almost all individuals of all species on record have a sexual aversion to closely familiar others; they prefer to mate with strangers." So, however you can, keep it strange. Be mysterious, unavailable; surprise him with what he still doesn't know about you. And make sure you create and maintain a "space between" in your relationship. Do things separately, have your own friends and interests, so you'll have something to talk about when you do spend time together. And when you can, do novel, fun things together. Travel to new territory, try new activities, and incorporate a competitive spirit when it's appropriate. Competition reliably raises testosterone levels, as does intense cardio exercise. So have fun out there. It may lead to great sex, which can help solidify the bonds of great love.

Remember that you're on the same team. Let go of the need to be right, and banish judging, controlling, blaming, shaming, and criticizing. Negativity is invisible abuse that is toxic to the relationship. It ruptures your connection to each other. So avoid these behaviors and you're more than halfway to your dream partnership. Also, heed your own sage advice to others. It's usually projection, and the person most in need of following your wisdom is you. We tend to give others the things we ourselves actually need. We lead by example. In writing, it's "show, don't tell," but in relationships, it's the opposite. Better to specifically verbalize what your needs are than to demonstrate what you need by giving your partner what they're not even asking for. Understand?

Also, only one of you gets to be a baby at a time. Two passive, irresponsible people cannot run a household or raise children. If you insist on being two children, neither of your needs will be met. You can decide between you, and it can be fluid, but one of you needs to be an adult in any given situation. If you're emotionally incapacitated, triggered by something in your history that is adding an extra charge, tell your partner so he (or she) can take the reins.

When you do talk, keep a few things in mind. No one can speak rationally when their limbic system is on fire. The emotional brain will short-circuit the rational brain. Wait to talk till you're both calm and can look each other in the eye while dialoguing. (Talking in the car or in your darkened bedroom is not as good as face to face.) Frame your speech with "I feel" instead of "You did." Mirror what's being said so your partner feels heard. Empathize with your partner so he or she feels validated. "You make sense, and I'd feel that way if it were me." This technique works with children and colleagues, too. Mirror, validate, and empathize.

Even though we may be physiologically built for multiple partners, we're actually happiest when we commit to one. For most of us, monogamy is hard, but staying with one partner for decades has innumerable benefits. Getting to truly know and accept someone, and being known and accepted, allows for tremendous growth, like budding flowers in the sunshine. Long-term love is the best environment for us to flourish and blossom. Cultivating and maintaining rich emotional relationships with family and friends is what life is all about, and it will feed your soul, or at least make you happier. The goal: making your spouse, who is the bedrock of your family, your friend.

Five

Motherhead

otherhood affects our bodies and brains in profound ways that stay with us for a lifetime. Like the massive neuronal reorganization that occurs when falling in love, in the early stages of pregnancy there are countless changes in the brain. Well, one number did come up in my research: neurons multiply at a rate of 250,000 per minute, as motherhood improves learning and memory. It's true some women feel themselves getting stupid during pregnancy; "baby brain suck" can sap your concentration and ability to multitask. Simply put, your brain is being reorganized. The increased estrogen levels put neuroplasticity into overdrive in the brain's memory center, the hippocampus, as new behaviors are prepared for, such as feeding, protecting, and caring for offspring. Our verbal and emotional memories need to be sharp to continue to catalog potentially threatening behaviors in our mates, like abandonment or violence, but spatial learning is particularly affected, as it's important to recall where food was located when foraging.

(Again, this is likely why mothers can locate missing things better than anyone else in the house; it's left over from our days on the savanna.) Parental-induced neuroplasticity can last for years, possibly providing protection from age-related brain changes including memory deficits seen in dementia.

The hormone responsible for this neuronal reorganization is oxytocin. Monogamy, commitment, and child care are all driven by neuroplastic changes partially facilitated by oxytocin, the hormone that makes us cleave to our partners and devote ourselves to our children. During conception, oxytocin stimulates the uterine activity that helps guide sperm to egg. During childbirth, oxytocin drives uterine contractions to expel the fetus. During nursing, oxytocin helps to bring the milk into the nipple, called the letdown reflex. Oxytocin gets credit for solidifying the mother-infant bond, making us feel warm, fuzzy, and connected. But oxytocin isn't about bonding indiscriminately. It helps us distinguish who's in our tribe and who's not. In some experiments, with extra oxy on board, people are even more harsh against those they feel aren't in their group. Motherhood brings a whole new set of behaviors from those seen in other life phases. In the research setting, aggression is seen more commonly in female mammals that are lactating and protecting their young. So it may be that part of that mama grizzly protective aggression comes from the "hormone of love."

The hormone of mother love could also be called the amnesic hormone, because it can erase learned behavior and replace it with new patterns. Sometimes existing attachments are supplanted by new ones. This may be part of the basis for falling in love with your baby at the expense of maintaining your attachment to your mate. Couples who raise children together are bonded as family, but they also face new obstacles.

From conception and pregnancy to birth and nursing and beyond, motherhood is a time of tremendous change. It is a magical experience for many, but it's also draining, difficult, and demanding. Understanding some of the science behind different phases of life can help you to navigate the roller coaster, and maybe even enjoy the ride a bit more.

THE TICKING CLOCK

Women are creators. We make order out of chaos, whether we're cooking, folding laundry, or organizing our households. As creators, we make babies, and we produce milk. Not all of us choose to perform all of these tasks, but most of us do. Though we're starting later (age thirty today, from age twenty-three in the 1950s) and having fewer kids (two instead of three), most of us (around 80 percent) are still opting into the mommy track.

The biological clock is no joke. In my twenties, when I would see the women of the Upper East Side with their strollers and baby joggers, I would practically sneer and say to myself, *Not gonna do it* (à la George Bush the first). But somewhere around age thirty-one or so, I'd notice a sharp heartache happening in my pelvis when I'd see a baby, and I found myself aching for one of my own. It was as if my body were using chemical warfare to trick me into reproducing. For many of us, this sensation that our ovaries are hijacking our brains is overwhelming. Estrogen and testosterone levels conspire midcycle to make us act like cats in heat, and it becomes harder with every passing month to resist the tug to breed.

In major metropolitan cities, the age for starting a family is higher than elsewhere. I have plenty of patients in their late thirties and even early forties who are still hoping to start a family. Many of us are getting our careers in order before we choose motherhood, something that was nearly always reversed just a few generations ago. The quality of eggs produced by the ovaries drops off substantially when you get to the early forties. Because of waiting longer to get started, many of my patients go from being on oral contraceptives for a dozen years or more to taking fertility drugs to help them get pregnant, barely stopping in between these two poles.

Fertility drugs can be hard on moods. Clomid, a medicine used to encourage the ovary to pop out a few extra eggs, can trigger massive PMS-type symptoms, as can many other hormones and follicle stimulators being used today to help women conceive. Hot flashes, emotional lability, irritability, and depression are all possible. Rare cases of psychosis or mania have also been reported.

Nesting, the particular cleaning frenzy that occurs during late pregnancy, is a very real phenomenon. What's less clear is whether there is some biological process that happens even before pregnancy to help us get our house in order. My sister got herself into fantastic shape before she got pregnant. She quit smoking cigarettes (no easy feat), stopped drinking, and lost weight, getting her body primed as a vessel for a fetus. I've seen it happen in my patients repeatedly. They want to go off their meds prior to conceiving and they do. Gynecologists will sometimes recommend that their patients stop their SSRIs, as serotonin increases prolactin levels, which can impair fertility. I also recommend that my patients lay off their nightly melatonin tablets, which also increase prolactin and lower follicle-stimulating hormone, both of which interfere with fertility.

The decision to stay on meds or go off everything during pregnancy is difficult and complicated. Psychiatrists know that the high levels of stress and cortisol that accompany extreme anxiety and the poor self-care seen during depression are bad for a developing fetus, but what is less clear is how staying on psychiatric meds affects the baby. The risks are low but present. Depending on in which trimester SSRIs are taken, exposure is associated with preterm labor or miscarriage for the mother and cardiac defects, pulmonary hypertension, seizures, and withdrawal syndromes for the infant. There is some concern about a link between

SSRI exposure and autistic spectrum disorders. One study reported that boys with autism were three times more likely to have been exposed to SSRIs in utero, while another said it was twice as likely. But other studies don't bear this out.

All of my patients would prefer to be medication-free during gestation, but a few have had to stay medicated because their symptoms were completely unmanageable off meds. This is especially true for women with bipolar disorder, where the risk of severe psychiatric symptoms often outweighs the risk to the fetus. For milder depression or anxiety, pregnancy is a great time to substitute other means of treatment, like psychotherapy, acupuncture, transcranial direct-current stimulation, or light therapy.

When faced with an impending pregnancy, not only can my patients successfully taper off their SSRIs or ADHD meds, but they also can re-vamp their diet, exercise more, and stress less. Instinctively, we do things for our children that we wouldn't do for ourselves, even before they exist. So, yes, our ovaries do hijack our brains, but in a way that helps us to protect and care for our offspring.

During pregnancy, hormonal levels are actually more static than they've ever been in your life. You don't cycle every month, so there's no ovulatory horniness or premenstrual bitchiness. For many women, it's a time of stability and quiescence. I'd been taught that pregnancy was "protective" against psychiatric complaints. Rates of depression are lower during pregnancy than at other times in the reproductive age, though some women may experience an increase in their OCD symptoms. (My assumption is that this is tied into the nesting impulse and its chemistry.) However, in women who are younger, have a history of depression, have fewer social supports, or are ambivalent about their pregnancies, depression may still occur.

Certain symptoms, like fatigue or insomnia, are seen in typical pregnancies, as well as depression, which can make it hard to differentiate between the two. Many women report the worst sleep of their lives occurring during pregnancy. Insomnia comes toward the end of gestation as your mind races, worrying about everything that may go wrong with the delivery and all the years after, your bladder is being squeezed out by your uterus, and you're trying to roll over in your bed when you're the size of a manatee. It may be that your brain is trying to prepare you for what comes next. After delivery, life with your baby is punctuated by interrupted sleep, which may last for months or years. My advice to pregnant insomniacs: read a few books on nursing. It's not completely intuitive, and there are things that can go wrong that are good to learn about ahead of time, not when your boobs are killing you.

BIRTH AND NURSING

The way we give birth now is far removed from nature. It is medicalized, scheduled, and anesthetized, so that we've lost touch with the natural rhythm and timing of a normally progressing labor. We're given Pitocin to bring on an unnaturally acute and painful process that then requires an epidural so we can tolerate it. Or we're given an epidural that stalls the labor so we're forced to use Pitocin to accelerate it. Once again, we are out of touch with our own bodies and our intuition of how a completely natural process should unravel, according to earth time, not obstetrician time. A flower's maximal expression is in the fruiting, and fruit ripens at its own pace. This is why I, as a physician, chose midwives for both of my births. Doctors have a hard time doing nothing. It's not in our nature.

I know that medical interventions are sometimes necessary and lifesaving, and I also know this is a touchy issue for many women. There is a certain pride in how we deliver, and it's a shame and a disappointment when it doesn't turn out the way we planned. I delivered both my children naturally, and while it was intensely painful, things progressed quickly, thanks to my nicely wide "birthing hips," a part of my body I fully appreciated at least two days out of my life. During my short, sharp "natural" labor, I was pretty darn altered between the endorphins, endocannabinoids, and adrenaline. My pupils were dilated, and between contractions I kept remarking to my husband, Jeremy, how high I felt. (Endocannabinoids help to maintain a pregnancy, and they peak during labor induction.) Because there was no anesthesia involved, both my children were born awake, alert, and calm. I remember not quite connecting with the warm, slimy being placed on my chest in that birthing room. For a moment, I was at a loss. What have I done and what do I do now? But I placed her on my breast; she began to suck, and the oxytocin surge helped kick everything into gear. I was a mother all of a sudden, and I was all set.

But for many women, nursing is hard, and sometimes painful until you get it right, but it's important to remember, when you're listening to your third lactation consultant or reading your fourth breast-feeding book, that it does have tremendous benefits. Breast milk contains everything that a baby needs and many things that formula doesn't provide, like enzymes, antibodies, growth hormones, proteins, and bacteria. Because of this passed-down immunity, breast-fed babies have fewer infections. Also, the fatty acids in breast milk boost neural development; breast-fed babies have higher IQs than formula-fed babies. It's also better for *you*. Mothers who nurse have lower incidences of breast cancer and ovarian cancer.

They also have lower incidences of stress, due to higher oxytocin levels. But remember that oxytocin can mediate maternal aggression. Never come between a mama bear and her cubs, especially if she's still nursing. Oxytocin turns down the fear response when it comes to being aggressive, so we're not afraid to fight.

Breast milk has tryptophan, the building block for serotonin, which stimulates endorphin production in infants. Breast milk contains a collection of endorphins called galattorphins, and both baby and mother have higher endorphin levels just after nursing. Mammalian breast milk also contains cannabinoids, naturally occurring substances similar to cannabis, regardless of whether the nursing mother is or ever was a pothead. Goat milk has the highest levels of cannabinoids, but human breast milk definitely has them, too. Now you know why babies look so happy and sleepy after they nurse. Not only are cannabinoids in maternal milk, but the activation of the cannabinoid receptors is critical in priming the oral muscles necessary for suckling in newborns. When cannabinoid receptor antagonists are given to newborn mice, it completely inhibits suckling and growth in the pups, and they die within days of its administration. Formula-fed babies may get fatter for the same reason pot smokers have smaller waistlines than nonpartakers. Even though stoners might ingest more calories, it does not result in a higher body mass index. Cannabinoids in breast milk likewise help to regulate the baby's metabolism.

One downside of nursing? Because of our increasingly contaminated environment, our breast milk now has appreciable levels of pollutants like flame retardants and polybrominated diethyl ethers (PBDEs). These can interfere with thyroid function and cause masculinizing features in our girls and feminizing ones in our boys. I still believe that the upsides, particularly the substances found only in breast milk, outweigh this horrific fact. But one more upside: you burn about thirty calories for every ounce of milk you produce. I ate like crazy during those early motherhood years and managed to lose the "baby fat" fairly quickly. I'd be pumping breast milk into a bottle, counting the calories as the ounces accumulated. Ten ounces were as good as a three-mile run!

BONDING

Attachment is crucial for our mates and our children, hence the post-coitus bump in oxytocin as well as those sustained high levels when nursing. The bonding hormone oxytocin is the glue that keeps mother and child together, mother and father together, and even father and baby together. Babies have oxytocin just like moms. Cuddling and nurturing produce elevated levels of oxytocin, calming their stress response. And it turns out that dads have oxy too. During the early phases of parenthood, cohabiting parents share elevated oxytocin levels, which are often inter-related. Although some men may be more likely to cheat when their mates are pregnant or are new mothers, it could be that if you allow your partner more time with his baby, his bond will be stronger not just with his child but with you as well. Vasopressin is the biggest factor in paternal behavior, helping a dad to protect his child and bond with its mother. Men have prolactin as well, which elevates as they hear their baby's cry, just as a woman's prolactin levels do.

Like other animals, and especially primates, we thrive on attach-ment and perish without it. Monkeys reared without physical contact with their mothers become violent and socially impaired as adults, their brain chemicals imbalanced after only a few days of separation from them. In laboratory animals, if a mother doesn't respond to her pup's dis-tress call, the pup will die even if it's fed. The type of attachment we re-ceive early on will affect our emotional functioning thereafter. Maternal care in infancy affects anxiety regulation in the brain of the offspring. Any disruption of attachment in infancy can lead to exaggerated stress reactions down the road in adulthood. Unmet emotional needs will trig-ger a stress response not just in childhood but potentially throughout adulthood as well. This is important to remember not just in mothering but also in being an attentive wife or partner. Disrupting the attachment bond causes all sorts of heartbreak and behavioral upheaval whenever it happens.

Attunement to our children's emotional states and needs helps us to fine-tune our relationship with them. When we give our children loving attention, we not only influence their brain circuitry but also affect their future relationships. When we're distracted, stressed out, or unavailable, our children suffer for it. Down the line, they may choose partners who treat them similarly, reenacting those early separations.

A tuned-in parent can help produce a healthy child. What our kids need most is our genuine presence. For children today, it is confusing and traumatizing to have a parent's face on a computer or smartphone screen most of the day. We may be physically present, but we are not emotionally available. It's hard for toddlers to wrap their heads around that paradox, called proximate separation. I'm here, but I'm not really here for you. We need to engage deeply and authentically with our kids, provide an anchoring gaze, mirror their communications, and validate and empathize with their emotions and experiences. This takes attention and focus, which can't be divided between their faces and our glowing devices.

POSTPARTUM DEPRESSION

The biggest disrupter of early infant-mother bonding is severe depression, which may occur after delivery. I have a colleague whose mother committed suicide when he was four months old, convinced he'd be better off without her. It has colored his entire narrative; that attachment disruption was forever wired into his stress response and temperament.

Postpartum is a vulnerable time for women both pharmacologically and psychologically, and it's common to be down. As many as 50 to 80 percent of women report a milder form of depression, sometimes called the baby blues, which may last a week or two. But roughly 10 to 15 percent have a true postpartum depression, disrupting functioning in a number of areas for at least two weeks: energy, appetite, sleep, and libido. More rare is a syndrome called postpartum psychosis, occurring in one out of a thousand deliveries, often accompanied by dangerous thoughts. I've interviewed new mothers in emergency rooms at Mount Sinai and Bellevue with a similar delusion, that their baby was the root of all evil, and if they could smother the baby, they'd save the world. Scary stuff, and those women had to be hospitalized and treated with antidepressants and short-term antipsychotics and were separated from their infants temporarily. This is why I do recommend that a psychiatrist get involved to assess whether you need treatment if your mood is down more days than not after you've delivered.

Prolactin, the hormone responsible for milk production, reaches its highest levels when we're nursing. Good news for a hungry baby. Not always great for the mom. Prolactin can make us sleepy and depressed. Sometimes the postpartum blues are associated with higher prolactin levels. Other times, the culprit is a quick drop-off of estrogen that occurs after delivery. Although there are massive changes in hormones that occur during pregnancy, they tend to occur gradually. Many of these changes quickly return to baseline right after delivery. Because of this, you can go from being blissed out to being an anxious mess in a matter of days. If you think about it, you can see why it would be biologically advantageous to be a bit jumpy and hypervigilant after your baby is born. Nature sets you up to be a hovering mother so you can keep your baby safe and attend to its every need. These hormonal drop-offs can be an uncomfortable and rocky time for many new mothers. Add being sleep-deprived and in constant need of a shower, and it's understandable why you'd be irritable and weepy.

The peak time for postpartum depression isn't right after the baby is born, but rather at ten weeks. Depending on when you wean your baby off breast milk, you may end up with a delayed postpartum depression as the oxytocin wanes. Breast-feeding reliably reduces the risk of postpartum depression, but in women who wanted to nurse but couldn't, the rate of postpartum depression is actually higher. So these women need more emotional support. Also, if your baby is colicky or has prolonged inconsolable crying, your odds for depression increase significantly. A history of a previous depression, or bad PMS, may also increase your risk for postpartum depression. It's challenging but important to remember good self-care after your baby is born. Sleep when you can, eat as healthfully as possible, and go outside for walks to keep your sanity.

THE TERRIBLE TWOS, THE F#*!ING FOURS, AND MOODY LITTLE BITCHES

This isn't a parenting book, and I'm not mother of the year, so I'll be brief. Kids' brains aren't done cooking yet. The rational frontal lobes don't fully inhibit the emotional limbic circuits of the brain until the midtwenties. Children, and especially adolescents, typically have poor control over their impulses and their emotional outbursts. They're not naturally mindful. That's your job. You need to be their holding environment, containing their emotions. The easiest way to do this is to mirror to them their concerns; don't minimize them. "You really wish you could have a cookie right now!" works better than "You know you can't have a cookie until after lunch." They also want to feel in control, so offer choices that you can live with, like "Do you want your bath before or after story time?" Also, for your teenage daughter, try being a helicopter pad, not a helicopter parent. Be a loving sanctuary where she can pause to catch her breath. She still craves attachment and connection with you, though she's not always acting that way. And keep track of her cycle. It'll help you immensely to anticipate and make space for her moody bitchiness.

The mantras for marriage hold for mothering. Same team. Conflict is growth trying to happen. You each have the blueprints for the other's development. Your children have valuable lessons to offer you as they push your buttons. Our demons surface when we're reminded of their existence, and we lash out. That moody little bitch is your yoga, a trigger for self-reflection, not a reason for you to go on psych meds. First of all, Do Not Take the Bait. She knows how to get your goat, and you need to consciously decide not to engage. Ignored behavior will extinguish itself more rapidly than behavior that is met with a big response, even if it's negative. Just stay connected to her as best as you can while maintaining your integrity. Mothering is as much about raising yourself to be an authentic, empathic woman as it is about raising your daughter to become herself.

IT DOES TAKE A VILLAGE

Since the 1970s, when I was growing up, the prevalence of nuclear families has slipped from 45 percent down to 23 percent. The rate of babies born out of wedlock has risen four-fold. Another new feature: unmarried couples living together and raising a child fathered by another man. This number has jumped 170 percent in the past twenty years or so.

My private practice is full of women in their late thirties or forties who really want a baby. They're desperate to find the right man for the job, aware that time is running out. I've gotten in the habit of exploring with these women just what it would take to go ahead and have that baby, man be damned. There are plenty of ways to get sperm, whether purchased or gifted, and there's no guarantee that the baby daddy is going to stick around or provide everything you and the kids need anyway. If you want a baby, I say gather your sisters, mothers, girlfriends, and mentors and make yourself a village. There are plenty of cultures that do it this way, and examples abound in nature, particularly among primates, that show it can be done just fine if sisters are doing it for themselves.

Three-quarters of women today are working mothers, a number that's quadrupled since the 1950s, and even though 40 percent of us are the primary breadwinners, the bulk of the child-rearing responsibilities still falls to us. And unlike long ago, when we had plenty of help nearby in the form of extended family and clan members, now we're going it mostly alone. We are overwhelmed by the responsibilities and the tedium that alternates with the power struggles when it comes to raising kids.

Children used to spend more time around different nurturing adults, and multigenerational homes and gatherings were the norm. Now kids are warehoused with other kids, whether in day care, school, or summer camp. They learn from their peers instead of their elders, and they are starved of the intimacy and attachment they require. Peer orientation puts them at risk for drugs and promiscuity, so my advice is to attend to your kids' attachment needs if you don't want them to fill those holes on the Internet or elsewhere.

Our ancestors were "cooperative breeders." We evolved in groups where all the resources and responsibilities were shared, including food, sex, and child care. In tribal societies, everyone chips in to raise the children. In some aboriginal groups, there is partible paternity, meaning the men aren't entirely sure which children are theirs. This not only reduces conflict in the tribe, as men are bound by the shared paternity with other men, but also benefits the children, who receive special interest from multiple male members. There are several nursing mothers, infants are shared, and each man works hard for all the members of the village. Parental exhaustion is "inappropriate for our species" and is likely a relatively new phenomenon because we're doing it alone.

We are all exhausted. Our fatigue is a huge issue, and it affects our ability to be there for our kids, our spouses, and ourselves. Unfortunately, when the baby comes, all of our energy seems devoted to child care. But if we don't devote time to self-care, we're going to feel even worse than we already do from sleep deprivation. And there's one more thing you need to fit into your schedule:

SEX DURING MOTHERHOOD—HAVING LITTLE KIDS MEANS HAVING EVEN LITTLER INTEREST IN SEX

My life is very full, my to-do list long. Buy milk, make sure Joe's homework is done, shop with Molly for her semiformal dress, and then one last expenditure of energy when I plop into the marital bed. Some nights, it feels like just another chore to be checked off my list. (I'm thinking of those pads of lined paper that say "Another Dumb Thing I Gotta Do...") I don't know about you, but by the time I get done in my office, having spent the day gratifying my patients, and come home to the kids, who need my loving attention, a dishwasher that needs emptying, and laundry that needs folding, there are other things that come to mind once I finally lie down. In a survey of married women, 63 percent said they'd rather watch a movie, read, or sleep than have sex with their husbands.

When my kids were younger, they were all over me—on my lap, playing with my hair, nursing. It was very hard for me to switch gears and interpret touch in a different way just because it was coming from someone I married. I remember wondering, *What happened to the horny girl I was in high school when I wasn't supposed to be having sex?* Is it Mother Nature's cruel little hoax that when I can finally appreciate and celebrate the intimacy of my relationship, I have lost interest?

Although there are exceptions, women in early pregnancy or early postpartum report significant reductions in sexuality. A major predictor of sexual satisfaction is relationship satisfaction. We know that marital satisfaction plummets during the first two years of parenting. Fatigue and depression are important throughout the perinatal period, but at six months postpartum, the biggest predictor of sexual happiness is "the quality of the mother role." So how you're doing as a mom matters, but let's not forget about hormones.

After the baby, you may be nursing for an extended period of time, and your sex life will likely be minimal because of this. The first three months postpartum are the worst. There are quite a few reasons for lackluster libido. Prolactin levels are up, which suppress testosterone secretion. Also, women who are nursing have less vaginal lubrication due to lower estrogen levels. The biggest issue: you may not be ovulating yet. Nature tries to help you out while you're nursing a little one, making sure you have plenty of time between your babies. Once the nursing ebbs, you're more likely to ovulate, and when your period comes back, the horniness will, too, a bit, at least midcycle when you're fertile. When you wean the baby completely, your libido comes back even more, but not necessarily to baseline. Having little kids climbing all over you can keep your oxytocin levels up, which will keep your testosterone down. Mothers of young children have lower testosterone than those with older children, who have lower testosterone than women with no children. And married women have lower testosterone than unmarried women. So that horny girl from high school? Gone, Daddy, gone.

Women's magazines and blogs talk about being "touched out." You have so much physical intimacy with your kids—they require a substantial amount of cuddling, holding, and physical soothing—that when you finally climb into bed with your partner, you're sick of it. It may be that you've filled your quota. Your experience with your children is so sensual and emotional, and there is a euphoric melding of mother and child much like that seen between lovers. So it may not be that you have nothing left to give at the end of your day, but rather that there is nothing more you need. Your children end up being the primary source of your physical and emotional gratification.

There is also the issue of body autonomy. This means it's yours, not anyone else's. When you have little kids, it's easy to feel like your boundaries are completely disrespected. With all that loss of control, it's simple to see why you may exert some when you finally get into your own bed with a curt "Don't touch me." (If you were physically or sexually abused in your childhood, you can expect these issues to be even more prominent. Because your body autonomy was violated in your youth, it might be a trigger for you when your children show you the same disregard.) No matter how assertive or dominant we are out in the world, some of us turn passive and reactive once we're finally in bed. He wants to, and it's up to us to say yes or no. Sometimes, just like a toddler asserting autonomy over Mommy by saying no to anything she requests (even "Do you want a treat?"), we deny him his requests because we can. We have the power to refuse and we want to exercise it.

Don't discount the loss of psychic autonomy, the "virtual annihilation of the self" that accompanies motherhood. If you have no self, you're certainly not entitled to fight for what you desire. As our roles change from independent working woman to mommy who subordinates her desires to her toddler, it's easy to feel lost in the shuffle. Some mothers learn to hide or deny their own needs, choosing to gratify those of their children instead, anticipating their kids' every whim so that they want for nothing. I often joke that the word *mother* is based on the word *martyr*. We spend our evenings feeding the mouths that bite, balancing work and family with no time or space left for ourselves. Once we finally get into bed, we're not just tired, we're tired of giving.

Our frustration about doing more nightly housework in addition to our day jobs can be a major cause of diminished sexual desire. And until nonsexual issues get resolved, many women have minimal interest in or motivation for sex. Resentment isn't sexy. When it comes to partner sex (not lust for a stranger, a different matter entirely), many women need to feel safe, cared for, and connected. Women are much more likely to reject their husbands if they're feeling unsupported, underappreciated, or misunderstood. Men, however, seem to be able to put aside all sorts of issues if it means they can get it on.

Pat Love, in her book *Hot Monogamy,* says that more men than women complain to her that they don't get enough touching, both sexual and nonsexual. Daddies are not touched out. For men, sex can be the only way they access emotional vulnerability and establish intimacy. The problem is, you might respond to those needs as if he were one more child to be taken care of instead of realizing that he is offering you something that both of you require.

A desire discrepancy in a marriage is normal. I have patients who routinely complain about the drudgery of attending to their husbands' sexual needs when they'd rather do anything but. But parents seem to know sex is important and may go ahead anyway, even if they're not in the mood. In an iVillage survey of two thousand women, those with two or more children were more likely to have sex out of obligation than those without kids.

I often talk to my patients about the difficulty of transitions. Toddlers aren't the only ones who have trouble moving from one activity to another. Coming home from work and transforming into mother mode is hard enough. What's even trickier is to switch gears from "mommy" to "wifey." If you can't turn off the mom radar, you're not going to be able to focus on your own physical sensations.

Motherhood may be all about giving, but sex is often about taking what you need, and maybe even being a bit selfish. You have a right to receive pleasure and release after all the caretaking you've been doing, but that's a pretty big mind flip. I find that transitions require rituals. You're supposed to warn the kids two minutes before leaving the park, so at least give yourself that buffer. After the kids go down, take a shower, have a cup of tea, meditate for ten minutes, or even just take a few deep breaths and a good stretch. Any one of those may be enough to help you focus back on your body and your relationship. Even better: have him give the kids a bath and put them to bed while you prepare yourself, mentally and physically, to reconnect with your lover and yourself.

Sometimes the only way for you to focus fully on yourself and your partner is if your children are asleep or out of the house. You may need to be locked in a room far away from theirs. The book *Sexy Mamas* recommends that you stock a lockable guest room with sex toys and lubes, sexy outfits and props, to have an exciting quickie getaway in the "playroom." I recommend, at the very least, that parents get a lock on their own bedroom door. The days may be focused on the kids and their emotional needs, but the nights are a time to turn to each other. This is an adults-only zone.

Children need to learn about the concept of privacy, that Mom and Dad need private time for adult conversation and adult activities. They should also learn that sex is a natural part of life and relationships. If they see you as "sex positive," happy and sexually fulfilled, it helps them have healthier sexual relationships in adulthood.

"DATE NIGHT" VERSUS SPONTANEITY

There are two ways to go here, and you don't have to choose. Establishing a predictable night when you promise to hook up with your spouse has its advantages. You mutually agree that it's valuable and important, intentionally affirming your bond with each other. You have days to prepare, fantasize, and tease each other with sexy e-mails or texts. That's a lot of foreplay. Anticipation can be a great aphrodisiac. Good sex doesn't have to be spontaneous.

But many do complain that any sort of routine or ritual kills the excitement that comes from unpredictability. Sometimes what's hot is a loss of control, or the risk of being caught. Enter the quickie. Your time is limited, I know. Scarcity is the watchword for young parents. There's not enough time, not enough energy, not enough space or privacy. But a lot can be done in a short period of time if you're game to be creative. And if you both agree that shared pleasure and connection are your goals, instead of intercourse or orgasm, you may find yourself even more in the mood. Follow your sexual intuition and do what your body tells you. What would you desire right now? *Men Are from Mars, Women Are from Venus* author John Gray encourages his readers to differentiate between gourmet sex and fast-food sex. Sometimes you just want small fries and that's it. Make those wishes ultraclear to your partner, who doesn't always know exactly what you want or when.

MILFS

Guys with babies always look hot, right? They're nurturing, and they've shown they're capable of commitment and stability. Why is it such a surprise that a mother would be sexy, too? Biologically, it makes more sense to invest your genetic material in someone who has shown she's capable of reproducing. Of course a mom should make a man horny.

Until very recently, mothers got a pass on the "hot or not" game. They weren't expected to be sexy, and for some women, that was just fine. It was nice to not have to worry so much about appearance and desirability. In most traditional cultures, motherhood is more saintly than sexy. It's often taboo to fetishize mothers. My pet theory: mixing our potency as mothers and as sexual beings may be too much for men to handle, making them uneasy. It's too much power all in one place. Or it may be a defense born of fear. Men may have difficulty eroticizing their baby mama because it tickles the boundaries of some very sensitive areas, like the Oedipal complex. And if you buy into these Freudian theories, then the MILF idea makes more sense. Lusting after someone else's mother is a safer way for you to project all your taboo sexual energy for your mother onto another sex partner.

One thing is for sure: as we mature, so does the quality of our sex. We need to reinvent sex now that we're mothers, building a bridge between being a mother hen and being a fox. With experience and maturity comes sexual sophistication. Optimally, we know what works for us, and we're more confident about sharing that information with our partners. Call it "authentic eroticism." Maybe the reason MILFs are such a turn-on is that mothers simply make better lovers. As we blossom and ripen, nurture and mentor, we are likely more capable of integrating intimacy and spirituality into our sexuality. And that is deep, and hot. So go ahead and be sexy, Mama.

Six

Perimenopause: The Storm Before the Calm

The ups and downs of the your menstrual cycles, relationship drama, and family responsibility may seem like enough to manage, but just at the moment you might begin to think you have everything under control, there comes another curveball: perimenopause. And it comes earlier than you may have thought.

Actual menopause lasts one day. It is the one-year anniversary since your periods have completely stopped. The average age for menopause is fifty-one, but anywhere from the forties to the midfifties is considered normal. Perimenopause, however, is the long, drawn-out transition from fertility to infertility, which begins seven to ten years prior to your period stopping. Things don't usually get problematic until the late forties, but this is a marathon, not a sprint. As you near the finish line, things will likely get intense. You learn to expect the unexpected: worsening PMS that seems to come earlier every month, flying off the handle for no good reason, feeling horny one day and completely turned off the next, and periods that come and go unexpectedly.

We've got an entertaining situation here in my house. Just as my teenage daughter, Molly, is entering into her cyclical moodiness, her mother is ungracefully exiting. Don't you wish you were my husband, sandwiched between a cadet just joining the ranks of the menstruation nation and a retired general who's bowing out? Both of us are having fits and starts of our ovaries, but only one of us gets a pass on her pimples and emotional outbursts. Puberty gets an allowance. Perimenopause gets bupkis.

Nearly a quarter of women with teenagers are in their fifties. Not only are we feeling terrorized by our moody little bitches, but many of us are also caring for aging parents. We are torn between two generations that compete for our attention, accommodation, and care. I marvel that my mother did not go completely batshit while raising three daughters and driving an hour a day to check on her parents to make sure my grandfather gave his wife her insulin and she his meals. Perimenopausal women today are not just balancing work and family; they're also trying to avoid putting their parents in a nursing home. It's not only stress inducing or anxiety provoking, it's depressing. We all have fears around aging and becoming "infirm." Watching our daughters blossom in the springtime of their fertility as we fade out in the autumn of ours, plus seeing what lies ahead as our mothers wither and weaken, is poignant and painful and very nearly too much to handle.

Hormonal surges and cycles are a major part of being a woman. Once those cycles finally stop, after we've weathered the hot flashes and mood swings, then how will we feel? According to plenty of older women, great. I cling to one Gallup poll from 1998 that asked older women when they felt happiest and most fulfilled, and a slim majority chose the years between fifty and sixty-five. So hang in there, baby. Fifty's coming. In the meantime, forewarned is forearmed. Just knowing you can get a little crazy and angry can help the whole process not get the better of you, and there are real ways to harness the powerful changes your body has in store for you.

NUTS AND BOLTS: SYMPTOMS AND COMPLAINTS

During perimenopause, symptoms change month to month, and day to day, as they gradually pick up steam, crescendoing right before your periods stop. And then start again, out of the blue. The absolute hormone levels matter, but what affects the brain most are the abrupt changes in those levels. Every little fluctuation triggers a symptom. Complaints during this stretch include weight gain, fatigue, low libido, and vaginal dryness and irritation. No, wait, it gets worse. Because collagen is estrogen sensitive, it becomes less elastic as you age, so say hello to wrinkles and good-bye to dry underwear; three-quarters of women between forty-five and fifty-four have some episodes of urinary incontinence. Weakened sphincters with less collagen lose their elasticity. Insomnia is the biggest issue, coming early in the transition and lasting for years. It can occur on its own or result from night sweats—the hot flashes that hit you while you sleep.

Hot flashes affect 80 percent of women in perimenopause, last between one and five minutes, and occur over a span of nearly a decade, starting years before, and continuing years after, your periods stop. Sudden dips in estrogen levels cause a drop in the set point of the hypothalamus, the brain's temperature regulator. Your brain then tells your body that it's overheating and goes about lowering your body temperature the only way it knows how, with sweating and bringing blood to the skin. Your face flushes as the blood vessels dilate, and the whole upper body breaks out in a sweat, sometimes followed by chills. Some women experience an "aura" before a hot flash, a sense of dread, suddenly feeling weak, or heart palpitations, all thanks to spiking norepinephrine levels, your brain's adrenaline. If this happens to you, it's normal. Your brain is trying to give you a heads-up that you're about to overheat, like a warning light on your dash.

ESTROGEN DOMINANCE: TOO MUCH OF A GOOD THING

For most women, perimenopause has two phases. At first there is a relative overabundance of estrogen due to rapidly falling progesterone levels. Because these two hormones balance each other out, this is referred to as unopposed estrogen, or estrogen dominance. Later in the transition, estrogen levels finally fall and you get a slightly different cluster of symptoms.

In early perimenopause, when you're still ovulating, your cycles may shorten, perhaps going from twenty-eight or thirty days down to twenty-one or twenty-four days. This is your body's way of giving you more opportunities to become pregnant one last time before the shop closes down. The first half of your cycle, the follicular phase, shrinks from fourteen days down to ten. This is when you feel halfway decent and may even be attracted to your partner, thanks to estrogen and testosterone levels being relatively high. Then you ovulate, the egg dies, and it's all downhill from there in terms of mood and libido.

Around the early forties, the quality of the released egg starts to fall precipitously, as does the leftover part that makes progesterone, the corpus luteum. Lower progesterone levels become the norm. Progesterone is what stabilizes the uterine lining, so expect heavier, longer periods with more cramping. Weight gain, water retention, headaches, breast tenderness, cysts, moodiness, and disrupted sleep cycles all characterize this high estrogen / low progesterone state. The closer you get toward menopause, when your periods stop, the more likely you are to have longer cycles where no egg is released at all, called anovulatory cycles. Then you're stuck in the follicular phase, where there's a buildup of unopposed estrogen. Your boobs hurt, you feel bloated, and, man, are you moody. This is PMS for the big girls.

Both estrogen and progesterone levels decline with age, but progesterone goes first, and the slope is steeper. A menopausal woman has 5 percent of the progesterone she had in her twenties, but perhaps still 40 percent of her estrogen thanks to her fat cells, which continue to pump out that hormone throughout her life. This means estrogen dominance is a bigger problem if you're overweight. As usual, there's a vicious cycle. Estrogen promotes fat storage and weight gain, and the fat cells make more estrogen. Add to this the xenoestrogens, external sources of estrogen coming from meats, plastics, pesticides, and soaps, which are stored in fat cells, and you have a recipe for disaster. Unopposed estrogen is not just uncomfortable, it's dangerous, putting you at risk for uterine, ovarian, breast, and colon cancer.

In the second stage of the perimenopause transition, your ovaries finally poop out and estrogen levels take a nosedive. Estrogen dominance is gone, and you have a new set of symptoms due to low estrogen, not low progesterone, but still topping the list are moodiness and irritability, even "rages." Lower estrogen levels mean memory loss and decreased concentration, bone loss (osteoporosis), and a lot more hot flashes and night sweats. Your appetite for food goes up. For sex, it goes down. The urge to mother or nurture, reliant on estrogen all those years, starts to give way to thoughts of *Why do I have to do everything around here? When is it my turn?* More on this later. First, let's talk about my belly.

THE MENOPOT: ABDOMINAL OBESITY IN PERIMENOPAUSE

I can't get rid of my menopot and it's driving me crazy. I always had wide hips and thighs, but my belly used to be relatively flat. No more. After two kids and waning hormones, I am now the not-so-proud owner of a "muffin top." I can grab a handful of flab and cop a *Scarface* accent. "Say hello to my little friend." In the fertile years, estrogen dictates that fat gets deposited at the breasts and hips, forming the hippy gynoid shape. The waist stays small, creating that low waist-to-hip ratio every (heterosexual) man goes gaga for. In the nonfertile forties, it's all about belly and back fat.

Women between thirty-five and forty-four gain weight faster than at any other time in their lives. By their late forties, a majority of women are overweight or obese. The biggest reason is that by menopause, our caloric requirements are about 65 percent of what they were when we were in our twenties. And it's not a gradual decline but a fairly abrupt shift. You'll need to learn how to eat all over again. Your risk for diabetes rises as your hot flashes worsen, and carbs, more than ever before, can make you fat. So can stress. As estrogen levels fall, the pelvic paunch becomes more sensitive to cortisol-stimulated fat accumulation. Menopausal women have an increase in abdominal fat, increasing their risk for cardiac disease.

Where's progesterone when you need it? Progesterone can help with weight loss and enhances the action of thyroid hormones, which help to keep your metabolism revving along. In pregnancy, women commonly feel overheated because progesterone signals the hypothalamus to run hot. Perimenopause, with its low progesterone levels, does the opposite. The metabolism downshifts and slows way down, so you're cold when you're not burning up.

If you don't ovulate, you're going to feel even fatter, because unopposed estrogen means more water retention and bloating. Worse still, high estrogen levels signal the liver to make a protein called thyroid-binding globulin, drastically lowering the available free thyroid hormone. You need this to keep your metabolism humming. So if you're feeling sluggish, your thoughts are slowed down, you feel cold all the time, your skin is dry, and your weight is up, make sure your doctor measures your free thyroid hormone levels and not just your TSH, which is the typical test to order when looking for thyroid troubles. An underactive thyroid is seen fifteen times more often in women than in men. It is quite common for my female patients to have undiagnosed thyroid problems at any age, but especially at perimenopause. Fifty-year-old women produce half the thyroid hormones that twenty-year-olds produce. Many of the complaints of depression are also seen in hypothyroidism: low mood, low energy, low libido, and problems concentrating. This is another reason not to jump on the SSRI bandwagon right off the bat. Have your thyroid checked first.

To compound the effects of a sluggish metabolism, welcome your new companion, a ravenous appetite. Rats that have their ovaries removed, mimicking menopause, have an increased desire to eat and drink, which is normalized when they are given estrogen supplements. You know how you get hungry during PMS? It's a bit like that, only it's not just for a day or two every month.

REPRODUCTIVE DEPRESSION REVISITED

Somewhere along the way in my psychiatric training I heard a term for perimenopause that I just loved, "climacteric psychosis." *Climacteric* is an older term for the menopausal period, and psychosis, well... in effect, perimenopause can make you crazy. This is a prime time for psychiatric complaints. I will often get a patient in her late forties or early fifties coming into my office. She's never seen a psychiatrist before, but she's at her wits' end due to insomnia, panicky sweats, crying at the drop of a hat, or just not giving a shit anymore. Often, one of the first symptoms of perimenopause, before the hot flashes, before the disrupted sleep, is depression. Your risk of depression nearly triples in the perimenopausal transition. The prevalence of depression is highest in women aged forty to forty-nine and lowest in women older than sixty; hence, the storm before the calm.

When you remove a female rat's ovaries, depleting her of estrogen, she shows increased anxious and depressive behaviors, which can be reversed by administering estrogen. Lower estrogen levels will lower overall serotonin activity. Remember, if you're prone to reproductive depressions—if you get significant PMS or if you've had postpartum depression—you're more likely to have mood complaints with your perimenopause. Reproductive depressions are responsive to hormones. Once you're past menopause, major depressions need to be treated with antidepressants because hormones won't work as well.

INSOMNIA AND ANXIETY

I was on the phone with a therapist talking about our mutual patient. The conversation quickly turned to the therapist's own issues and struggles. She's fifty and miserable, not depressed so much as she is agitated. She gets anxious during the day, and then her sleep is interrupted by frequent panicked awakenings.

The estrogen-dominant phase of perimenopause can be an anxious, depressed time for a couple of reasons. High estrogen, when it tamps down the thyroid function, ends up inhibiting the activity of a calming neurotransmitter, GABA. Lower progesterone levels also lead to lower GABA activity and therefore more anxiety. In the later transition, when estrogen levels fade, anxiety can become even more of a problem. There are estrogen receptors on the amygdala (the brain's fear and panic center) as well as the hippocampus (memory) and limbic system (emotional control). When the brain's hormone control center, the hypothalamus, sees lower levels of estrogen, it seems to panic, decreasing production of serotonin and dopamine but ramping up norepinephrine. The end result: low mood, insomnia, and fatigue, but with a touch of anxiety and agitation thrown in. It's not an anxious fear so much as it is irritation, often aimed at partners. Any little thing can set you off and make you angry. This is "roid rage," truly: agitation brought about by a change in steroid hormones.

Insomnia is a biggie during perimenopause. Throughout their lives, women experience insomnia more than men do, but it jumps from 36 percent of women at age thirty to 50 percent at age fifty-four. A few issues are at play here. Cortisol helps to establish circadian rhythms (your body knowing when it's day and night), so when cortisol levels drop during perimenopause, not only is your ability to cope with stress severely limited but also your sleep cycle is a mess. High estrogen levels in early perimenopause can deplete magnesium. For many women, magnesium supplementation can treat insomnia and anxiety, and it's also great for restless leg syndrome. While progesterone is calming on the brain, estrogen is more excitatory. Estrogen dominance exacerbates insomnia; progesterone replacement can help restore sleep. In early perimenopause, supplementing with natural progesterone can help with insomnia. Once you hit the waning estrogen phase of the transition, you'll probably see better effects on sleep by using estrogen.

THE AGING FEMALE BRAIN: ESTROGEN, TESTOSTERONE, AND COGNITION

Women describe a mental "fog" that comes with menopause, which makes sense, given that the brain is full of estrogen receptors. Estrogen is involved in learning and memory, motor coordination, and pain sensitivity. Estrogen helps maintain levels of acetylcholine, a neurotransmitter that is depleted in dementia. When estrogen wanes, expect some trouble with your memory and concentration. Giving women estrogen can improve verbal functioning, vigilance, reasoning, and motor speed.

Testosterone is essential for learning and memory as well, particularly spatial cognition. Testosterone can directly influence cognitive performance by acting on the brain's androgen receptors, or indirectly by being converted to estrogen. Postmenopausal women score better on long-term memory and logical reasoning tests when given estrogen alone, testosterone alone, or a combination of the two. Estrogen helps to regenerate damaged neurons and prevents the beta-amyloid and plaque buildup seen in Alzheimer's disease. Postmenopausal women who take estrogen are half as likely to develop Alzheimer's as those who don't. Testosterone also reduces beta-amyloid buildup, and it plays a neuroprotective role in aging.

BDNF, you may recall, is the brain "fertilizer" that helps you make new brain cells and underlies learning and memory. Animal studies show that if you have high estrogen levels, you have more BDNF and therefore more neuroplasticity in the brain. In women, estrogen increases BDNF levels in the brain's learning and memory areas. This may be one reason why estrogen replacement therapy in the menopausal years may forestall or prevent dementia.

COUGARS AND DESPERATE HOUSEWIVES: A BLIP OF (RELATIVELY) HIGH TESTOSTERONE

My younger patients who are on the Pill and antidepressants may be complaining about not being horny, but my forty-year-old friends most definitely are not. It's been said that a woman's sexual peak is at forty, while a man's is at eighteen. When I hit forty, it did seem as though something had shifted, and I was experiencing this "sexual peak" for myself. When I chatted with my girlfriends, they were going through this, too. Hornier and flirtier than ever, many of them were either having affairs or fantasizing about them. This was not how we'd behaved in the decades prior.

One thing seems clear: our reasons for sex changes as we mature. In the under-thirty-five crowd, 61 percent say their primary motivation for sex is emotional rather than physical. Over thirty-five, that number drops to 38 percent. When surveyed, women over sixty were the least likely to endorse making a long-term commitment to someone who had everything they were looking for minus the sexual attraction. Part of the cougar explanation is likely psychological, not biological. Women in their forties are empowered and no longer confused or shy about what they want sexually and how to go about getting it, and that confidence is sexy.

Just as women in their early thirties start to feel the tug of their ovaries telling them they need to have a baby soon, women in their early forties are feeling that clock ticking down. There's just enough time left to have one more baby, and it's "all hormones on deck" making one last-ditch effort to get pregnant before the machinery shuts down. The ovaries do what they can to stay in the game, and the brain tries harder than ever to make sure one last egg gets squeezed out, month after month.

You might remember a scene from *The Last Picture Show* in which Ellen Burstyn, playing the mother, explains a cougar/boy-toy matchup to her daughter, played by Cybill Shepherd, by saying, "It's an itchy age." Forty is an itchy age, and it's also dangerous. Because for many of us, the target is not our preselected mate but rather a newer model. Women, like men, are fired up by a new partner. New relationships are sexy, and sexy thoughts can trigger testosterone surges. Sexual function may rely more on a change in relationship status than on hormonal levels.

We're programmed to seek out an alpha male with the best possible genes, not the prince who's charmingly slumped at our side. We've all seen older men seek out younger women when they take a lover or start family number two. Younger eggs are more likely to make healthier babies. Well, we are no different. Older women are more likely to get aroused when in the company of younger, novel, pheromone-secreting men. We naturally pursue youthful specimens because there is less chance of genetic damage in younger DNA. The risk of autism and schizophrenia rises with older sperm.

What confounds this problem is that our men are becoming less attractive to us just as we're perking up to see who else is around. Men's testosterone begins to wane at age forty, muting motivation and libido. Women and men both can convert testosterone into estrogen, so older men end up having twice as much estrogen as postmenopausal women. These hormone changes affect not just body composition (less lean muscle and more body fat) but also sexual function (less firm and less frequent erections and lower libido). Our guys are going through "andropause" just as we're going through "andro-surge." Many of us simply aren't getting enough at home, whether sex or love, and so we turn into desperate housewives, craving connection with others.

In early perimenopause, testosterone levels are relatively constant while other hormone levels wane, resulting in something called testosterone dominance. Women in their early forties might notice they are getting pimplier and hairier, with a few more rogue hairs to pluck around the nipples, mustache, and chin, thanks to these higher androgen levels. As usual, it's all about balance. Usually testosterone's horndog effects are muted by estrogen and oxytocin, keeping you feminine and faithful. Because testosterone is the last hormone to fade out of the picture several years after menopause, this relative excess of androgens over estrogens can last for several years. A steep decline occurs between twenty and forty, cutting testosterone levels in half, but between forty and sixty there is virtually no change in testosterone.

When estrogen levels are high, especially if extra is taken orally, the liver produces the protein SHBG, which binds to testosterone, reducing the amount that's available for use. As estrogen levels wane in later peri-menopause, SHBG levels decrease, freeing up the bound testosterone. So there may be a libido bump not just at forty but somewhere around fifty as well. Testosterone not only affects sexual behavior but also influences thoughts. My patients who are using testosterone supplements say they're having more sexy thoughts and fantasies and are getting more easily aroused by these thoughts. Orgasms are easier to achieve and are often longer and stronger. One caveat when dealing with testosterone gels or patches: testosterone does not care what you promised your husband on your wedding day. Testosterone is the hormone of novelty, not fidelity. Androgens will make you horny for anyone—the gardener, your hus-band's cousin, your kid's teacher. When I talk to my patients about the potential side effects of using testosterone, I mention acne, increased fa-cial hair, infidelity, and one more: masturbation. I had a patient who called me from work once, laughing that maybe her testosterone dosage was too high because she had just locked her office door to give herself an orgasm. High testosterone levels in women correlate positively with an urge to masturbate, but not necessarily an urge to merge with a part-ner. As for testosterone's influence on mood, it seems to be bimodal, with complaints of depression at both ends of the spectrum, whether the lev-els are too low or too high.

LOW LIBIDO IN PERIMENOPAUSE: WHAT GOES UP MUST COME DOWN

Not everyone experiences the cougar phase, and if you do, it may not last very long. Many more women will have a waning libido during the meno-pausal transition. As many as 15 to 20 percent of American couples have sex fewer than ten times a year. Plenty of my patients are in sexless mar-riages. Perimenopause isn't always to blame, but it's often in the mix.

Lack of interest in sex is the number one sexual complaint among those ages eighteen to fifty-nine, voiced by nearly 40 percent of the respondents in surveys, with sexual complaints increasing among the older women.

What arouses women is multifactorial. Some of the dying sexual energy may be due to the pressures of raising children, caring for aging parents, or the monotony of the same nightly partner. Women have sex for any number of reasons, from a desire for emotional and physical closeness to knowing it's the only thing that's going to get your husband off your back (literally) so you can get some sleep. Sometimes partners are together for so long, they feel more like siblings than lovers. An aversion to the overly familiar is likely a reflection of our biological drive for novelty, nature's way of avoiding incest and genetic stagnation. This may be an echo of something called the Westermarck effect, seen in cohorts of children who grew up together, as on an Israeli kibbutz, where members won't wed others in their group if they were playmates when younger. If you feel like you've grown up with your husband, you may be less interested in having sex with him.

But clearly there are also biological influences. First of all, if your libido is low, you may want to have your thyroid checked. A badly functioning thyroid can definitely cause sexual complaints. Then there's magnesium. That worn-out cliché "Not tonight, dear, I have a headache" is a stereotype for a reason. When magnesium levels are depleted by estrogen, headaches are a common result. Also, estrogen keeps blood vessels open wide; vessel constriction causes headaches. So in the later stages of the transition, when estrogen levels are low, migraines can result. One more hormone-headache connection: synthetic progestins such as Provera or those found in oral contraceptives can cause headaches, especially in the first few months of taking them. Natural, bioidentical progesterones are less likely to cause headaches.

Later in the transition, when estrogen wanes, you see decreased blood flow to the vagina and surrounding area. This translates to less responsiveness of the nerve endings in the clitoris and thus decreased sensation. As the menopause transition progresses, orgasms become weaker or nonexistent because the estrogen receptors are not being adequately stimulated. Nipple sensation wanes as a result of aging and these hormonal changes as well. Later in perimenopause you also may have more anovulatory cycles where an egg isn't released. Hormonal imbalances are common in this situation, which lengthens the time between periods compared to typical ovulatory cycles. For libido, the big difference is that no ovulation means no spike in testosterone midcycle.

The most likely culprit if your libido has tanked is testosterone. Testosterone levels begin to wane in a linear fashion in women at around age thirty, and they reach their nadir at age forty-eight, the age I am as I type this. My cougar phase is a distant memory by now. Testosterone supplementation increases genital sensitivity and intensity of orgasms, but it's important to note that libido is not just a function of testosterone. Low estrogen will douse your fires as well. A study of menopausal women showed that half of them had improved libido from estrogen supplementation alone. In the remaining half researchers added testosterone, and 90 percent of them improved.

For women, testosterone is the forgotten hormone. Since it's not involved in the menstrual cycle, many women and their doctors don't know whether they're having low levels. With lower testosterone you see not only a lagging libido but also depression, fatigue, and lower motivation. Dr. Irwin Goldstein is a sex researcher who feels strongly that testosterone needs to be part of hormone replacement therapy along with estrogen and progesterone. "If women care about their bones, muscles, vaginas and brains, they should take this drug," he says. Testosterone supplementation reduces osteoporosis and the risk of bone fractures, enhancing estrogen's effects on bone density. It also increases muscle mass. Testosterone may help reduce the risk of dementia and prevent vaginal atrophy as well (see below). If you want to keep more of your testosterone, here are a few tips. Ditch the oral contraceptives or oral estrogen replacement therapy, as they both reduce free testosterone levels by increasing the binding protein SHBG. Also, synthetic progesterones drive down testosterone levels, which means that most birth control pills (since they have progestins) and the progesterone-only injection, Depo Provera, aren't going to help your libido one bit. And go easy on the alcohol. Testosterone gets converted to estrogen by an enzyme called aromatase. Drinking more leads to more conversion. This is a big reason why postmenopausal women are encouraged to drink, in moderation, to keep their estrogen levels up. Alternatively, men with breast formation are encouraged to quit drinking. And there are many scientists, myself included, who believe strongly that the xenoestrogens in plastics, pesticides, and many other chemicals disrupt the production of testosterone or antagonize its effects in the body. So you may want to do a little natural housecleaning, getting rid of these products where possible.

THE SENILE VAGINA

Hot flashes and night sweats will pass eventually. Your aging vagina is another matter. Vaginal atrophy, the thinning of the walls, drying of the mucous membranes, and general collapse of structures including the lower urinary tract are often progressive and require treatment. I came across one paper that referred to this situation as the "senile vagina," which tickled me, but only at first. A senile vagina is no laughing matter. One sex therapist warned me that there comes a time for many women when intercourse is definitely uncomfortable, when she'll want to shout to her sex partner, "Get out of me!"

Again, I refer you to estrogen, the hormone of accommodation. Less estrogen means less lubrication, less elasticity and accommodation, and a whole lot less pleasure during sex. In perimenopause, a common complaint is vaginal itching, dryness, and burning that can result in uncomfortable intercourse. Menopausal changes include alterations in vaginal pH and decreased blood flow to the vagina. Sex is one way to guarantee increased blood flow, so, once again, use it or lose it. Regular sex may help to maintain higher levels of perimenopausal estrogen and delay the onset of menopause, possibly via pheromone signaling. If lubrication is a problem, coconut oil or water-soluble lubricants can help, and sometimes estrogen-fortified creams, like Estrace, will be required. There is also Estring, a soft silicone ring that goes around your cervix and releases a continuous dose of estrogen. Vaginal estrogen is superior to oral dosing for vaginal symptoms. Local hormone treatment applied directly to the vagina via creams or suppositories is not associated with the same risk of strokes and heart attacks that oral hormones are. Progesterone and testosterone can also relieve painful intercourse and enhance lubrication. If you'd like to try an herbal remedy, I recommend maca for lubrication issues (see below).

VIAGRA AND VENIS

As men age, they have more trouble getting and maintaining erections. Anything that interferes with blood flow, like diabetes, cardiovascular disease, or blood pressure medication, is going to make things worse. Having sex standing up can help, but that's not for everyone. Another choice is to use medications like Viagra. The problem here is that sex becomes more goal oriented and the focus becomes penetration only. We all heard about how K-Y started flying off the shelves when Viagra became available. A lot of menopausal women were back in the saddle, like it or not.

Is what's good for the gander good for the goose? Yes and no. In prescreened women who had low blood flow but not low desire, Viagra did help them achieve orgasm and feel more genital sensation. So if you're an aging woman with diminished blood supply to the vagina and uterus, Viagra won't get you horny, but sometimes improved sexual functioning, more lubrication and blood flow, will in turn improve your sexual response, and good sex will get you horny. Another option is the kind of sex taught by the Berman doctor-sisters, called VENIS (very erotic, noninsertive sex). No erections are necessary for this kind of full-body contact, playfully called erotic wrestling, which includes massaging each other, manual stimulation, mutual masturbation, and body kissing. Clearly there needs to be a renegotiation and a reexploration of sexual life when both men's and women's bodies age. Why would you be having the same kind of sex you had in your twenties when virtually nothing else about your life is the same?

HORMONE REPLACEMENT THERAPY

There are whole books on using hormones to treat perimenopause and menopause, and the medical literature is ever evolving on what the best strategy is. As with most things in medicine, one size definitely doesn't fit all, and whatever treatment you choose, it's important to monitor all your levels every few months with blood tests, physical exams, and talks with your doctor.

We all need to understand the challenge and the many possible choices here. On one hand, we are likely overmedicalizing a natural transition, and in many cases we're probably better off leaving well enough alone. On the other hand, women are living to eighty-five, on average, and thirty-plus years with no sex hormones are going to take their toll. Both estrogen and testosterone supplementation can prevent dementia, bone loss, muscle loss, and artery disease in the heart and brain. And they can both help to prevent vaginal atrophy.

In terms of weight and metabolism, hormone replacement therapy (HRT) can be life saving. Taking estrogen lowers the risk for diabetes and gives diabetic women better control over their blood sugars. HRT attenuates the accumulation of belly fat, lowering the risk of cardiac events and helping to normalize weight and appetite.

Early in perimenopause, when estrogen-dominant symptoms are problematic, progesterone can help immensely. Later, when hot flashes get bad, estrogen will be helpful. Some doctors prescribe low-dose oral contraceptives early in perimenopause and full-on HRT once menopause hits. Most recommend bioidentical hormones; synthetics can cause weight gain and bloating and are more likely to cause mood problems. Provera and other synthetic progestins commonly cause depression, for instance, in about 30 percent of their users. Synthetic hormones can also deplete the body of vitamin B_6 and folic acid, vitamins needed for mood maintenance.

There's also a relatively new class of medicines being added to the hormones called selective estrogen receptor modulators, or SERMs. Drugs like tamoxifen and raloxifene are SERMs. These can work as well as progesterone for protecting the uterus without the progestin side effects of depression, anxiety, and sedation. It may also be possible to use SERMs derived from botanical sources like flaxseed, hemp, or soy, called phytoserms.

For estrogen supplementation, there are pills, patches, creams, and sublingual drops. Pills get broken down by the liver and can increase the risk of blood clots, while the other three go directly into the bloodstream and bypass the liver. For testosterone supplementation, there are time-released capsules of micronized testosterone, sublingual drops, or trans-dermal gels and patches. Again, avoiding oral doses and the liver is probably best.

Some gynecologists feel that the ideal time to start hormone supplementation is when you're still menstruating, prior to menopause. As

soon as hot flashes begin, steady doses of hormones get rid of the fluctuations that cause most symptoms. Others feel strongly that you should
take hormones only if you're struggling with perimenopausal symptoms.
What we do know is that starting too late misses the window not only for
protecting against Alzheimer's, but also for reaping the cardiovascular
benefits.

The cancer issue is particularly complicated and warrants conference with your physician. The Women's Health Initiative (WHI) followed
nearly forty-two thousand postmenopausal women aged fifty to seventy-
nine. Roughly half were given Premarin and progestin, two synthetic
hormones. While there were benefits to using these hormones, such as
decreased incidences of colon cancer and bone fractures, the study was
aborted three years early due to worrisome accumulating data showing
an increased risk of breast cancer, coronary heart disease, stroke, and
pulmonary embolism in the study participants. The breast cancer rate
was .42 in the control group and .6 in the hormone-taking group, which
really isn't that huge considering that every American woman is now
afraid to go on hormone replacement therapy for fear she'll develop
breast cancer. The "million women study" in the United Kingdom used
these same two medications and found similar results. The women who
started the hormones within months after menopause had a three-fold
higher risk of breast cancer than those starting ten years later. If a
woman has her uterus removed and takes estrogen without progesterone, she does not have the same increase in breast cancer risk. It may be
that the synthetic progestin is the culprit.

Estrogen dominance puts you at risk for breast cancer. Progesterone
deficiency does as well. A study of infertile women with progesterone deficiency showed a 540 percent greater chance of breast cancer. Many
researchers and practitioners I interviewed felt similarly, that the WHI
study was a great disservice to women everywhere. The data was blown

out of proportion, and millions of women stopped their hormone replacement therapy abruptly, so their menopausal symptoms came roaring back. Since the WHI study, millions more women have opted to not begin HRT.

Here is what we know. Postmenopausal women taking synthetic hormones is a problem. We need more data on perimenopausal women taking bioidenticals. The longer you're exposed to unopposed estrogen, the higher your risk for breast cancer. But for primary prevention of heart disease, it's not effective if you start ten years too late. The party line is that v   none replacement therapy for the shortest peri   at does that mean? At what point do we not w   nse and brain function, vaginal health, and st   One sex researcher I interviewed is still menstr   ks to her sublingual hormones.

THE GOVERNMENT DOESN'T WANT HORNY WOMEN, ONLY HORNY MEN

If you're going to replace sex hormones in perimenopause or menopause, testosterone should be in the mix. So why isn't the FDA on board with this? Testosterone products for men are readily approved with minimal long-term studies. There are now twenty-six products available, from patches to injections, sublingual drops to nasal sprays, to make sure that men stay horny and hard. Compare that to the zero products FDA approved for women. Despite long-term studies showing the safety and efficacy of testosterone in women, doctors are forced to prescribe testosterone for women "off label," which means insurance companies won't pay for it. Many physicians are uncomfortable straying across that line, so millions of women don't get treated as they should.

The Intrinsa patch for women is a good example. Procter & Gamble invested millions of dollars to develop an effective testosterone-containing product for women. Despite excellent efficacy and a four-year safety study, unheard of for most drugs in development, the all-male FDA committee told the researchers, "Women don't need this." Not that it is unsafe or ineffective, just that it's not necessary. And they're wrong. Currently, the FDA is asking for data stretching five to ten years to look at risks of breast cancer, strokes, or heart attacks in women using testosterone, even though there is no evidence for any of these risks, especially at the tiny doses women require. Don't hold your breath for an FDA-approved testosterone medication for women at this point. The likelihood of any company pouring millions into developing a drug where the institutional gender bias is so strongly set against it is minimal.

SELF-CARE: EXERCISE, DIET, AND HERBAL THERAPIES

Perimenopause is a time of great changes and heightened stress, so it's important to do all you can to stay healthy. Please refer to the survival guide to help you take better care during this challenging transition. I always remind my patients about good nutrition and exercise, but in perimenopause, it really becomes crucial. Obesity increases your risk of anovulatory cycles and hot flashes, so you have two good reasons right there to watch your diet and hit the gym. Yoga and Pilates can help improve pelvic floor strength, important for sexual pleasure and urinary continence (always sexy), and moderate exercise may help with hot flashes. Exercise helps immensely with depressed mood and insomnia, and don't forget that it also helps to make you horny. Try for thirty minutes of cardio three times a week, in the first half of the day. (Exercising too late in the day can interfere with falling asleep.)

We know exercise helps to make sex better, but it turns out that you can also count sex in the category of exercise. So you may want to start looking at sex not just as something you do for your partner, or for the relationship, but as a healthy activity that you do for yourself, your cardiac status, and your vagina. Having sex may help you to live longer, and there is a correlation between orgasms and decreased mortality.

As for foods to eat or supplements to take, here are a few suggestions. Vitamin D is crucial for your ovaries to make estrogen and testosterone, so make sure you're getting sunshine or taking a D_3 supplement. Soy milk has components that bind to estrogen receptors without creating a spike in estrogen levels. If you're estrogen dominant, with heavy periods and cramping, it would be best to avoid soy products. They can lengthen the luteal phase and cause heavier menstrual bleeding, especially if you're low on progesterone, which helps to maintain the uterine lining. But later in the transition, after your periods have stopped, soy can help. Phytoestrogens—plant compounds that weakly mimic estrogen—are found in soy, licorice, red clover, thyme, turmeric, hops, and verbena. The highest-binding herbs for progesterone-like activity are oregano, verbena, turmeric, thyme, red clover, and damiana. Sprouts, particularly broccoli sprouts, are a good source of phytoestrogens. Cannabis also has estrogenic activity, and I'll talk more about that below.

In the land of herbal studies, there are more scientific papers showing black cohosh efficacy than for many other supplements out there. There are randomized, placebo-controlled trials showing that it works to reduce hot flashes and night sweats, and one study found that it worked even better than the prescription estrogens. Pine bark extract, also known as pycnogenol, has also relieved a multitude of symptoms in clinical trials. Evening primrose oil and vitamins B_6, B_{12}, and folate can also help with hot flashes, and sometimes women will respond to natural progesterones instead of estrogens for this.

Then there's maca. This is a root cultivated in the Andes and used to treat perimenopausal complaints in Peruvian women. Many studies have

found it helpful in balancing hormones and relieving various perimenopausal symptoms. It's well tolerated and may also be used to alleviate
SSRI-induced sexual dysfunction, improving libido. Maca can help to
make you horny and frequently improves vaginal lubrication. It's important that maca works its wonders without changing hormone levels, so
none of the risks from HRT are an issue. Another reason I like it: its ability to protect against brain damage likely acts via the endocannabinoid
system.

Chasteberry, also known as vitex, is good for PMS and early perimenopause, as it helps to support progesterone levels.

CANNABIS FOR PERIMENOPAUSAL SYMPTOMS

The female cannabis plant bears flowers that have been used as a medicine for thousands of years. There are compounds in cannabis that show
estrogen-like activity and historical reports of its effectiveness treating
a variety of perimenopausal complaints. Cannabis increases luteinizing
hormone levels in perimenopausal women, which might help improve
progesterone levels in the early part of the transition. Hemp seeds added
to the diet of rats who'd had their ovaries removed decreased anxiety and
improved cholesterol levels.

I have patients, friends, and colleagues who swear by pot to treat
their hormonal complaints, whether PMS, menstrual cramps, or perimenopausal insomnia and hot flashes. Cannabidiol (CBD), the component of cannabis that can yield medicinal effects without getting you
high, does bind to the estrogen receptor, and apigenin, a phytoestrogen
in cannabis, also binds to the receptor.

There is a vaginal ointment made out of coconut oil and cannabis
called Foria, though there aren't any clinical studies showing its efficacy
in enhancing sexual response or rehabbing a senile vagina. What we do

know is that there are cannabinoid receptors on the cells that make bones, called CB2 receptors, and that when something locks onto those receptors it stimulates bone formation. Animal studies show that a synthetic CB2 agonist rescues bone loss in animals with their ovaries removed. Also, people who have a genetic problem where their CB2 receptors aren't working well are more likely to have menopausal osteoporosis. Does this mean ingesting cannabinoids will help you keep your bones strong? It might, indeed.

VITAL AGING: LIFTING THE VEIL

Because women's average life expectancy is currently eighty-five years, we're easily spending a third of our lives being postmenopausal. The largest demographic in America is women in their forties to sixties, and by 2020 there will be nearly 60 million peri- and postmenopausal women living in the United States. I'm hoping that most of us will succeed in our attempts to age with health, vigor, and vitality.

It seems damn near impossible for a woman to grow old in America while keeping her dignity. Face-lifts, Botox, hair dyeing, mustache waxing—the upkeep is exhausting. It is a slippery slope once you head down that path. Botox needs to be maintained every few months, and synthetic fillers like Restylane start to move around over time. It's hard to grow old gracefully in our changing bodies, but ladies, we have to. My rule for myself is just don't start. No plastic or synthetic anything in my body. I will have earned each wrinkle and gray hair, and I want to proudly display them like trophies of a life well lived.

So much emphasis and worry are put on physical aging in women and their appearance that the emotional maturity and freedom that can come at this time are given short shrift. The most interesting thing about menopause is what happens after. Women come into their own. It's a time of redefining and refining what it is we want to accomplish in our time left. The cyclicity that dominated the first half of our lives has been replaced with something more solid and consistent, though I still advise keeping the sanctity of the cycle by having some delineated downtime on a monthly basis. I wish we had some sort of red tent, where women could gather to learn from one another and grow together, to hang out when they're menstruating or nursing or delivering. I hate that there is so much shame and secrecy around menstruation and menopause. It's not fair, and it's not healthy.

Menopause is a time for pruning. It is our version of the midlife crisis, where we weed out those who are "toxic," prioritizing and further honing our mission, whatever it may be. Yes, your ovaries may have signed off, to a large extent, but your adrenals are still plugging away. That means cortisol, the stress hormone, is still handy for when you need a little gas, but the hormone of accommodation, estrogen, has waned. And because estrogen triggers oxytocin receptors and production, we're going to slip out of our tend-and-befriend response a bit more. In the mating years, it seems as though we live for our family, and "whatever you want, honey" is the mantra we chant to our partners and children. Most of us learn to love it. We thrive by cultivating relationships and nurturing those around us. The estrogen years have us keeping the peace, giving to others, and doing it ourselves instead of delegating, because at least it will be done right that way.

When estrogen levels fall, we start to slowly transition from the self-sacrifice of "Okay, sweetie, I'll just take care of this" to a more assertive "Do it yourself, why don't you?" Less accommodation isn't just better for us; it's probably good for our kids, too. This may be the time when children—adolescents, in particular—are ready to take on more responsibility, so perhaps there is a benefit for everyone in changing that family dynamic. If you have your kids early enough and they haven't boomeranged back to the nest, then this is a time when it's just you and your beloved, if you can still call him that with a straight face now that the hormones that were lubricating communication, caretaking, and conflict aversion are on permanent vacation. This is prime time for late-marriage divorces, or else it's time to really sit down and do some major reworking of your relationship. The majority of divorces in America, 60 percent, are initiated by women in their forties, fifties, and sixties. Again, this may be a reflection of less accommodation and more "It's my turn, pally." Optimally, there is some middle ground between destroying the family you've created and maintaining the status quo. The trick is to turn the anger and assertiveness into action, making changes that will benefit not just you but possibly your whole family.

For working women, there's another opportunity. These changes come at a time when most women will have a fair amount of experience under their belts. Perhaps this is the moment to push: take more of a leadership position, enter a new arena, or strike out on your own. My mother was a great role model in her perimenopause, taking her symptoms in stride and referring to her hot flashes as "power surges." She got another degree and switched careers; that appealed to me as a teenage girl. Now I see this rise in power as a way to channel new energy and even new anger, putting it to good use to make changes that should've been made decades ago.

I dedicated this book to Jeremy's mother, Sara, who ran an older women's group at her community center and wrote about her experience in *Vital Aging*. I have seen the third act of aging women time and again in my private practice. Sara, in particular, was inspirational, continuing her work as a therapist and becoming an author in her eighties. I'm also noticing more women in the media showing us how to age well, and I thank them. I hope that because of them the new standard for aging women will be about vitality, strength, and assertiveness. Forget accommodation; struggle for authenticity.

This goes for appearance as well. As we age, our looks change, and this is natural. Lately I'm noticing more older women wearing less makeup, not more. Dropping the beautification agenda is liberating, allowing you to look more relaxed, natural, and even more beautiful. Trade in dewy naiveté for glowing intelligence. It is our time to shine, as our essence is distilled. In folklore, the older woman typically embodies mystical or magical powers, a quantum shift in knowledge and potency that accompanies aging.

There is tremendous wisdom embodied in a menopausal woman. If you aren't one, then seek out your elders. Wise women mentoring others is a powerful chain of teaching and healing.

PART THREE

THE MOODY BITCHES SURVIVAL GUIDE

Seven

Inflammation, The Key to Everything

We all know that inflammation and injury go hand in hand: smack your knee into the coffee table and watch it swell. But inflammation happens deep inside the body, too, and understanding how it works is key to maintaining your mental and physical health. When the body identifies an intruder, armies of white blood cells converge to attack. One invader, like a virus or a bacterium, and the immune system stays organized and focused. But when the triggers are everywhere or are constant, the immune response mutates into something no longer helpful or healthy, inflaming or destroying important machinery of the body. This sort of chronic inflammation is how many illnesses start. Heart disease, asthma, Alzheimer's, obesity, arthritis, diabetes, autoimmune diseases, and more are all inflammatory illnesses.

Inflammation influences the functioning of diverse systems within the body and brain, and once it is triggered it can be difficult to prevent the chain of responses. This would be simpler to address if there were one cause of inflammation, but that is not the case. Inflammation has many triggers and partners. Stress and inflammation fuel each other. Ditto for obesity and inflammation. Sleep deprivation exacerbates inflammation and obesity. Even inflammation and depression are codependent. For women suffering from these issues, it can be a nightmare to sort it all out. So it's important to understand that inflammation is a common denominator for a host of problems that plague women.

Keeping inflammation down may be your single best form of health insurance. But how do we do that? The chapters that follow address diet, sleep, exercise, and sex, all powerful practices for building resilience and combating inflammation.

INFLAMMATION, STRESS, AND DEPRESSION

Anytime there is a stressor, cortisol—a stress hormone released from the adrenal glands—surges in the bloodstream, suppressing the immune system and causing inflammation to go down. Because responding to an acutely stressful situation may require you to be on your toes, adrenaline is released from the adrenals as well, increasing the heart and respiratory rates. Occasional acute stress keeps us vigilant and primed for action. Our body deals with the situation and then returns to normal.

Like many things in the body, a little is fine, but too much is a disaster. Acute stressors and resulting bursts of cortisol briefly tamp down the immune response, and then it bounces back. Chronic stressors are another story entirely. Cortisol becomes deregulated with chronic stress. Autoimmune diseases (like lupus, rheumatoid arthritis, and scleroderma) reflect an exhaustion and disruption of the normal stress-control mechanisms. So chronic stress ends up enhancing immune reactivity, creating chronic inflammation. In the modern world, the stress never stops. Because of this, we are all more inflamed than we should be. And all this inflammation can create depression and more. Chronic stress can precede or exacerbate depression and is a risk factor for both medical and psychiatric illnesses.

If you induce inflammatory reactions, you also create symptoms of mood disorders. Chronically stress a laboratory animal and its behavior mimics that of a depressed person, normalizing when antidepressants are given. People who have inflammatory illnesses are more likely to show signs and symptoms of depression than are those who have other illnesses, and interestingly, anti-inflammatory agents have antidepressant effects.

Depressed people, even though they may be medically healthy, often have elevated markers of inflammation. These markers, called cytokines, are higher in depressed patients and lower in those who've been successfully treated. Depressed patients with more intense suicidal ideation have significantly higher levels of proinflammatory cytokines. Stressed-out patients with anxiety show heightened cytokine levels as well. The hepatitis drug interferon is actually a cytokine that sometimes creates psychiatric side effects like depression, anxiety, irritability, and even suicidality.

Certain areas of the brain are implicated in the neural circuitry of depression. The anterior cingulate cortex, sometimes called the "neural alarm system," is responsible for emotional regulation and processing. Giving proinflammatory cytokines activates this area, and once it's overactive, treatment-resistant depression results. Normalization of activity is seen in patients who respond to treatment with antidepressants, cognitive behavioral therapy, or deep brain stimulation.

Stress causing inflammation makes sense, but why would inflammation lead to feeling stressed out, anxious, and depressed? Inflammation is the body's way of encouraging "sickness behavior." You need to hunker down and conserve energy to fight off an infection. Also, if you lie low, you don't contaminate others. Fatigue, apathy, social withdrawal, reduced appetite, and increased sleep are nature's ways of helping you to get better faster. Sickness behavior sounds an awful lot like depressed behavior, right? Typically, once the infection is gone, the body should reset and resume normal activity. When this process goes awry, inflammation persists after the infection is gone and keeps you in a depressed state. Prolonged sickness behavior can progress to depression.

Until a few hundred years ago, many people died before the age of sixteen, primarily from infections. It's crucial for the brain to know when the body is or may become infected and act accordingly. Even looking at sick people coughing and sneezing can promote an inflammatory response. A body that runs hot, inflames easily, and can kill an invader expeditiously will survive to pass on genetic material coding for higher inflammatory states. A brain that quickly assesses danger of contamination would be selected for, which may explain why anxiety disorders have persisted in our gene pool. The amygdala, our fear and anxiety center, springs into action when we are in danger, and it causes us to go into avoidance mode if negative social cues exist. The amygdala is also involved in sickness-induced social withdrawal. If you inject bacterial toxins into human volunteers, the resulting inflammation leads to greater amygdala response to socially threatening images and greater feelings of social disconnection. More research papers are connecting the dots between anxiety and inflammation.

But it's not just anxiety. Inflammation creates changes in the brain that are bound to make you feel terrible. First, cytokines target and sabotage the brain's mechanisms for preventing depression. They enhance replication and activation of the serotonin reuptake transporter (SERT), the site on the receptor that SSRIs block. This leads to increased reuptake of serotonin, so less is available in the synapse. This is the exact opposite of how antidepressants work. Cytokines also break down tryptophan, the main building block for serotonin, diverting it into the production of something called kynurenine. The problem with kynurenine is that it is further metabolized to products that can induce more inflammation. So here we have a vicious cycle of pathological inflammation. More cytokines, less serotonin; more kynurenine, more inflammation; the exact combo platter you don't want if you're battling anxiety and depression.

To make matters worse, some cytokines diminish motivation and desire. They also antagonize glutamate, the neurotransmitter required for making new brain cells and encouraging their growth, neurogenesis, and neuroplasticity. Less neuroplasticity means less learning and growing. People who respond to antidepressants typically show more neuroplasticity, so here the brain is moving in the wrong direction, fueled by inflammation and getting stupid.

Nearly a third of depressed people typically don't respond to antidepressant medication. Those nonresponders in particular have been found to have higher levels of proinflammatory markers, which implies that testing for cytokines prior to treatment may help predict who will and who won't respond to antidepressant medications. Some researchers have used anti-inflammatory medications, like those used to treat autoimmune disorders, to relieve many depressive symptoms, like anxiety, fatigue, disruptions in sleep, slowed movements, and an inability to feel pleasure, called anhedonia.

Inflammation makes cell membranes leaky. Particles that would typically be kept out of certain areas of the body end up oozing through barricades. Leaky barriers play a role in inflammation and the creation of depression and anxiety. The "leaky gut" theory proposes that poor nutrition and other factors can inflame the gut, allowing toxins to enter our bloodstream. So anything we can do to decrease gut inflammation will help our brains function better. Like the gut, the brain has its own immune barrier and is intensely picky about what it lets across. Once there's inflammation, all bets are off. Infections and autoimmune diseases make the blood-brain barrier leaky, just like the gut. This allows antibodies to cross into the brain, causing inflammatory reactions.

When the body's immune system starts to attack itself, you're in trouble. Increased inflammatory reactivity like this has been observed in subgroups of patients with severe depression. Several autoimmune diseases, like multiple sclerosis and lupus, are associated with excessive inflammation in the brain and mood complaints. So if you have infections or autoimmune disorders, you're at a higher risk for becoming depressed.

EMOTIONAL STRESS AND HEALTH

When I was in medical school, I would study like crazy, take my exams, and then go on break. Inevitably, while away somewhere to recover, I would get a cold. While I lay on my hotel bed surrounded by used Kleenex, I joked with my parents that my immune system was on vacation as well. Turns out I wasn't joking. Chronic stress increases the risk of acquiring infections and can throw a wrench into immune functioning. Natural killer cells are anti-inflammatory cells; these are the good guys. Depression and stress lower their activity, while antidepressants augment their invader-fighting abilities. Immune defenses and natural killer cell numbers are suppressed in medical students under the pressure of final exams.

Stress creates inflammation, and the most important stressors are emotional. People under extreme stress are four times more likely to suffer exacerbations of inflammatory illnesses like multiple sclerosis. In asthmatic kids, you see a strong association between their ability to move air through inflamed airways and their emotional states. In premenopausal women who have heart attacks, it is more often an emotional stressor that triggers the event, not a physical stressor, as it often is with men. Unfortunately, women have greater coronary artery reactivity to stress than men do. The connection between stress and illness is particularly important for women to grasp. The take-home message: stay calm to save your life.

The main factors that can trigger a stress response are uncertainty, lack of information, a loss of control, and a sense of helplessness. Inescapable shocks, but not escapable ones, suppress immune function. If you block a rat's ability to respond to a stressor, its artificially created autoimmune disease will worsen. People who develop a greater level of control over their health-care issues experience a reduction in depressive symptoms over time.

Feeling powerless imperils your health. Subordinate female monkeys secrete more cortisol than dominant ones, and if you switch their positions, their chemistry changes. The higher your social position, the healthier you are, regardless of socioeconomic status. Where you think you fall in the hierarchy matters. This is one reason why social networking like Facebook may be unhealthy. When you compare your inner, insecure self with others' external, self-assured posts and come up feeling like a loser, it's not just bad for your mood and stress level; it may affect your immunity and longevity.

Being a "good girl" will take its toll, too. Certain repressive behaviors in women that are considered self-abnegating, like compliance or conscientiousness, can create or exacerbate illness. Suppressing emotions like anger or neediness negatively affects hormonal balance, immune status, GI functioning, and skin, to name just a few. One study reports that the greatest risk factor for death, especially from cancer, is "rationality and anti-emotionality," that is, denying or repressing the emotional components of the illness. In breast cancer patients who are able to express anger and adopt a fighting stance, the natural killer cells are more active, leading study authors to conclude that emotional factors are potentially more important to survival than the degree of the disease. The message here: survival of the bitchiest. Let your true feelings show, and save your sanity and your health. Being authentic in your actions and in line with your emotions, doing what you feel instead of what you think you should, can lead to improved health.

RESILIENCE: WHO'S YOUR MOMMY?

Resilience is a key component of mental health. It is your ability to bounce back, to adapt to adversity, and particularly to recover from trauma, whether physical or psychic. More resilience means staying healthy in the face of tragedy and stress. Less resilience means becoming overwhelmed, getting stuck, breaking down, and getting sick.

How do we foster resilience? Like anything else, it takes practice. Exposure to mild or moderate stressors in early life provides opportunities for mastery in adapting a stress response and helps to boost resilience. This is known as stress inoculation. You need a few minor triumphs growing up to prepare you for major hardships as you age. Students cocooned by protective helicopter parents in their childhood are less resilient because they're less prepared for the inevitable failures that occur during their college experience.

Rat pups separated from their mothers for fifteen minutes grow up to become more resilient than nonseparated pups; they are less anxious and their cortisol levels return to baseline more quickly after a stressful event. Separate a pup from its mum for too long, though, and you have trouble.

A secure early attachment is crucial for establishing higher levels of resilience in humans. While moderate amounts of hardship and stress improve resilience, chronic trauma will destroy it, causing a sustained activation of the panic/stress circuitry. People who've been traumatized repeatedly have overactive amygdalae, more baseline inflammation, and higher inflammatory responses.

Research on resilience shows that, as with most behaviors, both genes and environment play a part in the outcome. Nature, your genetically determined sensitivity to stress, is influenced by nurture, the number and intensity of unfavorable events you encounter growing up. Number one nurture priority: how much actual nurturing you get as a baby. The quality of early parenting is key in developing resilience. Limbic circuits are programmed in childhood, as are the links between the brain, endocrine system, and immune system. How a mother cares for her infant programs the stress response in the offspring by altering the development of the neural systems that mediate fearfulness. Adult rats who had been licked and groomed more by their mothers had more calming benzodiazepine receptors in their amygdalae than those who had received less nurturing. Early parenting can also influence inflammation. A recent study showed definitively that children who get more nurturing in their infancy have lower levels of markers of inflammation as many as eight years down the road.

Interestingly, if you take a pup of a low-nurturing mother and adopt it out to be raised by a high-nurturing mother, it will eventually develop the markers seen in the adoptive group, even though its genetics didn't start out that way. So the early parenting environment can strongly influence the gene expression that leads to greater resilience once a child is an adult.

Nurture may even be able to win out over nature. In studies of rhesus monkeys, the ones who were high reactors because of separation from their mothers could have their behavior modified by changing the environment. If they were adopted out and reared with especially nurturing foster mothers, they rose to the top of the hierarchy. In subsequent generations, adopted females took on the maternal style typical of their especially nurturing foster mothers when it was time to raise their own young. So nurture can triumph over nature, and a mother's love conquers all.

But don't count out genetics just yet. Anxious mothers are likely to rear anxious offspring. Mothers with severe PTSD have children with greater impairment in their cortisol regulation. Children, and even grandchildren, of people who have suffered major stressors show hormone and behavioral changes as if they had experienced these stressors personally. I have several patients who are children of Holocaust survivors. Every one of them is incredibly anxious, and many are depressed, even though they weren't directly exposed to the trauma. You see this in laboratory animals as well; the effects of a long-ago stress get handed down to subsequent generations. If you mate a stressed-out rat with a nonstressed rat, you can see changes in the second and even third generation that come from this pairing, particularly when measuring exploratory behavior, how curious and novelty seeking the rodent is. The more stressed out, the more they hide out and don't explore.

How reactive you are to stress is genetically dictated. If you have inherited particular copies of genes that code for serotonin production, your risk for depression, suicidality, or aggression is increased, especially after you've been stressed out. If you inherit the wrong genes that control the SSRI docking space, SERT, you're less likely to be resilient and adaptable, and your levels of optimism, happiness, life satisfaction, and impulse control will be affected. Because of inherited genes, the same patients who are more vulnerable to depression are also more vulnerable to inflammatory illnesses and to getting depressed when they're medically ill. There is a strong correlation between being emotionally reactive to stressors and being medically reactive to triggers of inflammation, and this is primarily driven by genetics.

DON'T STRESS ABOUT STRESS AND IT WILL ALL BE OKAY

How you think about stress matters. If you were faced with a hungry tiger in the jungle, you'd be grateful for your rapid breathing, delivering oxygen to your blood, and for your pounding heart, pumping that blood to your brain and muscles. That's exactly what you need to wisely and quickly escape. If you can reframe your attitude to your body's natural reaction to stress, you'll remain significantly healthier. A typical stress reaction increases heart rate but constricts blood vessels. This is a setup for high blood pressure, heart attacks, and strokes. Change your mind about stress and you can change your body's response to it. If you welcome the stress response, reminding yourself that your body is helping you to rise to this challenge, then you can keep your blood vessels relaxed and dilated, not constricted. Decreased anxiety over stress can then translate into increased confidence or courage. One study showed a whopping 43 percent risk of premature death in subjects who not only experienced a lot of stress but also believed that stress was bad for them. You lower your risk if you can reframe your attitude. Reappraise a stressor as a challenge, not a threat, and see how you feel.

Thank goodness for psychiatric research proving the obvious: feeling good makes us less likely to feel bad. Positive emotions prevent or undo the effects of stress, helping with cognitive flexibility and improving coping. Develop your ability to experience positive emotions and you buffer against both stress and depression. Women with more day-to-day positive emotions are less reactive emotionally on their higher-stress days. If you grin, you'll bear it more quickly. Positive emotions *during* the stress exposure contribute to a faster recovery. More resilient folks are more likely to experience positive emotions alongside the anxiety that accompanies stressful experiences, and they also show a faster cardiovascular recovery from stress. For patients with depression, focusing on strategies or activities that improve positive emotions may be key to preventing re-lapses of depression. I make a point of asking my patients what brings them joy and what makes them smile. "Then do more of that!" I say. (It's the opposite of "Doc, it hurts when I do this." "Then don't do that.") Whether it's walking your dog, tap dancing, or playing guitar and sing-ing, follow your joy to enhance resilience and reduce stress.

STRESS AND INFLAMMATION AGE THE BODY

Chronic stress chips away at the ends of our genes, the tips known as telomeres. As cells reproduce themselves, these telomeres get shorter, a normal sign of aging. In a study of women taking care of a chronically ill child, the longer the woman had been caring for the child, the shorter her telomere length. Perhaps more important than the time spent caring was the perception of the hardship. The women with the greatest negative perceptions of their stressful situations had the telomere length of women a full decade older.

Chronic inflammation can shorten telomere length. If your immune cells have to keep responding repeatedly, they divide more and start to show their age. You get an old immune system in a young body. Less re-pairing and patching up goes on, and it's harder to identify pathogens. As immune cells age, they also tend to produce proinflammatory cytokines, which feed the inflammation cycle.

Short telomeres are a sign of aging and stress on the body, helping to predict the onset of diseases such as cancer and dementia; we want to find ways to lengthen our telomeres, or at least slow down the shorten-ing. Abdominal obesity shortens telomere length, but exercise will help to keep them long. Less stress and better sleep help to lengthen telo-meres, as do omega-3 fatty acids and other antioxidants. More studies are suggesting that mindfulness-based practices will induce telomerase activity, lengthening the telomeres. Mindfulness also improves inflammatory marker levels. Expert meditators, after eight hours of mindfulness practice, show multiple molecular and genetic differences compared with controls, including decreased expression of proinflammatory genes and faster physical recovery from experimentally induced stress. One extra benefit of mindfulness and meditation practices is that you learn to not stress about stress.

OXYTOCIN IS A STRESS HORMONE

My friend Jay is "battling" testicular cancer. It's so easy for us to get into a military mind-set when it comes to illness, and there are pros and cons to that mental framework. What has impressed me most about Jay and his lovely wife, Katie Rose, is their call to arms via e-mail and Facebook to allow their friends and family to help out with visits, bringing soups, taking Jay to chemo, and just being a therapeutic presence. They've knit together a healing network of friends, and it's been beneficial for all of us involved, not just Jay. Stress has the potential to make you social, to reach out for support. It can strengthen close relationships and make you more supportive and inclusive of the people you care about. The chemical that makes all this happen is oxytocin, the hormone that underlies bonding and cuddling. Remember that stress reactions don't just involve cortisol and adrenaline; it's not just fight or flight. Especially for women, a stress reaction often includes tend and befriend, mediated by oxytocin.

Social support keeps you healthy, buffering the effects of the stress response. Social connectedness improves resilience and prevents mental health problems. Positive social interactions have stress-protecting effects, and oxytocin can fuel these social interactions. Social support can lower cortisol levels and lower cardiovascular reactivity in response to stress. It can also ameliorate symptoms of depression. Oxytocin has anti-inflammatory activity and it relaxes blood vessels. Frequent hugs are associated with higher oxytocin levels and lower blood pressure. There are even oxytocin receptors on the heart to help it heal from stress-induced damage.

ISOLATION IS CRUEL AND UNUSUAL PUNISHMENT

Isolation is a stressor in and of itself, with disastrous medical complications when combined with other stresses. Isolation can exacerbate both the stress response and the intensity of physical illness. Socially isolated adults suffer higher rates of mortality, dying sooner than those who have a stronger social network. Lonely people have worse sleep, higher blood pressure, and poorer heart function than nonlonely subjects, as well as more depressive symptoms and a diminished sense of well-being. Isolation also impairs immune functioning.

Isolation is stressful, stress can cause inflammation, and inflammation can make you dumb. Therefore, isolation can make you dumb. Studies of stress, isolation, and neuroplasticity in rodents found that isolation interferes with learning and memory formation. Isolation also leads to impaired top-down emotional control, so you can add "stay social" to the list of what keeps you from losing your cool. Social support is a primary resilience mechanism, helping you to recover by keeping inflammation down and neuroplasticity, and therefore learning, up. Making strong social connections allows the brain to blossom and form new neural connections.

GOING GREEN HELPS WITH STRESS RESILIENCE

Cannabis and naturally occurring cannabinoids in the body can help counter the effects of stress and enhance resilience. Not only are cannabinoids anti-inflammatory, but you can think of the whole endocannabinoid system as anti-inflammatory. Cannabinoids alter immune reactions in the body and in the brain, influencing white blood cells and cytokine production. Immune cells can synthesize their own endocannabinoids, or they can be influenced by administrated cannabinoids, as many immune cells throughout the brain and body have cannabinoid receptors on their cell surfaces.

Anandamide, our main internal cannabis molecule, helps to tamp down the stress response and return our hormones and nervous system to a normal balance, or homeostasis. Higher anandamide levels are associated with better stress tolerance. When cortisol is released, anandamide levels rise, trying to put things back in order. This is an example of the endocannabinoid system "righting the ship" after it's been rocked.

It is true that pot affects memory. Short-term memory function is depressed when you're high, and that can actually be a help. Endocannabinoids are necessary for the clearance of negative emotional memories in the brain. Boosting anandamide can promote this forgetting process, while lower levels of anandamide promote the retention of negative emotional memories. Disrupting endocannabinoid signaling may cause overactivation of the stress response. This heightened sensitivity to stress is a major feature of anxiety disorders and depression. Many of my patients "self-medicate" with cannabis in an effort to destress. Veterans with PTSD may smoke cannabis to forget what they've seen overseas, attempting to rebalance a dysfunctional endocannabinoid system.

Many psychiatric disorders, as well as inflammatory illnesses, have a basis in deficient functioning of the endocannabinoid system. Endocannabinoid levels are significantly lower in depressed women than in controls. Mice raised to have no cannabis receptors have brain and behavior changes similar to what you'd see in someone who is chronically stressed, and they may represent a good animal model for depression. Animal studies show that enhancing endocannabinoid receptor signaling produces effects similar to what is seen following conventional antidepressant treatment.

Because the endocannabinoid system helps to regulate anxiety and fear responses, some drug companies are looking to it to treat anxiety. One potential site of action is the enzyme fatty acid amide hydrolase (FAAH), which metabolizes anandamide. When we're exposed to acute stress, FAAH is mobilized to break down anandamide, helping our body become excitable and ready for action. Inhibiting FAAH, which raises anandamide levels, helps to calm anxiety and mitigate the effects of traumatic stress. Variations in the human FAAH gene may help to explain individual differences in how the amygdala processes threats and in how we cope with stress overall. People with a gene variant causing lower FAAH levels, so anandamide is broken down less, show lower scores on stress reactivity; their amygdalae bounce back more quickly in reaction to threats.

The cliché of pot smokers being mellow couch potatoes makes sense if you think about it in terms of reactivity to stress. If you smoke a lot of pot, you enhance resilience, and you may be thrown off course less by slight traumas. Stoners don't sweat the small stuff because their endocannabinoid system has been primed to be resilient.

Women and cannabis enjoy a special relationship. Anandamide levels fluctuate throughout the menstrual cycle, peaking during ovulation. This may help to explain how great most of us feel midcycle. Peaking estrogen is also responsible, but it may act indirectly through the endocannabinoid system. Estrogen inhibits FAAH activity, thereby increasing anandamide signaling, keeping us calm. This same estrogen/FAAH interaction happens in the uterus, which is full of cannabinoid receptors. This helps to explain the oldest known recommended use for cannabis: an Egyptian papyrus from 1550 B.C.E. detailed treatment of menstrual cramps with a vaginal suppository of cannabis and honey. Queen Victoria was prescribed cannabis by the royal physician Sir Joshua Reynolds to help her with her royal cramps. Another long-standing use of cannabinoids has been to treat the nausea and vomiting of pregnancy.

Learning more about cannabis and the endocannabinoid system is a no-brainer. This is an ancient medicinal plant that is a potent anti-inflammatory drug as well as a stress modulator, and it has particular relevance to women. Medical marijuana laws are being passed with accelerating frequency by more states and countries around the world. For its positive effects on energy metabolism and its stress-relieving properties, most people smoke or vaporize the dried flower. If you don't want to get high, you can juice the whole plant or ingest only the CBD, the component of cannabis that won't make you feel out of it but does yield many of the same beneficial effects on metabolism and inflammation. Whether or not you choose to partake, your body runs on cannabinoids, helping to keep you healthy. It's hardly the only anti-inflammatory remedy, however, and in the chapters that follow you'll find diverse techniques for combating inflammation and fostering health and well-being.

Eight

Food: A Drug We Can't Resist

Many women are struggling with their weight or their relationship to food as much as they are with their moods. Of course, for women, food and mood are directly linked. Most women have stopped using food as a fuel and started using it as a drug, to soothe their anxieties or to transport them away from their stressed-out lives. What they don't realize is that food, when used properly, can be the best medicine, helping to stabilize blood sugar, brain chemistry, and moods. This chapter will teach you how to feed your head—relying on a fat-friendly, plant-rich diet that combats inflammation and boosts the feel-good neurotransmitters in your brain. It's simple, but it's not easy. Eating is tied in with strong emotions, and we were all soothed orally as babies, whether with breast, bottle, or binkie. My patients drown their sorrows in comfort foods; many times these are the same foods their mothers would offer them if they'd had a hard day. Being loved, cared for, and fed is our first formative experience in infancy and childhood. Food and love become intimately associated in nearly all of us, which leads to a lot of calorie-laden self-soothing behavior in adulthood.

These bad habits are hard to break, but the first food rule needs to be energy in, energy out. If you eat nutrient-dense foods, you will have more vitality.

WIRED TO GORGE

Our bodies were designed to hoard calories now for hard times later. What we have now is a genetic mismatch—old genes that tell us to feast whenever we can to prepare for the oncoming famine, when there is no longer any food shortage. Our bodies and metabolisms have not changed much since we were hunter-gatherers, ten thousand years ago, but our food sources have completely morphed. We've gone from cooking bison legs over an open fire whenever the hunt was successful to eating burgers and burritos at a thousand calories a pop on a daily basis.

On the savanna, if you saw a food source, you would immediately mark it as important (salient) and either hunt it down or gather as much as you could. The dopamine circuitry would light up like a pinball machine to help you remember where you got this food, motivate you to forage, and to reward you with pleasure so you'd keep eating, all in order to survive. Flash forward to the modern day, when high-calorie foods are abundant, but just looking at them triggers this same dopamine circuitry. Remember that dopamine is the molecular cornerstone of addiction. Just hearing the words *chocolate brownie* or looking at pictures of high-calorie foods can activate dopamine reward centers, especially if you already have food issues.

Processed foods, with the perfect symphony of sugar, fat and salt, are explicitly designed to exploit our innate food preferences and end up acting just like drugs. Junk food is literally addictive, changing your brain chemistry much as it would if it were crack or speed. Indeed, in a study pitting Oreos against cocaine, the Oreos won, triggering a bigger dopamine response in rats. And not only do junk foods get us hooked, but we get tolerant and require higher doses, and they leave us hanging when we quit them.

Sugar creates a "bliss point" that lights up the reward circuitry that keeps us coming back for more. Fats trigger overeating by giving us a pleasurable mouthfeel, and salt further boosts the appeal of processed foods. Fat content is difficult to discern when it is not easily visible in foods, as in a marbled steak. When sugar is added, it's even worse. As more sugar is added to processed foods, the bliss point is constantly being moved upward. If kids grow up on fruit juice and soda, water tastes boring to them. Processed foods are so salty, broccoli might as well be cardboard. This is a learned behavior, and eating healthier is going to involve retraining your (and your kids') taste buds.

Even artificial sweeteners can get us hooked and, unlike with cocaine and methamphetamine, offering a mate or a running wheel doesn't interfere with self-administration. Basic research on feeding behaviors shows that our internal morphine receptor system, the endorphin circuitry, is activated by certain foods. Rats fed a high-sugar diet that is then abruptly discontinued show brain chemistry consistent with opiate withdrawal, with classic symptoms like chattering teeth and the shakes. Giving women who are binge eaters the opiate blocker naloxone damps down their compulsion to overindulge in high-sugar and high-fat foods. This makes it clear that the endorphin system acts a bit like the engine of the runaway train known as the binge.

We know that food affects our physical health. What's becoming clearer is the connection between food and mental health. What we eat affects how we're feeling, and, of course, how we're feeling affects the way we eat. Stress and emotions affect your gastrointestinal system, and vice versa. Nerves from the gut to the brain actually outnumber those from the brain to the gut. This two-way communication may help to explain having a gut feeling about something, or having "butterflies in your stomach." Also, neurotransmitters are made in your gut as well as in your brain. This means that what you eat can directly affect your mood.

When stressed, we are often triggered to eat carbs, which can enhance our levels of dopamine and serotonin, neurotransmitters that not only make us feel good but also lower cortisol levels. This is known as a negative feedback loop. High cortisol leads to eating sugars and starches, which leads to higher serotonin levels, which then lower cortisol levels. Tasty treats also increase endorphin and endocannabinoid levels. So there's a reason they're called comfort foods. With all these feel-good neurotransmitters circulating, fattening foods make us feel great.

Not only are we stimulated by this rewarding neural soup, but we can't stop once we've started. Foods with just the right ratio of sweet, salty, and greasy trip our brains into euphoria, and the brakes for overeating come right off. Research in stressed-out monkeys that overeat shows that they have compromised dopamine systems. They self-medicate with food to stimulate their dopamine reward pathways; they have less inhibitory control in response to these reward cues from eating, and they show a reduced satiety response. More reward and less control are hallmarks of addiction. The brain's ability to register dopamine surges is significantly lower in obese individuals, in much the same way that it is in the brains of cocaine addicts.

So why is it that we stage interventions when people are ruining their lives with drugs or alcohol, but no one steps in when the abused substance is food? Food addiction is a critical health issue in this country, where two-thirds of adults are overweight or obese. I joke in my office about sugar being "the other white powder," as addictive and unhealthy as cocaine and heroin. Turns out it isn't that much of a joke. The brain reacts to sugar much as it does to drugs.

It's not unusual for an addict to get clean or sober only to gain a tremendous amount of weight. Drugs and food compete in the brain for the same reinforcement sites. So when manufactured food is specifically designed to hit your addiction sweet spot, what's a girl to do? You may want to approach overhauling your eating behavior much as you would tackle an addiction. There is solid evidence that twelve-step programs are a great way to reorganize disordered eating. If your eating is drug-like, use the twelve-step approach and start at step one. Admit that you're powerless over your drug of choice. Willpower has nothing to do with it.

One creative end run around the binge involves using your mind to satisfy your stomach. Different parts of the dopamine reward pathway are recruited in anticipation of—as opposed to experiencing—a reward, and it turns out both are pleasurable. Your brain's chemistry changes just as much by anticipating pleasure as by experiencing it. If your brain squirts out that happy juice just by thinking about your favorite foods, go ahead and imagine eating a huge sundae or a hunk of cake. Think about how it smells, looks, and feels as your lips pull it off your silverware and onto your tongue. Take all the time you want, and enjoy the food fantasy instead of opting for the actual sugary mess. First, it's never as perfect as you can imagine it to be. And, more important, once you start, it may be hard to stop.

THE MUNCHIES, WHETHER YOU'RE STONED OR NOT

The endocannabinoid system is one of the reasons humans are still alive. It plays a vital role in regulating feeding behaviors. Just like stoners who'll hoover up anything in sight, when this system is triggered, you get hungry and don't stop eating. It's the job of this system to encourage you from the first bite to keep it up. This is great news for painfully thin medical marijuana patients with cancer or AIDS, whose medicines make them feel nauseated, but it's not so great for everyone else.

The hormone leptin helps you to stop eating. Leptin tries to keep you thin by signaling the brain's hypothalamus to reduce appetite because you feel full, and also to burn more calories. The more fat cells you have, the more leptin gets secreted. In this way, it acts as a sensor, telling your body just how fat you really are—a true friend. But here's where it gets tricky: the more body fat you have, the more leptin you have, and at some point, the body's receptors just stop listening. You become tolerant of the signals to stop eating and, more important, to the high leptin levels. This is leptin resistance, and it's bad news for you, because fat cells in the belly generate all sorts of chemicals that you don't want in your body, creating a low-grade inflammatory condition that further deranges metabolism.

Low leptin levels signal the endocannabinoid system to get to work and make you hungry. High leptin levels reduce endocannabinoid levels in the brain's hypothalamus, turning off the munchies. When you binge, your brain is flooded with endocannabinoids. So why not block these receptors so that the weight will just fall off? Maybe the endocannabinoid system can be harnessed to combat leptin resistance. Great idea, except that it didn't turn out so well in real life. The medication rimonabant works by blocking the cannabis receptor CB1. By antagonizing the endocannabinoid system, it is the antimunchie medicine. Rimonabant was researched and marketed as an appetite suppressant. The problem was that when this medication was used in humans, people became so depressed and suicidal that eventually rimonabant was withdrawn from the market.

It turns out that the endocannabinoid system does a lot more for you than just encouraging feasting. It helps to keep you happy. Newer research suggests that the focus might be shifted to endocannabinoid receptors in the gut, which could alleviate overeating without creating psychological side effects.

HORMONES AREN'T JUST FOR SEX

The endocannabinoid system is just one of the smart feedback loops for our appetites. Our bodies are calibrated to manage our appetite and our weight. Three main hormones work together to affect our blood sugar, hunger, and overall energy metabolism. Understanding how these hormones affect your hunger can help to arm you in your quest to eat for health. You've already learned about leptin, so let's continue with insulin, which helps to regulate carbohydrate and fat metabolism. Insulin keeps you insulated, preventing the breakdown of fat to be used as an energy source. Instead, insulin preferentially makes sure that sugar is used by the cells. As you eat, your blood sugar goes up, then insulin gets released from the pancreas (located beneath and behind your stomach), driving sugar out of the bloodstream and into the cells, and so your blood sugar goes down. All is well. The problem comes when your pancreas overreacts and releases too much insulin, resulting in lower blood sugar levels than when you started. This happens when you eat simple carbohydrates that quickly turn to sugar. Or drink them. Sweetened drinks made rats more hungry, not less.

Sweet foods trigger the insulin response, and they also make you hungry. Artificial sweeteners do not satiate the way sugars do, but they do cause an insulin spike that further triggers your appetite, and can make you fat. Feeling like a moody bitch? It may be that your blood sugar has bottomed out, called hypoglycemia, making you cranky, grumpy, shaky, sweaty, nauseous, and ravenous. Sometimes these symptoms are interpreted as anxiety or panic. With lower blood sugar, you start craving sugar and carbs to normalize those levels. Carbs beget carbs. Start the morning with sugary foods and you'll be chasing that high all day long as your blood sugar levels keep dipping to new lows.

Since simple carbs tend to drop your blood sugar eventually, you're better off sticking with things that will trigger a slower release of insulin, like complex carbs, protein, or fat. Complex carbs are whole-grain foods like oats, quinoa, farro, and millet, which not only help to stabilize blood sugar but also help to improve your serotonin levels and your memory. Most complex carbs are high in the B vitamins (B_1, B_6, and B_{12}) needed for your brain to function. So be smart; eat your fiber-rich grains. It'll help your mood.

A high-protein, low-carb diet will not only help you lose weight and lower your risk for heart disease, it will keep your blood sugar as stable as can be. Anything with a low glycemic index (easy to look up online) will help to stabilize your blood sugar, as will cinnamon and the supplement chromium picolinate. Sugar in excess is bad news. It gets stored as fat and can increase your risk of heart disease and diabetes. Type 1 diabetes is typically diagnosed in childhood. The pancreas doesn't produce insulin, and so it must be injected as a lifelong medication. Much more prevalent is type 2 diabetes, a resistance to insulin or a relative insulin deficiency given the demands of a high-sugar diet. Over time, the cells become less sensitive to insulin's signal that they absorb the sugar in the bloodstream. Type 2 diabetes is treated by adjusting the diet and exercising more or by taking medicines that reduce blood sugar. Injected insulin is given only in the advanced stages.

Insulin resistance is a huge problem when it comes to health and weight management. If you are insulin resistant, you typically will have symptoms of increased hunger, abdominal fat, and sleepiness after meals. You may also have "brain fog" and depression. Obesity and inactivity are risk factors for insulin resistance, as is a diet high in refined sugar and carbohydrates. Exercise combats insulin resistance, improving the body's sensitivity to insulin. It also helps the muscles absorb sugar from the bloodstream without insulin. Numerous studies suggest that the omega-3 fatty acids in fish oils also combat insulin resistance. What

else reverses insulin resistance? Cannabis. It turns out that the cannabinoid system is intimately involved in sugar and energy utilization.
Chronic pot smokers have smaller waistlines, better cholesterol and fatty
acid levels, and less insulin resistance than people who don't use the
drug. The endocannabinoid system is crucial to maintaining your metabolism, and insulin sensitivity and resistance are critical when it comes
to weight management.

The third hormone, ghrelin, is made in your stomach. Ghrelin triggers hunger, food seeking, and consuming by increasing gastric motility
and secretions, making your stomach ghrumble and ghrowl. Ghrelin levels rise in anticipation of eating; just thinking about what's for lunch is
enough to stimulate your appetite. Ghrelin also slows metabolism and
decreases the body's ability to burn fat. You may be able to suppress the
ghrelin secretion a bit by drinking a glass of water before you eat a meal,
or having an apple beforehand. Ghrelin levels rise at night, just in time
for your bingeing needs, thank you. And sleep deprivation increases
daytime levels of ghrelin and reduces leptin levels, which is why the current thinking is that you need to sleep more if you want to weigh less.

In obese people, eating doesn't affect the ghrelin or leptin signals the
way it does in lean research subjects. Weight is primarily genetic. Twins,
whether they grow up together or are separated at birth, maintain nearly
exactly the same body mass index, and children adopted out have the
BMIs of their biological parents, not their adoptive ones. Everyone has
their own set point and feedback loop when it comes to these hormones.
As you may well know, after you've lost weight, it's an uphill battle. Australian researchers tested fifty overweight adults after they had lost an
average of 14 percent of their body fat. Their levels of leptin and ghrelin
had changed dramatically, slowing their metabolism and intensifying
their feelings of hunger. These altered levels lasted up to a year, and most
of the research subjects gained back nearly half the weight they had lost,
despite sticking to their diets. This is the set point in action. But there are

still choices you can make that will benefit your overall health, like what you eat and how you eat it.

WHAT TO EAT

Your meals are the only fuel your machine gets. Your food should look good and taste good, of course, but it also should be good for the machinery. You wouldn't put cake frosting into your car's engine, I'm betting, so maybe you shouldn't be spraying that can of whipped cream directly into your mouth either.

Only about a quarter of us eat three servings of vegetables a day, and the truth is that we need way more than that. Out of convenience and time pressures, we don't prepare fresh vegetables as often as we opt to buy Big Macs. The trend of eating processed foods is life threatening. Countries like ours, with the lowest percentages of calories consumed from unrefined, whole foods, have the highest rates of cancer and heart disease. The longer immigrants live in America, the worse their rates of diabetes, high blood pressure, and heart disease become. American-born children don't live as long as their foreign-born parents.

Here's what I tell my patients to keep it simple. Choose vegetables over fruit, natural foods over processed foods, and proteins over starches. This diet might be your best bet, not just for stabilizing your weight and appetite but also for maintaining your mood. One study that divided people into two diets, whole foods and processed foods, found a 58 percent higher risk for depression in the second group.

Nature is smarter than corporations. Once the food industry has separated the components of food and processed it, you're going to get into trouble. We're not designed to ingest sugar without fiber. We are designed for raw, whole, natural, balanced foods. There is an entourage effect in food, where components in the plant work together to keep us healthy. Plants turn sunlight into energy. This energy provides the fuel to run the chemistry experiments of your body. Vitamins and minerals are also necessary for these chemical equations. It is better to find them in your food than on your bathroom counter. (I have a patient who jokes about how healthy her medicine cabinet is, because all the vitamins are in there instead of in her body.)

The paleo diet, heavy on protein and fat and light on carbs, is gaining in popularity and is a good option for both weight and mood maintenance. You may want to ask yourself, *What would a cavewoman eat?* One thing's for sure. The war on fat is over. We tried to go low fat in the nineties, and we got fatter and more diabetic as we substituted in more carbs and sugars. Fat is filling and satisfying; most of us are more likely to binge on sweets than on steak. And here's the kicker: diets high in fats and low in carbs cause more weight loss, and in particular belly fat loss, than low-fat diets do. They also lower blood sugar and insulin levels and lower your risk of diabetes. Newer research is contradicting the advice we got for decades. Saturated fat and cholesterol don't increase our risk for heart attacks or cardiovascular disease. Sugar does. The countries eating the most saturated fat have some of the lowest rates of heart disease, thus the "French paradox."

Low-carb diets can lower cardiovascular risk factors, improving your cholesterol numbers and triglyceride levels. As for good fats and bad fats, the advice has changed there, too. Saturated fats, like those found in butter, meat, and dairy, used to be bad, but now they're okay again. Trans fats are still bad. They're man-made, toxic, and strongly linked to heart disease. This includes margarine, Crisco, and anything partially hydrogenated that's added to processed foods like cookies, crackers, chips, and doughnuts. French fries and movie popcorn are often cooked in trans fats. Monounsaturated fats, found in nuts, are still good. Nuts are also high in protein, fiber, and omega-3 fatty acids—three reasons to make them a regular (and satisfying) snack.

I'd grown up hearing that palm oil and coconut oil were bad for you. Now, it turns out, coconut oil is the hot new thing. It's a way to add a bit of sweetener without inducing an insulin spike, and it may even reduce belly fat while improving your cholesterol levels. You can cook with it at a high heat without its breaking down the way olive oil can, and it doesn't go rancid as quickly as other oils. I like to sauté dark green vegetables in coconut oil. The mild sweetness helps to counterbalance bitter greens. When that taste doesn't work, use extra virgin olive oil if it's low to medium heat, and grapeseed oil for high heat.

Every day, if you can, eat a big salad. Raw vegetables are important. People who eat seven servings a day have a lower chance of getting sick or dying from cancer and heart disease. If you don't want to stop eating carbs, at least add more vegetables to each meal. I've learned to really love salads, not resent them. For a long while, I went with lemon and olive oil as a salad dressing. Lemon can help alkalinize your body, and there's suggestive literature on the health benefits of staying on the alkaline side, including maintaining bone health and lowering your risk for obesity, diabetes, and heart disease.

These days, I'm convinced that apple cider vinegar (ACV) is an even better way to go than lemon for alkalinizing, so that's my go-to salad dressing now. There is strong evidence that ACV lowers insulin responses and glucose levels after a meal and can help keep diabetes in check. It also helps to drive weight loss, improve cholesterol levels, and reduce inflammation. The acetic acid in vinegar inhibits the digestion of starches and sugars, so more of them pass through the digestive system as indigestible fibers. Also, because vinegar helps you digest, you won't be so bloated after you eat. Many cultures eat pickled foods as appetizers, a smart way to go. It may be that some of the benefits seen in a Mediterranean diet are due to eating pickled products, especially early in the meal.

Your body needs sugar to function, but not all sugars are created equal. Though many of the body's cells can use fat or protein as a fuel source, the brain is picky and uses only the sugar glucose. Glucose does not need to be broken down by the liver; it is absorbed from the stomach, and as long as insulin is around, it will be picked up by the brain cells. The sugar fructose is unique in needing the liver to break it down, and fatty triglycerides are created in the process. Fructose, more than other sugars, causes fatty livers. Research shows that consuming fructose in particular induces insulin resistance, lowers leptin levels, impairs glucose tolerance, elevates fatty acid levels, and causes high blood pressure in animals. Chronic consumption of fructose can lead to increased caloric intake, weight gain, and obesity. It can also increase blood triglycerides, LDL cholesterol, and a fat-binding protein, all markers for heart disease.

In the old days, fructose was consumed only when fruit was eaten, which meant that plenty of fiber and antioxidants were part of the package, buffering the effects of the triglycerides. Now, thanks to high-fructose corn syrup, which is in nearly every processed food, we're getting huge amounts of fructose minus the fiber buffers, and our bloodstreams, livers, and brain cells are being deluged with fat as a by-product of its metabolism. High triglycerides create fatty livers and heart disease and also put you at risk for cognitive deficits and Alzheimer's disease. Estrogen may blunt some of these effects; male lab rats are more affected by high-fructose diets than female rats are. Moody bitches beware: high triglyceride levels from high-fructose diets not only put you at risk for memory problems but also interfere with neurotransmitter production and function and can increase your risk for depression.

The solution is to cut out fruit juices and high-fructose corn syrup completely and consider limiting fruits in your diet. One smart move: eat only what is in season, not what's been flown in from South America.

Melons in summer, apples and pears in fall. Mangoes year-round aren't natural. It's not what nature intended, and we weren't designed to eat that way.

Obesity, diabetes, high blood pressure, strokes, and heart attacks are often referred to as "lifestyle illnesses," meaning if we could alter our unhealthy choices, we wouldn't have the pathology. Unfortunately, in our pill-popping culture, we don't tackle the harmful behavior so much as we simply opt to take a medicine to negate its effects. We don't alter our nutritional intake as readily as we take a cholesterol-lowering or blood-sugar-lowering medication. A quarter of Americans are prescribed statins. If you've been told your cholesterol is high and you should take a statin, please consider cutting out carbs and fructose in particular before taking a medicine that could cause memory loss, increased blood-sugar levels, muscle damage, and tingling and numbness in your extremities. Statins also deplete key nutrients, and, perhaps most alarming, new studies suggest that people taking statins develop a false sense of assurance and eat more unhealthy foods.

And while we're on the topic of cholesterol, eggs are a great source of protein and have all the B vitamins you need. Eggs raise your HDL level (the good cholesterol) and are not associated with an increased risk of heart disease or stroke. Our bodies make cholesterol, and in most cases, if we have healthy livers, our livers will make less cholesterol when we eat more. Also, eggs are high in choline, which is a nutrient that is easily depleted when you're stressed and your cortisol levels are high, so eggs are a way to defend your body against your jam-packed lifestyle. Many women aren't getting enough choline in their diets, necessary for neurotransmission and to make cell membranes throughout the body. Another moody bitch alert: low choline levels are associated with anxiety and depression in women. My point here is simple. Eat eggs.

When I start my day with protein, like eggs, instead of carbs, like pancakes, I have more energy and focus and my hunger stays in check.

As mentioned earlier, carbs beget carbs. Simple carbohydrates (doughnuts, muffins, pancakes, croissants—any combination of flour, sugar, and fat, basically) spike your insulin levels, which causes your blood sugar to drop, which makes you hungry... for more carbs. This is a main reason to not drink sugary soda.

WHAT TO DRINK

I try to minimize flour, sugar, and dairy in my own diet, and I encourage many of my patients to join me in that endeavor. There is mounting evidence that the protein in milk, casein, wreaks havoc with our bodies and brains. When we are babies, we are designed to grow and develop by ingesting our mothers' breast milk, not that of a cow. There is no other species on the planet that sucks on the mammaries of another. We are not baby cows, and so we are not genetically engineered to benefit from their mothers' milk, and certainly not through adulthood. Cream, butter, cheese... I know these things all taste amazing and make your life worth living, but I tell my patients to pretend they are lactose intolerant. It's the only intolerance I encourage. If you are going to drink milk, make it 1 percent or 2 percent fat, because skim ends up creating a bigger spike in insulin due to its relatively higher percentage of sugar.

Unsweetened almond milk is a better alternative to dairy, because it's got more protein than rice milk, which is high in sugar and carbs. Unsweetened coconut milk and soy milk are other options. Avoid soy if you are estrogen dominant (see the perimenopause chapter), have a sluggish thyroid, or are taking Synthroid. The phaelates found in soy interfere with iodine absorption, which your thyroid needs to do its job.

Diet soda? Nope. Artificial sweeteners trigger insulin release as much as or more than real sweeteners. Plenty of studies show that giving diet drinks to research subjects ends up causing more weight gain and potentially causing insulin resistance from chronically high blood sugar. Rats given aspartame in their chow have higher blood sugar levels than those given regular chow, and rats given saccharine water end up fatter than rats given sugar water. Also, liquid calories don't tend to trigger satiety the way that solid calories do, so be especially careful with non-diet drinks. Our bodies are less aware of excessive calorie intake in liquids than in solids.

The solution is simple. Drink water.

FOOD AS MEDICINE: UNDERSTANDING (AND PREVENTING) INFLAMMATION

Not only is what we eat important, but how we feel has a huge impact on our appetites. Welcome to the Bermuda triangle of mood, obesity, and inflammation. Stress creates inflammation; stress triggers overeating; body fat creates inflammation; inflammation feeds obesity and depression; and they all imperil our health.

Inflammation gums up the works in your stomach, which is bad news for your brain. Some neurotransmitters, such as serotonin and dopamine, are primarily made in your stomach using vitamins and amino acids (protein building blocks) from your food. If there is inflammation, the manufacturing of these basic neurotransmitters will suffer. Not only will you have digestive issues, like bloating and diarrhea, but you may be cranky or depressed as well. Eating foods that aren't right for you can drastically alter how you feel, both mentally and physically.

Feeling kind of blah and bloated? Try an anti-inflammatory diet and see if you don't feel better. Indigenous cultures with no processed foods have minimal prevalance of dementia, heart disease, and arthritis. If you want to prevent many of the medical illnesses that await you as you age, avoid the unhealthy white powders like sugar and flour, and eat your colors. I joke with my patients, "Be a food racist. Nothing white." Think of it as an affirmative-action diet. Bright red and orange foods like beets, peppers, and squash; dark green leafy vegetables like kale and spinach; and deep purple fruits like pomegranates and blueberries have anti-inflammatory benefits. Avoid all processed foods in favor of fresh, or, even better, eat raw foods, vegetables, nuts, and seeds. Refined white flour and sugar can trigger an inflammatory response, as can fatty red meats, sweetened drinks, and diet sodas, so these should all be avoided. In a Harvard study, women who ate bread and pasta (white foods) had higher inflammatory markers and depression scores than those who didn't. So start by changing your "go-to" breakfast. Ditch the bagels, doughnuts, and cereal. Try eggs with vegetables, but no toast. Or have yogurt with seeds and nuts instead. Above all, choose nutrient-dense foods that are high in fiber and low in calories, a.k.a. vegetables. Nearly all of them have anti-inflammatory benefits. Ginger and turmeric are two spices with anti-inflammatory activity, so be liberal in their use.

The body's machinery produces waste products from metabolism, called free radicals, which build up, setting off a chain reaction that can damage cells. This is called oxidative stress, and it leads to inflammation. Antioxidants, like beta-carotenoids (found in yellow and orange vegetables), lycopene (tomatoes), anthocyanins (blueberries), catechins (green tea), theaflavin (black tea), and polyphenols (red wine, green tea, and chocolate), all protect the body's tissues from oxidative stress, thereby earning the label "anti-inflammatory." Vitamins C and E and selenium are all antioxidants, and cannabis is, too.

Omega-3 fatty acids are antioxidants that lower inflammation. Nearly 70 percent of Americans have omega-3 fatty acid deficiency, because many of us don't eat enough fish, especially the cold-water, carnivorous fish, like wild salmon, black cod (sablefish), and halibut. Omega-3s are found in algae and fish, flaxseed, hemp seed, and their oils. Fish has long had a reputation of being brain food, and for good reason. Anxious and depressed patients have lower levels of omega-3s, and supplementation improves symptoms.

There is a growing body of literature that says fish oils can be used to decrease impulsivity and lengthen a short fuse, perhaps being helpful in treating ADHD and bipolar disorder and even some schizophrenia symptoms. Omega-3 fatty acids may also slow down telomere shortening, combating the effects of stress and aging. One more reason to ingest them: omega-3 fatty acids can form endocannabinoids that latch on to both CB1 and CB2 receptors, helping to keep inflammation down. Hemp seeds (great by the handful) and hemp seed oil (fabulous in a vinaigrette) are tasty sources of omega-3 fatty acids as well as complete vegetarian proteins, suitable not just for birdseed or animal feed but for all of us. I add hemp seeds to my morning muesli, which keeps me full all day long.

PROBIOTICS CAN SOOTHE INFLAMMATION AND MAY HELP WITH DEPRESSION

Our bodies host a diverse community of bacteria called the biome. Only one out of ten cells in our bodies is mammalian; bacterial cells outnumber human cells, nine to one. Trillions of bacteria in our GI system produce chemicals that help us not only to digest our food but also to modulate our appetites. How do you get a fat mouse thinner or a thin mouse fatter? Transplant it with the intestinal bacteria of the other. Gut bacteria have a lot to do with obesity. Obese people and thin people have different levels of certain bacteria. In humans given a lean donor's microbes (called a fecal transplant; don't ask), insulin sensitivity improves as the gut microbes repair disordered metabolism. Probiotics help stop the weight gain and insulin resistance sometimes seen with administration of the antipsychotic olanzapine (Zyprexa), so they may work with other psych meds that cause weight gain as well.

People who have gastric bypass surgery tend to lose around two-thirds of their excess baggage. There are many reasons for this. Smaller stomachs fill up more quickly, and the surgery reduces levels of the appetite-inducing hormone ghrelin. A recent discovery, though, is that this surgery changes the balance of gut bacteria as well. When gut contents from animals that had undergone bariatric surgery were transferred into other animals, the nonsurgical recipients also lost weight.

Unfortunately, our typical Western diet of processed foods heavy on sugars and low on fiber alters the gut bacteria we were born with, reducing its diversity. (Rounds of antibiotics typical in childhood and overexposure to antibacterial products disrupt our normal flora as well.) Artificial sweeteners such as Splenda, Equal, and Sweet 'n Low also kill off beneficial gut bacteria, deranging glucose metabolism. Healthy gut bacteria are promoted and maintained by eating vegetables and other high-fiber foods and fermented foods like yogurt, kimchi, and sauerkraut. There are also fermented drinks, like kefir and kombucha. Fiber feeds the fermentation process in your gut, so adding bran, oats, beans, and nuts to your diet can help to tamp down inflammation as well.

Probiotic supplements are capsules filled with beneficial bacteria that can lower inflammatory cytokine levels and improve nutritional status. They can relieve diarrhea, bloating, gas, and irritable bowel syndrome, and reduce allergic responses by modifying the immune system. Some recent studies suggest that taking probiotic supplements along with eating prebiotic foods will encourage weight loss. Probiotics are foods that feed the bacteria. Onions, artichokes, asparagus, and sunchokes along with probiotics will not only assist weight loss but will also help to keep down inflammation even more.

Our gut bacteria also play a role in the manufacture of substances like neurotransmitters (including serotonin), enzymes and vitamins (notably Bs and K), and other essential nutrients, including important amino acids and short-chain fatty acids. Short-chain fatty acids, a by-product of fermentation, can also act to prevent inflammation, which is why adding fermented foods to your diet can be so beneficial. Some of these compounds may play a role in regulating our stress levels and even our temperament: when gut microbes from easygoing, adventurous mice are transplanted into the guts of anxious and timid mice, these mice become more adventurous.

Everyone has a balance of good and bad bacteria. Yeast and bad bacteria grow out of control when there are no good bacteria to keep them in check. One product that is produced in this situation is lipopolysaccharide (LPS), an endotoxin that can make you sick. In animal studies, LPS administration creates symptoms similar to the clinical symptoms of depressive disorders: poor appetite, slower movements, fatigue, malaise, and loss of interest. A person's immune response to LPS may increase her risk of chronic depression. Also, LPS breaks down tryptophan, the precursor of serotonin, and elevates cytokines associated with depression that can further deplete tryptophan. This is one way that the wrong balance of bacteria in your system can have a negative effect on your mood.

Ingesting probiotics may improve depression and anxiety. Patients with depression have elevated levels of proinflammatory cytokines and limited nutrient absorption due to altered gut bacteria. By manipulating the bacteria found in the stomach and intestines, brain function, mood, and behavior can be altered. Treatment with probiotics lowers scores in three areas: somatization (complaints about aches and pains), depression, and anger/hostility. Probiotics may even help you be more rational, enhancing top-down control and frontal inhibition. Women who eat probiotic yogurt twice daily have stronger activity in the neural network connecting the prefrontal cortex (involved in decision making and emotional control) with the brain stem (involved in responding to pain and emotional stimuli). This means that probiotics can help to keep you chilled out. They affect GABA, a neurotransmitter that helps to calm the nervous system, lowering anxiety, promoting sleep, and helping us to be more resilient in the face of stress. There is a new watchword in nutrition: psychobiotics. The idea that bacteria can decrease anxiety and depression is catching on, but remember, you heard it here first.

LEAKY GUT SYNDROME

Given the link between inflammation and depression, it makes sense to avoid certain foods that trigger allergic reactions or other inflammatory responses. Different people have reactions to different foods. Perhaps due to something called regional genotyping, certain intolerances show up in populations in the same area. Generations of native Americans grew up on corn and now become inflamed when flour or sugar is added to their diets. Other populations grew up on wheat, and their inflammation occurs due to corn. So moving to a new country and adopting its diet can sow the seeds for inflammatory-based illnesses like diabetes, heart disease, and cancer.

Gluten, the protein found in wheat, barley, and rye, is an allergen for many people even if they don't have the official celiac diagnosis. Lactose, the sugar found in dairy foods, is another. It's not binary; everyone falls on a spectrum of how well they can tolerate these food components. For many, ingesting bread, pasta, or dairy products creates inflammation that makes the gut lining leaky, letting across particles into your bloodstream that normally wouldn't have gotten through.

Your intestines cover miles of ground, all coiled up tightly in your belly. Their lining composes a barrier that lets only properly digested particles through to the bloodstream. The cells decide what passes through and what doesn't, but if the junctions between the cells are too loose, unwanted substances can squeeze between the cells. Certain undesirable bacteria that have a corkscrew shape and the yeast candida can push apart intestinal cells, making junctions more leaky. Again, if your balance of good and bad bacteria is off, this is going to be an issue. If you have gut inflammation, you're likely to have a leaky gut. And once it's leaky, it leads to more inflammation, which can lead to obesity and depression, as well as other symptoms.

If the gut is leaky, then things like bacteria, undigested food, and other toxins can sneak into the bloodstream. This triggers an antibody reaction that causes even more inflammation. Besides intestinal cramps and bloating, inflammation can cause chronic fatigue, compromised immune status, migraines, and mood swings. When your gut is leaky, you can't properly make or absorb the neurotransmitters your brain needs. Food allergies, rheumatoid arthritis, and many other autoimmune diseases may have a basis in a leaky gut. This is one theory for why going gluten-free can help not only with autoimmune diseases and GI complaints but also with mood and metabolism.

Stress, obesity, poor diet, and a leaky gut can all conspire to create a proinflammatory state that can create or worsen depression. I encourage my patients who have depression, arthritis (achy joints), fibromyalgia (muscle aches), chronic fatigue syndrome, or irritable bowel syndrome (characterized by bouts of diarrhea and constipation) to consider an anti-inflammatory diet. The biggies that can trigger an allergic, inflammatory reaction: gluten, dairy, eggs, corn, soy, nuts, shellfish. Corn and soy products are in nearly every packaged food, and it's amazing how often wheat flour is listed as an ingredient, so you're going to have to read long lists of ingredients to successfully cut out some of these potential allergens if you're eating premade foods. This is another advantage of cooking and preparing your own meals from whole, recognizable plants: less reading of the fine print.

I've had many patients and quite a few friends and colleagues tell me how miraculously their gloomy moods lifted when they went gluten-free. But it may be tricky to do so. The two main groups of proteins in gluten are considered exorphins. You've heard of endorphins—your body's internal morphinelike substances that can keep you blissed out and pain free. Exorphins are things you ingest that trigger your endorphin system. And gluten can do that. There is a specific compound in gluten that crosses into the brain called gluteomorphin, which hits the endorphin receptors. So, yes, I totally get that steaming bread and chewy pasta make you happy—high, even—but just because you're addicted to wheat doesn't mean you can't kick it cold turkey. There are more whole-grain breads being made without flour all the time, and more gluten-free products are being created daily to accommodate this new way of eating. The problem here is that they're often heavily processed. Again, it's simpler to eat whole, real, recognizable food.

HOW TO EAT

As a child, I started out sneaking forbidden foods from my mother, but somewhere along the way I ended up sneaking them from myself. I would scarf down taboo foods quickly so that I wouldn't notice, eating in a dazed, fuguelike state so that I wouldn't be present. Many of my patients who binge-eat (the medical term is hyperphagia) report feeling like they are in an altered state as they chow down. Eating like this is a way of hiding, not from just others but also from the self.

When I got to medical school, convenience foods, an addiction to my own fresh-baked bread, and sitting down to study colluded to make me truly doughy. I ended up about thirty pounds overweight by my third year, which is when I discovered two important things: exercise and vegetables. I finally figured out that certain foods made me feel awful, not just emotionally but physically. I was nearing thirty, the time cell metabolism goes from building up to breaking down. Growing children and teenagers can get away with eating like this, but I could not.

What eventually helped me more than anything in my quest for *Thinner Thighs in 30 Days* (a book I remember owning) was learning to understand and accept my own hunger. My discovery of Geneen Roth's books was hugely important. Her advice is simple: eat when you're hungry, eat *exactly* what you want, and then stop before you get too full. To anyone who has been easily slim all her life, it sounds a bit like saying, "Breathe in and breathe out." But to millions of women, eat when you're hungry is exactly what we're *not* doing. We're afraid to trust our bodies and our hunger, and so we search for pills to kill our appetite. The gateway to healthy eating is making peace with your appetite. Here are a few tips to get you started.

Remain conscious while eating. Be present and accounted for. Pay attention to the food as it is going into your mouth, to the texture as you chew, to the taste as you savor each morsel slowly and thoroughly. Eat at a table, sitting down, with no distractions—no television, no magazine, just you and your food. Then you won't "wake up" after you've eaten a plate full of something and wonder whether you enjoyed it.

Truly savoring what you're taking in accomplishes two things. When you're actually present and enjoying every bite, you're more likely to ingest a smaller amount of food. If you shovel food into your mouth quickly so no one notices, including yourself, you taste nothing. You're left with guilt and shame at having binged, with none of the satisfaction of true nourishment. This will only make you physically and psychically uncomfortable, and what do you do with those bad feelings? You medicate them away with more food. And when I say you, I mean me, too.

Like three o'clock at the Hilton, check in. Get centered, take a few deep breaths, and then eat a small amount of whatever it is you are hankering for in a mindful way. To enhance your consciousness, sit down and make yourself a plate; don't grab and go or eat standing up in front of an open refrigerator. The worst: mindlessly munching while hypnotized in front of the tube. Make a sanctified place, physically and mentally, for eating. Use visible boundaries, like a placemat and napkin and maybe even a candle. If you can leave your workplace for lunch, that's wonderful. If you must eat at your desk, turn off your phone and computer and just eat, nothing else. Look at your food. Make a concerted effort to taste it, notice the texture, and pay attention to lunch only. It's fifteen minutes out of your day; your computer can manage without you.

Slow the fork down! Seriously. If you key in to how you're feeling, there is often tension or unease in your abdomen, like butterflies, a tightened belt, or a rock. If you are stressed, your stomach is in no shape to take on a big responsibility like digestion. Your parasympathetic nervous system is primarily responsible for digestion. When the competing sympathetic nervous system is engaged, as when you're anxious or rushed, your heart and muscles require all the blood supply and cellular energy, so digestion gets put on the back burner. Would you fill up your gas tank while barreling down the highway? At the gas station, you turn off the engine. Your body cannot refuel properly if you are in fight-or-flight mode. Slow down and stop before you eat.

The simplest way to kick your body into parasympathetic mode is through the respiratory system. Slow, deep breathing through your nose will signal the brain to flip the switch. (My Bikram yoga teacher is always reminding the class that mouth breathing triggers the sympathetic system and exacerbates panic.) Even if you spend all day flitting around like a hummingbird, try to go into three-toed-sloth mode when you finally sit down to eat. Calm down, slow down, and, again, remember to come back into your body. When you do this, your whole body can relax, including your abdomen.

The calmer you are, the thinner you'll be. Stress, whether physical or emotional, triggers high-calorie food binges. It makes sense to fuel up in a crisis. High-calorie foods enable you to fight or flee from a predator. The problem is, most modern-day stresses don't actually require us to move a muscle, so we fuel up for no good reason. Stress makes you pig out by triggering cortisol release. Cortisol surges cause ghrelin levels to rise, leptin levels to fall, and a protein called peptide Y to trigger carbohydrate cravings. That's a hormonal trifecta for gorging.

Acute stress gets the ball rolling, but chronic stress makes it hard to stop. Subordinate, bossed-around monkeys have excessive cortisol. Monkeys lower in the dominance hierarchy eat their pellets in an uncontrolled manner. Lower-ranked British civil servants are more obese than higher-ranking bosses. People who are more stressed out eat more fat-laden, sweet snacks throughout the day. We eat, and eat, in order to comfort ourselves. Studies are mounting that reducing stress through meditation or yoga can help you lose weight even if you don't change what you're eating all that much, because not only does stress make us binge, but the high cortisol levels associated with stress cause higher blood sugar levels and excess abdominal fat storage.

Put your fork down between bites and go slowly. It really *does* take twenty minutes for your stomach to signal to your brain that you're good to go. So if you inhale a thousand calories in five minutes, you're losing out on nature's wisdom. Try to aim for stopping when you are about two-thirds of the way to full. Your body will catch up soon after, and you'll realize you don't need to eat more food. If you're anything like me, you eat when there's food around, even if you're not that hungry. Like compulsively packing for a trip, planning for every eventuality, I eat now in case I can't eat later. Psychologically, this is masking a fear of being in a state of need. Biologically, it is something bigger, the genetic mismatch. Now that food is consistently plentiful, this panic to eat whenever possible has to be consciously tamed. We must learn to heed that tiny, distant voice saying "Enough!" even though there is plenty more on our plate and in our cupboards.

Eat intuitively, not emotionally. As girls growing up, we're given the message that we cannot trust our bodies, that our hunger is insatiable and we need to learn to curb it, lest we blow up like balloons. We are taught to ignore our desires, and so we grow out of touch with our hunger, treating it like a traitorous saboteur. And because we deny ourselves so frequently, when we finally do get around to eating something that tastes good to us, it's nearly impossible to stop. So we don't eat when we're hungry, and we don't stop when we're full. And "eat exactly what you want" is tantamount to heresy. As girls and young women, we're endlessly told what to eat and what not to eat. Advice on dieting is implicit in our mothers' disapproving glances, explicit in large font on the covers of magazines, and traded among girlfriends at the gym.

My advice: Listen only to your body, and honor what it is telling you. Once you truly allow yourself anything you're fantasizing about eating, with no foods forbidden, you can settle down to nourishing yourself with the foods your body is actually craving. After reading those Roth books, I went through a short period of eating ice cream sundaes for dinner and fettuccine Alfredo for brunch, testing the boundaries that no food was off limits, before my stomach started informing me that what it really had a hankering for were salads with salmon and sautéed kale or spinach. No joke.

Intuitive eating means really listening to that inner voice that will tell you honestly what your body requires to stay healthy. It means trusting and believing your hunger, and making healthy choices. When you give your body what it needs, not what your mouth wants, it's not deprivation; it's nourishment. The quality of the fuel affects the machine. Notice how you feel after you've eaten pasta versus vegetables; gauge your energy level after a Danish versus an omelet. Try to give yourself what will make you feel good later, not just taste good now. To do that, you need to focus on what you're feeling and really get into your body, listen to its signals, and then act in a way that makes you feel better physically.

It's easy to misinterpret those "pings" your body gives you. Sometimes hunger is really thirst. You might open the fridge before you've thought through what's really going on. Have a cup of water or tea and sit down for a moment before deciding on a snack. It's also possible that you're neither hungry nor thirsty. You might just need a "time-out" that doesn't entail chewing, be it a walk in the park or a moment in the sunshine and breeze. If you don't pay attention, you're going to miss the information.

If you truly honor your cravings, give yourself *exactly* what you're imagining, and then fully experience it without turning it into an out-of-body experience, you will actually ingest a smaller amount. It's a bit like scratching exactly where the itch is instead of all around it. Also, food tastes best for the first few bites, so better to have those best taste experiences consciously and deliberately than one marathon of diminishing pleasure as you absentmindedly clean your plate.

Beware the witching hour. Many of my patients tell me about "being good" all day long, sticking to their meal plans, and even making it to the gym, only to lose it at night, in the no-man's-land between dinner and bedtime. In college, this was when we'd have a fourth meal, whether pizza or diner eggs. When I became a mother, it turned into something else. I had been giving to others all day long, doing for everyone else, and when I was finally alone, I'd graze, just like my patients. Nighttime is when we finally get around to giving to ourselves, but too often it's not in a healthy, nurturing, or patient way.

Often, our nighttime eating is distracted, dispirited, and destructive. We're zoned out in front of the television, or, worse, we're drunk. So much worse. Alcohol disinhibits many of our appetitive behaviors, like having sex and eating, so we end up breaking our diets or choosing junk-food sex partners.

The opposite of mindful eating is performed on autopilot, like an altered state of consciousness. The repetitive mindlessness of eating is soothing; it's hypnotic and rhythmic. It takes us out of ourselves, which is where we want to go when the going gets rough. Bingeing also releases dopamine, endorphins, and cannabinoids, your body's way of making sure eating is pleasurable, so that you'll keep doing it. Nighttime is also when we're finally less harried and distracted, so our emotions start to bubble up to the surface. Most of us are quick to distract ourselves with e-mail, television, or cleaning up the kitchen so that we don't have to feel anything, but my advice: sit down, shut up and FEEL, dammit! That trite phrase "It's not what you're eating; it's what's eating you" may be overused, but it is terribly true. The gal on her couch comforting herself with a pint of Ben & Jerry's is a cliché for a reason. Research shows that intense feelings can affect our taste buds; we're more sensitive to flavors like sweet, bitter, or salty, but less sensitive to how much fat or how many calories we're consuming when our mood is low.

We often eat because something is nibbling away at our insides. When I think, *I'm hungry,* I try to reflexively ask myself, *What is rising up to the surface that I'm trying to stuff back down?* For many of us, it is a feeling of isolation or loneliness. That Starbucks poster with images of caramel-drizzled lattes with the caption "Some Friends You Can Depend On" is genius, if you ask me.

Those stressed-out monkeys lower in the dominance hierarchy did most of their bingeing at night. Part of this urge is psychological, but there is an awful lot of biology to overcome. Ghrelin, the primary hormone that drives hunger, rises from afternoon through evening, and galanin, a hormone that makes us seek out high-calorie food, spikes at night, ensuring enough sustenance to last till morning. Make sure you're eating a healthy combination of protein and vegetables at dinner to keep your blood sugar in check, drink plenty of water, and then clear out of the kitchen until morning. Most important, find ways to reliably soothe yourself that don't involve food.

When you step away from that pizza, remember: You are not denying yourself anything, but rather giving yourself the gift of pleasure, joy, and good health for years to come. Emotional growth requires tipping the scales toward self-preservation and away from self-destruction and sabotage. When it comes to maintaining your physical and mental health, food is a big part of the equation. The quality of the fuel you put into your engine affects its performance. If you want to have more energy and vitality, you need to eat plants that have captured the energy of the sun while growing in the great outdoors. Animals that eat plants are a distant second, and factory-farmed animals fed antibiotics and corn, soy, and other animals are an even more distant third. Keep in mind that the balance of your hormones and gut bacteria dictates your metabolic health. And let's not forget sleep. It turns out that the more sleep you get, the thinner you can be. So on to the next chapter.

Nine

So Tired
We're Wired

W omen are more sensitive to sleep deprivation than men
and are more likely to wake up grumpier, angrier, and
more hostile if they haven't slept enough. Women are more
prone to insomnia than men, primarily due to hormonal fluctuations.
Becoming a mother, and the hypervigilance that goes with that responsibility, triggers insomnia in many women. The other problem area is
perimenopause, where one of the first and most persistent symptoms
is difficulty falling and staying asleep. Given these two populations, it
shouldn't surprise you to learn that three out of four insomnia patients in
sleep clinics are women, and twice as many women use sleeping pills as
men. Nearly 30 percent of American women report using some kind of
sleep aid at least a few nights a week, and 80 percent of women surveyed
reported being too stressed or worried to fall asleep easily.

Sleep is one of the body's most vital activities. Sleep quality is the
single biggest predictor of longevity, more than diet or exercise. It is

crucial to many bodily functions, including hormonal balance, immunity, and metabolism. When sleep is off-kilter, a host of problems can develop, including an increased risk of blood clots, cardiovascular disease, diabetes, autoimmune disorders, cancer, obesity and inflammation. "Not enough sleep makes you fat, hungry, impotent, hypertensive, and cancerous with a bad heart."

As usual, when one function is off in the body, the rest fall out of line. Sleep deprivation leads to more inflammation and less resilience in the face of stress. This can be a setup for depression. Even one night of poor sleep can affect your brain the next day, with higher scores on tests of anxiety, stress, and depressed mood. Higher resting heart rates accompany these higher stress levels.

Disordered sleep is often seen in people with depression and anxiety disorders, chronic pain conditions, and stress. Especially work stress. When my patients have trouble in the office, it inevitably gets played out in the bedroom, and not in a sexy way. Nights are spent stewing about the day's events and fretting about tomorrow's. The high cortisol levels that result from bilateral candle burning reliably disrupt initiating and maintaining sleep, and chronically high levels lead to more accumulated belly fat, higher blood sugar levels, and the possibility of diabetes. As you'll see below, sleep deprivation is intimately tied into weight management, so keeping stress down and sleep quality up is an important part of being physically fit.

As a culture, Americans are sleep deprived. In 1910, the average adult slept nearly ten hours nightly. In 1960, it was nine hours. Now we're lucky if we get seven. Just because we are sleeping less does not mean that we pass out immediately once we hit the pillow, either. Because chronic sleep deprivation yields higher evening cortisol levels, we end up wired at the end of the day. We can't wind down properly by bedtime and end up feeling like we need sedation. In the United States, sleeping pills are big business. One-quarter of American adults report occasional difficulty getting to sleep, and nearly half of them will reach for a pill to deal with it, with older, well-educated women topping the list. Almost 70 million prescriptions are written yearly for hypnotics like Ambien, the top earner with more than $2 billion in worldwide sales in 2011.

Feeding and sleeping are interconnected. Animals that are starved sleep less, and animals that sleep less eat more. If you haven't gotten a full eight hours of sleep, it's easier to put on weight and harder to take it off. Chronic sleep deprivation does three things you don't want when it comes to your metabolism. It increases your appetite, decreases your energy expenditure, and alters your body's ability to deal with glucose. Once you're tired, your body starts to crave carbohydrates to keep going. You're more likely to pound the sugar, not just the caffeine, to stay awake the day after an all-nighter. Animal studies and human studies both show that sleep restriction leads to hyperphagia, the medical term for eating a ton. Fewer hours of slumber lead to higher caloric intake, specifically from snacking between meals. Obese research subjects show a nearly inverse linear relationship between weight and sleep time.

Your body is fighting for energy when you're sleep deprived, and your hormones are its first line of defense against fatigue. Chronic sleep deprivation lowers leptin levels and raises ghrelin levels, making you hungrier and heavier. Even a single night of sleep deprivation is enough to pump up ghrelin levels and hunger, specifically for calorie-dense, high-carbohydrate foods. Sleep deprivation has been linked causally to increased insulin resistance and a heightened susceptibility to type 2 diabetes. Less than one week of sleep restriction can result in a prediabetic state in young, healthy research subjects.

Here's something else that might motivate you. That sleep you're missing can actually kill you, or someone else on the road. Yes, speed kills, but drowsy driving does, too. Sleep deprivation creates horrendous performance in driving simulations. Up to a third of fatal crashes may involve drowsy driving, and just over 4 percent of American drivers ad-

mitted they fell asleep briefly while at the wheel at least once in the previous month. Those most at risk are truck drivers, night-shift workers,
people with untreated sleep disorders like sleep apnea, and anyone who
didn't get enough sleep the night before, which could be any of us.

Understanding the science and benefits of sleep, and how a lack of it
might be the cause of more problems than you think, is key in maintaining your physical and mental health. Learning good sleep habits, paying
attention to light exposure, and making eight hours of sleep a top priority will go a long way toward reducing your moodiness and stabilizing
your eating patterns.

NORMAL SLEEP ARCHITECTURE

Seven to nine hours of total sleep time is an ideal amount, though there
are plenty of people who require more or less. Consolidated sleep is best.
I tell my patients who are exhausted in the afternoon to try not to nap
in order to guarantee that uninterrupted block of sleep at night. If you
must nap, you need to be strategic about it: either twenty-five minutes
or ninety minutes, nothing in between, and try to be done napping by
three P.M.

Typically, sleep cycles proceed through four stages of sleep. Stages
one and two are a lighter sleep that is easier to disturb. Stages three and
four are the deepest levels of sleep, where the brain is relatively quiet,
and are known as slow-wave sleep. Following stage four, there is the
dreaming phase, known as REM (rapid eye movement), and then you
progress toward wakefulness, through stages four, three, two, one. REM
is the only phase where dreaming occurs. During REM your eyes dart
around in your head and you are paralyzed, which is good; otherwise you
would act out your dreams.

Both slow-wave and REM-phase sleep are absolutely crucial, though it's not clear exactly why. Sleep is restorative to the body and the brain; the immune system uses sleep time to do a thorough housecleaning and repair work. Spaces widen between neurons, allowing the brain's immune cells, the microglia, to clean out debris from synapses and dead cells. In humans, chronic sleep deprivation creates a proinflammatory state and alters microglia function. This is bad for two reasons. Microglia are the only immune cells the brain has, but they also do double duty as the cells that help out with learning and neuroplasticity, helping to form new connections between neurons. As you'll see below, sleep deprivation can make you stupid. But it's more serious than that.

Sleep prevents seizures, which are more likely in sleep-deprived individuals. Lab animals die when deprived of slow-wave sleep. If you've been sleep deprived, once you finally do conk out, both slow-wave and REM phases become overrepresented (known as rebound). Usually, we bounce back and forth between non-REM and REM sleep all night long. There is more non-REM in the earlier part of the night and more REM toward the end, when your alarm clock will interrupt a delicious dream. Most adults spend a total of one and a half to two hours nightly in the REM stage of sleep, in four or five separate periods that lengthen throughout the night. About three-quarters of our sleep is non-REM. The elderly sleep fewer total hours and spend even less time in slow-wave sleep, which means they wake up more easily from the lighter stages.

Not all nighttime waking is considered insomnia. Some is perfectly normal. The more hours you're in bed, the more likely it is that some of that time will be spent in a nonsleep state that is more akin to meditation, which is also great for your brain and body. Most of us wake up in the middle of the night at the end of a sleep cycle. Sometimes you're barely conscious of this surfacing. Other times, you fully wake up, flip your pillows around, and maybe even go to the bathroom, but optimally, you dive back down into another cycle. The trick here is not to engage your brain. If you wake up between sleep cycles and start to think about everything you need to do in the morning, you're in trouble. What I've learned to do is jam the circuits. I don't let my brain get going. I think to myself, loudly, *Dive! Dive! Dive!* like the sounding bell of a submarine. I push my brain back down into phase-one sleep. Even if I get up to use the bathroom, I'll keep a mantra going in my head, *Don't think, don't think, don't think,* until I get back into bed and settle into another sleep cycle with *Dive! Dive! Dive!*

SLEEP AND DEPRESSION

Insomnia and mood disorders are interwoven. Missing out on sleep can make you cranky, irritable, and sometimes disinhibited. If you carry a bipolar diagnosis, even one night of sleep deprivation can trigger a manic episode. Insomnia can create relapses in mood symptoms, and major depression can create sleep disturbances. Early-morning awakening is specific to depressive disorders. People fall asleep with little or no problem but pop up at three or four A.M. and can't fall back asleep. This is often one of the first symptoms to resolve when a depression is adequately treated, whether with medication or with light therapy. Circadian manipulation and sleep deprivation are old-fashioned, nonpharmacological ways to treat depression that still work.

Early-morning awakening may be the brain's response to depression. It's encouraging you to get up early, go outside, make sure you see the sunrise, and maximize your exposure to sunlight during the day. Using bright light in the morning has been shown to reliably treat depression without the typical side effects of medication. Optimally, you then go to bed earlier the next night. Early to bed and early to rise is actually a great natural treatment for depression. Following the earth's natural rhythms for sleeping and waking, instead of imposing your own crazy schedule of staying up late and trying to drag yourself out of bed after you've hit the snooze button several times, is one easy way to improve your mood.

SLEEP AND COGNITIVE FUNCTION

When I was in medical school and would spend long days studying, I'd often wake up and roll over in my bed at night, aware that my brain was still processing all I had been memorizing. While we sleep, we consolidate memories, deleting older facts we no longer need and moving newer data into long-term storage. Both slow-wave sleep and REM-phase sleep are necessary to consolidate memory. This is why you need to sleep to really solidify new information—one reason I remind my kids to sleep well before a test. All-nighters are not going to help you memorize. As much as a ninety-minute nap is all you need for this reboot, and then the brain can soak up new material.

Many studies have found a decline in cognitive performance in proportion to sleep deprivation, which is why if you think you have ADHD, you'd better sleep on it. Losing sleep repeatedly results in reduced vigilance, a shorter attention span, more difficulty sustaining or dividing attention, and deficits in verbal memory. Cognitive testing also reveals more errors in judgment and impulse control.

Do you know how toddlers get when sleep-deprived? Not sleepy, right? Frazzled, cranky, with minimal frustration tolerance and even less focus. In some people, particularly children, sleep deprivation causes the opposite of lethargy, looking more like hyperactivity. Many kids diagnosed with ADHD are actually sleep-deprived due to disorders like sleep apnea or restless leg syndrome, in which slow-wave sleep is disrupted. One study showed that 100 percent of children with an ADHD diagnosis had slow-wave sleep deficits, as opposed to a handful of the control subjects. Half the children undergoing tonsillectomies no longer needed their ADHD meds once their sleep improved, after their snoring was surgically corrected.

CIRCADIAN RHYTHMS AND HEALING

Every plant and animal on the planet, including human beings, has a system for detecting light and dark, helping us know where we are on the planet, when a day has passed, and what season it is. Our body calibrates accordingly. We have light-sensitive cells in our eyes, on our skin, and even in our bones and bloodstream. We need to prepare for the rigors of each season, and the amount of light on any given day provides this information. Light exposure entrains our circadian rhythms, and much of our body's functioning takes its cues from this rhythm.

Our body cycles over the course of the day: temperature is lowest in the morning; blood pressure and liver metabolism are lowest overnight. Testosterone levels are lowest in the late afternoon, a bad time for the gym or your A-game at work, and highest in the morning. (Now you know why both of you wake up hornier than when you drifted off. A reason to set the alarm clock a little earlier?) Muscle strength and dexterity improve later in the day. This explains all the button fumbling that occurs when you're getting your kids ready for school. And speaking of kids, nighttime breast milk has more compounds to induce sleep than morning milk does.

Our circadian rhythms help to align our brains and bodies to nature, and maintaining them is crucial to health maintenance. Light and dark cycles turn hormone production on and off, activate our immune systems, and time neurotransmitter release. The most important circadian hormone, melatonin, surges in the evening in order to trigger sleep.

Melatonin is made in the pineal gland, a tiny organ deep in the center of the brain. We need to take in sunlight during the day to activate its proper release in the evening. Serotonin is the precursor to melatonin. Healthy serotonin levels will lead to healthy melatonin levels and better sleep. So will being outside during the day.

What disrupts our rhythms and our own melatonin production? Shift work, for one. Working nights and sleeping days is very tough on the brain and body. Jet lag is another.

Traveling across multiple time zones is a great way to induce insomnia and psychiatric symptoms. At Bellevue, we often had foreign travelers who were in a manic episode due to their circadian rhythm disruption. Another big disrupter is light at night. Sunlight dictates much of our rhythm, so exposure to nighttime light throws our circadian rhythm off significantly. Until the invention of the lightbulb, we spent at least twelve hours a night in the dark, depending on what season it was. Because of artificial light, we are out of sync with nature and with the seasons. And don't even get me started on changing the clocks twice a year. Few things have a more negative impact on my patients' moods than daylight savings time manipulations.

Ever since we started to extend our day length with artificial lights, we have been getting less sleep than we need and paying the price in pounds and our overall health. Nighttime light disrupts our melatonin secretion and resets the body clock. Breast cancer has been linked to nighttime light exposure; women who are blind have lower rates of breast cancer than those with even limited vision. Sleeping in a dark room and avoiding any exposure to nighttime light can potentially decrease your risk of cancers. It is also a crucial factor for getting good sleep and staying healthy.

ENDLESS SUMMER

We are now exposed to a lot more light than our ancestors ever were. This has repercussions for metabolism and weight maintenance. We are hardwired to store fat during the summer in order to prepare for food shortages in the winter. The longer light exposure warns our bodies that the famine is coming and that we'd best eat carbohydrates now or starve later. Excess light at night suppresses melatonin release and basically tricks our brains into thinking it's always August.

Think of insulin as an essential hormone for creating insulation. Fat storage through carbohydrate loading and higher insulin levels is a normal part of the cycle that prepares us for food scarcity and hibernation. It's natural to eat sugars and starches in the summer. That's when watermelon and corn are in season. The problem is, we're eating carbs year round. It would be healthier to eat carbohydrate-rich diets in the summer and fat-rich diets in the winter. Winter is the time when, if you eat fewer carbs, your body can burn its fat stores. In seasonal-breeding mammals, the brain's hypothalamus naturally becomes leptin resistant during longer days with more light and leptin sensitive during the shorter days. Remember, leptin helps you to stop eating, so leptin resistance means you keep going.

There is a complex relationship between sleep and the hormones that make you hungry and full. Unfortunately, our bodies are set up so that carbohydrate craving is a normal precursor to sleep. Rising ghrelin levels in the evening are one of the signals for our bodies to sleep, and so with sleep deprivation come higher ghrelin levels in an effort to promote rest. The problem is, this can also promote our late-night carb fests.

As melatonin levels rise throughout the night, so do leptin levels. Melatonin may enhance the appetite-suppressing effect of leptin. This is one reason why sleeping more helps to keep you thin. In lab rats fed high-calorie diets, melatonin helped to alleviate the resultant weight increase, high blood sugar and insulin levels, as well as improve leptin, triglyceride, and cholesterol levels. Sleep deprivation is associated with decreased leptin levels. Women with lower levels of melatonin secretion are more likely to develop type 2 diabetes. The take-home message is this: light exposure affects melatonin, and melatonin affects metabolism. In summer's longer days, we are supposed to eat well and prepare for the coming famine. In the winter, we're supposed to eat less and sleep more. As melatonin is secreted during sleep, and it helps to balance our hunger hormones, more sleep means a healthier metabolism.

Circadian timing and light have everything to do with obesity. The liver shuts down when it thinks we are getting shut-eye, so eating in the middle of the night leads to more weight gain than daytime eating does. In a study on mice fed during daylight or nighttime, the latter got fatter. Another vicious cycle: once you get fat, your timing is off. In obese mice, the genes responsible for regulating the body clocks are impaired and less rhythmic than those of thinner mice. Imposing strict circadian rhythms on eating and sleeping may help to prevent or treat obesity. Bright-light exposure in the morning increases leptin and decreases ghrelin concentrations in sleep-restricted individuals. So phototherapy— bright light in the morning and darkness at night—could be used to treat not only depression and insomnia but probably obesity as well.

SLEEP AND BACTERIA

A full night's sleep helps your immune system to function properly. While we sleep, our immune systems go on their nightly rounds, patrolling for pathogens. Our bodies kill bacteria and viruses while we doze. If you sleep less than seven hours nightly, you're three times more likely to get sick with a cold.

Melatonin is secreted earlier in sleep, and prolactin, a hormone also involved in sleep maintenance, is secreted later. Both melatonin and prolactin help to mediate immune function. The darker the environment at nighttime, the better for melatonin secretion and, therefore, for immune function. Your immune system and your gut bacteria need this light/dark pattern in order to function properly.

About 80 percent of your immune system resides in your gut, which makes sense, as many pathogens and toxins enter through your mouth. Your gut bacteria thrive during light exposure. When your temperature drops each night, it helps to kill off some of the bacteria in your body. Melatonin helps to lower body temperature while you sleep. This not only slows down your metabolism to thwart hunger but also slows down the metabolism of the bacteria. In the initial phases of sleep, melatonin rises, body temperature drops, and your immune system cleans house.

LIFE IN THE BIG CITY—CAFFEINE, SIRENS, AND SCREENS

My patients who live in Manhattan work long days, and many of them will go to Starbucks at three or four o'clock in the afternoon so they can keep at it for even longer. They get home late, eat, drink, or maybe hit the gym, and then spend hours on their computers, phones, or television screens in order to unwind. The caffeine they ingested in the afternoon can last a good eight hours or so, and those flickering screens mimic sunlight, impairing the brain's ability to secrete melatonin. And so my exhausted patients can't fall asleep. They're jazzed from their cappuccinos, and their glowing screens make it impossible for their brains to know it's nighttime.

Caffeine interferes with sleep induction. As women age, they metabolize and tolerate caffeine more poorly. It is not uncommon to hear a perimenopausal woman confess that she cannot drink coffee like she used to. It feels too stimulating and causes insomnia when it didn't in her twenties. Many medications or hormonal states can affect how long it takes your body to metabolize caffeine. Estrogen, in particular, is involved in caffeine metabolism. Because caffeine's half-life is up to eight hours, if you drink a second cup in the afternoon or evening, you'll have some caffeine in your bloodstream all the time.

Caffeine triggers adrenaline and releases stress hormones like cortisol. It also reduces REM sleep and slow-wave sleep. Whenever I have a patient with insomnia, the first order of business is analyzing caffeine use and getting rid of any after two P.M. Remember two things: decaf doesn't always mean no caffeine, especially if it's espresso, and green tea is not the same as herbal tea. Caffeine constricts blood vessels, and abrupt caffeine withdrawal dilates them, causing headaches. To avoid apoplectic pain, phase out your caffeine slowly.

If your sleeping environment isn't completely dark and quiet, you're going to have trouble initiating and maintaining sleep. In New York City, there are car alarms and sirens wailing, ridiculously loud predawn garbage trucks, and streetlights that never turn off. The answer to this does not have to be just popping a pill. I have quite a few patients who were able to trade in their Ambien prescriptions for a set of earplugs and eyeshades—a healthy swap. A white-noise machine can also work wonders in a noisy environment. And for my patients whose husbands snore, I recommend Breathe Right strips or a CPAP machine for him to eliminate that disconcerting noise for her. Sleep apnea is a major cause of insomnia, as is restless leg syndrome. Find a sleep expert in your area for a full evaluation if you think either of these diagnoses fits you or your bed partner.

We know melatonin is suppressed by light, especially sky-blue sunlight. Exposure to artificial light at night disrupts melatonin production and delays sleep onset. This is not just about lightbulbs. Just two hours of iPad use at maximum brightness is enough to suppress the normal night-time release of melatonin, and two hours of computer use not only lowers melatonin secretion but also enhances cognitive performance and sustained attention. So I get why all my patients are telling me about their second wind at night when they get home and log on. The problem is, we don't need a second wind. We need sleep. Growing research is backing up the advice I have been giving to my patients for years: no glowing screens at least one hour before sleep. Dim the lights and shut off your television. Do not bring your laptop to bed with you, and put down your iPhone. If you're going to read, books or magazines are the way to go, not backlit iPads. Even electronic readers can shift your circadian rhythm signals to later hours, prolonging the time it takes to fall asleep.

There's a program called f.lux that dims your computer screen depending on the time of day. There's also the option of wearing blue-blocking sunglasses at night to filter out the spectrum of light thought to stimulate circadian receptors the most. Blue blockers can significantly improve sleep quality, positive affect, and mood.

What? No computers or TV at night? Whatever will I do? Try getting out of cyberspace and back into your body. Breathe. Stretch. Wind down and relax. Take a hot bath. Drink some herbal tea and just sit down for a spell. Listen to music. Meditate. Write in your journal, especially about all the things you have to be thankful for. Gratitude is good for your mood. Most important, power down your devices and just be. (See more on this in the downtime chapter, page 267.)

CHRONOTHERAPY

Circadian rhythms can be powerful sources for healing in the body. Chronotherapy uses circadian rhythm timing as a way to treat or prevent illnesses. In sleep disorders, chronotherapy is used to shift the bedtime.

In people who have delayed sleep onset, who routinely can't fall asleep until three or four A.M., a doctor can perform sleep-phase chronotherapy. The sleep time is advanced later and later until a normal sleep time is established. There is also an advanced maneuver called controlled sleep deprivation with phase advance, where the subject forgoes sleep for one whole night, delaying sleep time as much as possible the next day, and then delaying sleep by a few hours each subsequent day, until the ideal sleep time is reached. These are experimental procedures that require clinical supervision, with a real risk of inducing a manic episode in bipolar patients. But for some patients it is a great prescription. Well-timed sleep deprivation can be at least a short-term treatment for depressive episodes.

Understanding your own circadian rhythms can improve your sleep and mood. Some people are owls; they get a second wind at night and are happy to sleep late the next morning. Others are larks, early to bed and early to rise. Toddlers and younger kids are natural larks. Teenagers tend to morph into owls, and senior citizens mature into larks, even if they were a bird of a different feather in their youth. Your natural rhythm will present a particular window of opportunity for falling asleep, and if you miss it or plow through it because you're binge-watching something on a glowing screen, it's going to be harder to fall asleep. As with catching a wave when surfing, timing is everything. Optimally your body's internal clock will jibe with the clock on the wall. When it doesn't, you can use bright light in the morning and melatonin at night to shift your circadian rhythm.

PRESCRIPTION SLEEP AIDS

You'll find lots of details in the appendix, but I do prescribe quite a bit of Ambien, a sleeping pill that helps my city folks turn off their minds, relax, and float downstream. Women need lower doses than men, 5 milligrams instead of 10. It doesn't work well on a full stomach, and you may build up a tolerance if you take it regularly. Some people have reported sleepwalking or sleep eating, but the most reliable side effect is "Teflon brain." Once Ambien kicks in, you won't lay down any new memories until it's out of your system. Also, because it has a short half-life, it's common to wake up once it's worn off, three to four hours later. A medicine I like a bit better is Lunesta. It's better on a full stomach, is more reliable, and lasts a bit longer, but around 10 percent of people who take it get a metallic taste in their mouth the next morning, often a deal breaker.

Magnesium can help immensely with insomnia. Calcium is great, too. Try those first, especially if restless legs are involved. Melatonin is worth exploring, and there are many herbs that make you sleepy, like valerian, hops, and chamomile.

Some tranquilizers (the benzodiazepine family of Xanax, Klonopin, Halcion, Ativan, Valium, and others) are more likely to be abused or create tolerance and dependence than other medicines (trazodone, gabapentin, or Benadryl), so I tend to avoid prescribing them for sleep. Many of my patients complain of depressed mood the day after they take Xanax for sleep, and it also has a higher potential for abuse because of rebound anxiety, which means when the drug wears off, you actually have more anxiety than when you started. If you've become dependent on sedatives, it's crucial that you taper the dose gradually to avoid withdrawal symptoms. Seeking the advice of a clinician would be the smartest move. To assist in the process, I often recommend that an herbal supplement like Deep Sleep (by Herbs, Etc.) or melatonin be used while the tapering is taking place.

There is mounting evidence that certain sleeping pills are riskier than you might think. A government study reported a tripling of ER visits related to zolpidem (Ambien) from 2005 to 2010—from 6,111 to

19,487—and women made two-thirds of those visits. Women take these pills more frequently than men, and the drugs can be even more potent in our bodies. In early 2013, the FDA recommended that women take half the typical dose of 10 milligrams of Ambien, as women metabolize the drug differently than men. I've been telling my female patients for years to take only 5 milligrams, and I felt relieved (okay, vindicated) to finally see it in the *New York Times* after the FDA's announcement. Seniors also need a much lower dose of Ambien. One-third of the ER visits involved adults aged sixty-five and older (10 milligrams is too high a dose for your mother; call her).

The chronic use of sleeping pills has been linked to an increased risk of injuries from falls, dementia, and a nearly five-fold increase in early death. In a study of more than twenty thousand various sleeping pill users in Pennsylvania, 6 percent died over a four-year period, compared with 1 percent of nonusers. And the more sleeping pills taken per year, the higher the risk. Heavy users weren't the only ones at risk—even people who took fewer than eighteen pills a year were three times more likely to die than nonusers. In addition to the 450 percent increased mortality risk, the study pointed out a 35 percent higher risk of developing a major cancer during the study for those who took sleeping pills. The risk was the same whether or not people were medically ill to start with.

Obviously, the makers of Ambien took issue with this study and were quick to release a statement that seventeen years of demonstrated clinical safety spoke for itself, but the results of this study did leave me pretty shaken. I prescribe these medicines commonly, and so do most doctors in the United States. I started recommending eyeshades, earplugs, herbal supplements, and melatonin more frequently after this study was released.

SLEEP HYGIENE AND NATURAL REMEDIES

There are plenty of ways to treat insomnia that don't involve a prescription. Acupuncture, aromatherapy, and various herbal remedies can all help tremendously. There are also cognitive behavioral therapy, mindfulness, meditation, and relaxation techniques.

The smartest place to start is with good sleep hygiene. This means sleeping in a quiet, dark, cool room and not bringing work into your bed. Only sleep and sex should happen in your bedroom. Also, it's crucial that you keep the same sleep schedule seven days a week. If you want to sleep an extra hour on the weekends, that's fine, but not more. Sleeping in on Sunday morning will make it tough to fall asleep that night, especially if you're worried about things you need to take care of on Monday morning.

Most crucial is to minimize your exposure to light one to two hours before bed. No Glowing Screens. No caffeine after two P.M. Exercise earlier in the day, not within four hours of sleep onset. Also, cigarettes at bedtime are a bad idea. Nicotine is a stimulant. It will not help you fall asleep, though sitting and taking slow deep breaths will calm you, which is why cigarettes seem so soothing. (For tips on quitting smoking, please see the drug guide in the appendix.)

Some of my patients use alcohol as a sleep aid, but this is a bad idea. Alcohol might help you pass out, but you'll wake up wired a few hours later, when the sugar finally hits your brain. Even low doses of alcohol reduce total sleep time and leave you feeling foul when you wake up. It can also worsen sleep apnea, one reason you might have a horrible hangover the next day. Alcohol also delays and suppresses the restorative REM-phase sleep, which destroys sleep quality, meaning your concentration will suffer the next day.

If you feel that you need to take something to help regulate your sleep cycles, please know that a lot of this is trial and error. If you have trouble falling asleep, start with one-half to one milligram of immediate-release melatonin at night and bright light first thing in the morning. If you have trouble staying asleep, you may want to try sustained-release melatonin. It's the same principle with the prescription medicines. Use the faster, shorter-acting ones for sleep induction and the longer-acting meds for targeting mid-night awakenings. There are many herbal and homeopathic remedies that you can try before you switch over to the prescription sleep aids, which should be your last resort. If you need pills from your doctor, please use them as a way to entrain your sleep back into a healthy cycle, and then slowly taper off your use while continuing with more natural means to maintain good sleep hygiene.

Ten

A Sex Guide
That Actually Works

G ood sex is good for you. Like all exercise, it helps you destress, lowers your blood pressure and risk of heart disease, and stimulates your immune system. The endorphins released during sex and orgasm can help diminish pain and enhance blood flow to the genitals, preventing vaginal atrophy, the thinning of the tissues of the vaginal wall that can accompany menopause. Remember the senile vagina? This is one reason why many gynecologists remind their older patients to use it or lose it.

Nearly all animals have sex for procreation only; they mate only when fertile, and then usually from behind. Remember, humans and bonobos, who have sex for other reasons, have vaginas tilted to accommodate face-to-face sex. In our species, sex is not only for creating life. It is a means of communication, a reflection of our relationships, a sign and measure of intimacy. And sex has a tremendous impact on our moods:

good sex can calm you down or elate you, and it can enhance your self-esteem.

Bad sex is a different story. We long for love, connection, nurturing, and cuddling. We want to be held, and we want to feel like we matter deeply to someone, so we sometimes trade sex for love, and nearly every time we come up short. As with drugs, junk food, and the Internet, if it doesn't fully satisfy us, we become compulsive consumers, hoping that maybe next time it will, or that quantity will make up for quality.

There are plenty of women who are either not enjoying sex or not able to have it at all; 43 percent of women have complaints of some sexual dysfunction, and that number climbs to more than 50 percent in women over forty.

What gets in the way of our sexual pleasure? When it comes to women, you name it. Stress, depression, anxiety, impeded blood flow, inadequate lubrication, tons of different medications, and changes in hormones throughout the menstrual cycle can all play a role in sexual dissatisfaction. Depression, anxiety, or chronic stress can decrease libido, sexual response, and the ability to climax. All of these mood states come with higher cortisol levels that inhibit sexual arousal, as these levels are supposed to fall throughout the sexual experience. With depression or chronic stress, a woman is more likely to choose sleep over sex. She's also less likely to put her needs first if her self-esteem is bottoming out, figuring she's not worthy of the time and attention her orgasm requires.

Arousal (lubrication and engorgement) requires adequate vaginal blood flow, so any medical problems that restrict circulation can cause or add to symptoms of sexual disorders. Here, a medication like Viagra that enhances genital blood flow can help. Other requirements for adequate arousal are genital lubrication, normal sensation, and healthy hormone levels. Both oral contraceptives and antidepressants can negatively affect lubrication, desire, and the ability to reach orgasm. Decongestants and antihistamines can dry up natural vaginal secretions, and other medicines can make it harder to climax, including those used to treat high blood pressure, seizures, and seasonal allergies.

Of course, if there are tensions in your relationship, there may be iciness in the bedroom. Anger and irritation decrease libido and sexual responsiveness. Men are more likely to forget any little spats if it means they can get it on, but women are like elephants: we never forget. We have more brain space devoted to memories of their behavior than they have for ours. Sex researchers joke that for women, foreplay covers the twenty-four hours before sex. Any lingering ill will, or feeling overworked or underappreciated, is going to have consequences when it's time for sex. Let your partner know: his doing his chores with you watching might be the best foreplay!

WHY THE F%&# CAN'T I COME?

There's good reason why so many women are faking it—orgasm can be difficult to achieve and is often impossible without honest conversation with your partner. First, your head needs to be in the right place. All it takes is a bad smell (maybe mismatched pheromones?), an insensitive remark, a sharp fingernail, and the magic is gone. While men can stay on the same steady trajectory toward orgasm, a woman's mission can abort at any step. Any interruptions (especially if it's the kids), insecurities, or a thought about what to remember to add to the shopping list can stop us in our tracks. Men reach a point of "no return" where ejaculation is inevitable, no matter what, but with women, there is no such inevitability. Once the thrill is gone, we need to start at square one, while men can pick up where they left off.

Varied neural mechanisms must fall into place, and in precise order, for climax to occur. A little bit of anxiety or fear, or even shame, can be arousing, but too much, and all bets are off. The calming parasympathetic system is in charge of lubrication and engorgement, then the panicky sympathetic system takes control for orgasm. Some people need more adrenaline than others to flip that switch. That's why some people enjoy sex in public places or cheating on their partners. The thrill of the fear of being caught may be just the spark they need. So a little adrenaline is good, but chronic stress means high cortisol. Cortisol blocks the actions of oxytocin in the brain, so when we're really under pressure, we may not want to cuddle or even be touched. It also tamps down testosterone levels, so we don't want any action, period.

As with many things in nature, timing is everything. Women, who inevitably warm up more slowly than men, tend to be nervous that they're taking too long and try to climax as quickly as they can. This stress and anxiety jams the brain chemicals necessary for climax, and all that tensing up constricts the blood vessels necessary for arousal. Many women need up to thirty minutes to go from desire to arousal to orgasm. Men are quicker to become aroused and reach orgasm than women are. Plenty of men can do it in five minutes or less. Communicating this basic discrepancy with your partner is a good place to start when talking about sex.

Menstrual cycle matters. We are naturally horny in the first half of our cycle, peaking at ovulation, when we're the most fertile. During the second half of the menstrual cycle, the egg is no longer viable and our interest in sex wanes, as does our natural lubrication. Some women have a bump in desire just before their period starts, when serotonin levels conveniently drop enough to increase libido and make orgasm slightly easier to achieve. For the same reasons that SSRIs, which increase serotonin levels, make women less interested in sex and make it harder to climax, PMS, with lower levels of serotonin, can do the opposite. PMS is a time of feeling angsty and needing soothing, and sex, for many women, seems to scratch that itch. But for the millions of women who take antidepressants that enhance serotonin levels, sex is something they can take or leave, all month long.

HOW ANTIDEPRESSANTS AFFECT SEX

Sexual pleasure involves a complex interplay of pharmacology and psychology. If you think of dopamine as the gas pedal and serotonin as the brakes, it becomes easy to see why antidepressant medicines that increase serotonin levels make it harder to be horny and climax. Serotonin is the chemical that comes in at the end of sex and tells you it's over: pack it up and get back to work. If serotonin levels are high to start with, you're finished before you've even begun.

Most serotonergic antidepressants (SSRIs and SNRIs) do two things: they make you less libidinous, and they make it more difficult to climax. Great, huh? Honey, my depression's gone, but you're on your own tonight. And tomorrow night. When the package insert says side effects may include sexual dysfunction, what they mean is this: when it comes to coming, either it takes significantly longer or it just doesn't happen at all. SSRIs are commonly prescribed by some doctors to treat premature ejaculation in men. They can also put a stop to compulsive masturbation. (My theory: men tend to soothe themselves with orgasms the way women do with food. The joke in my office is that guys on SSRIs now have much more time on their hands, so to speak.) Some SSRIs even make your pelvis feel numb, so not only is climaxing nearly impossible but it is difficult to even feel sexual pleasure.

During the plateau phase, a delicate balance of dopamine and serotonin helps to provide the proper propulsion and delay, respectively, to make sex exciting, to maintain an erection, and to intensify yet forestall orgasm. Dopamine enables erections and ejaculation, and serotonin tamps down the high dopamine to avoid premature ejaculation. Too much serotonin, and climax is delayed or impossible, thus SSRIs and their sexual side effects. But antidepressants that enhance dopamine transmission, such as bupropion (Wellbutrin, Aplenzin), are considered prosexual, improving sex drive and the ability to reach orgasm.

Prolactin and dopamine are on opposite sides of a seesaw. When one is up, the other is usually down. Some antidepressants cause high prolactin levels that lower dopamine levels and diminish libido. Prolactin is likely part of the negative feedback mechanism that lets you know that sex is over. After climaxing, when it's difficult to be aroused in the refractory stage, serotonin controls sexual inhibition and sexual satiety. Just like prolactin, serotonin lets your brain know you're done. It may be that people on SSRIs are already satiated, even without beginning the sex act. In laboratory animals, the SSRI fluoxetine (Prozac) disrupts measures of sexual interest, lordosis (the arched back / come hither posture?), and ovulatory cyclicity.

The sex act is a balance of lower animal urges and higher brain dissuasion. The planning, executive functions decide when to put the brakes on the impulsive motor functions. When you have too much on your mind, it's harder to focus on arousal and pleasure. That's serotonin's influence on your prefrontal cortex over your limbic system. If you can't get out of your head and into your body, blame serotonin. Sex researcher Jim Pfaus explains that too much serotonergic inhibition can numb feelings of intimacy and bonding and make having sex feel like "going through the motions."

One thing's for sure: it's definitely a dose-dependent phenomenon, so it's worth scaling back on the amount of SSRI you're taking to see what you can get away with in terms of balancing the desired antidepressant effects and less desirable sexual side effects. Obviously, you need to do this with your doctor's blessing and monitoring. What I usually recommend is something called the "sex holiday schedule." Don't you just love the idea of a sex holiday? A drug holiday is when you take a short break from your medicine for various reasons, such as to avoid tolerance. A sex holiday is stopping your meds briefly to enjoy sex a bit more. Another option is to switch from an SSRI to a nonserotonergic medicine, like Wellbutrin, which has the fewest sexual side effects of them all (and the least weight gain, incidentally). Women who are taking Wellbutrin instead of an SSRI don't typically complain about decreased desire or increased time to orgasm. In fact, some psychiatrists consider Wellbutrin to be prosexual. It is very common for psychiatrists to add Wellbutrin to an existing SSRI in order to cut down on the sexual side effects generated by the SSRI.

THE DOUBLE WHAMMY

We know that SSRIs cut down on sexual desire and response. We know that oral contraceptives do as well, because they prevent ovulation, and the longer you've been on the Pill, the lower your levels of free testosterone become. Also, keep in mind that artificially elevated levels of estrogen from the Pill will artificially elevate serotonin levels. The higher the serotonin levels, the tougher it's going to be to achieve orgasm. Many of my patients are on the low-libido double whammy, antidepressants and birth control pills. For anyone, this is a lot of pharmacology to overcome, but for a select few with a certain genetic vulnerability, it's particularly vexing. If sexual pleasure is a priority to you, but you absolutely need to be on antidepressants, please consider a nonhormonal form of birth control. If you require oral contraceptives for medical reasons, you should consider a nonserotonergic antidepressant or natural treatments that don't involve medications. (Or you can stay on this combination of medicines and become a nun. Your call.)

HOW DRUGS AND ALCOHOL MAKE SEX LESS PLEASURABLE

Anything that helps you relax might assist you in achieving orgasm, so a massage or a hot shower can be an excellent prelude to sex, but many sedatives, including alcohol, have a "therapeutic window." Too much, and it's not going to happen.

In addition to serotonin, the opioid and endocannabinoid systems help to inhibit sex. These chemicals are supposed to appear at the very end of sex to calm everything down and "close up the shop," but they can also shut down desire and sexual responsiveness. The right doses of our body's own natural opiates help to make us horny and help to quiet messages of pain or discomfort during arousal. The endorphin rush of sexual satisfaction that accompanies orgasm helps to ensure we'll pursue sex repeatedly. In rats given an opioid receptor blocker, sexual behaviors were interrupted. However, too much opioid receptor stimulation is not great either, which is what happens if you shoot smack or take one too many Percocets; it's a no-go signal for orgasm. One reason it's hard to climax on painkillers is that if you block pain, you also block some of the pleasure sensing required for orgasm.

Besides the endorphin system, our body's natural cannabis system is involved in sexual enjoyment as well. The endocannabinoid system helps to keep sex arousing and pleasurable, so a little puff might enhance your enjoyment, but smoke too much pot, and you've given the endocannabinoid system too much gas. There's a chance your orgasm will be impeded. THC, one of the active ingredients in cannabis, can have effects similar to alcohol, that is, lessening inhibitions. The problem is that THC can also act as an analgesic, lessening pain, or worse, blunting sensations and your awareness of them. When a patient tells me she's having troubling climaxing, I go down the list of possible medicines that can get in the way (antidepressants and oral contraceptives are the two biggest culprits in my office). If it turns out she's a pot smoker, I encourage her to not smoke on the days she wants to have sex or to switch to a higher CBD strain and see if that solves the problem.

However, I have plenty of other patients, both men and women, who swear by a little bit of cannabis or hashish to help put them in the mood. Cannabis can help you get into your body more, enhancing sensation and focus. In a study of five hundred women, 81 percent reported that cannabis improved their sexual experiences, crediting increased sensitivity when touched and improved relaxation. Women are more consistent in reporting beneficial effects of cannabis on sexual response than men are.

One last word about drugs and sex: disinhibition. Drugs like alcohol, cocaine, and speed may make you more aroused, sexually and otherwise, and more likely to engage in risky behaviors you'd think twice about if you weren't intoxicated. Please be careful out there. Keeping your wits about you and remaining sober are your best defenses against bad decisions that can have lifetime consequences, like not using a condom or choosing an inappropriate sex partner.

Sexual assaults, whether between people who know each other or not, are on the rise, especially on college campuses. Many point the finger at Internet porn, but I would also lay blame on a culture where bingeing on alcohol is the norm and drinking is rampantly promoted. Women are getting trashed and losing all responsibility for their behavior and bodies. The message "no means no" needs to be amended now to include this: the absence of a no is in no way the same as the presence of a yes. President Obama put it best when he launched the "It's On Us" campaign to fight campus sexual assaults: "Society still does not sufficiently value women."

PORN

One young woman in my office told me a story of sex with a new guy that involved a strange interlude of his whipping her face with his erect penis. "Why would he think I'd like that?" she asked me. "Porn," I answered simply. This is a case of life imitating art, such as it is. Internet porn has taught many men to ignore a woman's experience because often, in the world of porn, women are, at best, props moaning with pleasure no matter what is being done to them.

For men particularly, Internet porn is addictive. According to psychiatrist Norman Doidge, porn is a perfect setup for neuroplasticity, or rewiring the brain. Focused attention is one of the prerequisites for neuroplastic change, and staring at screens induces a mildly altered state akin to hypnosis. Feeding your brain images of intense sexual stimuli will change its triggers for sexual arousal. Neurons that fire together wire together: keep stimulating the same brain circuits, and networks start to form. Grooves get laid down, and those grooves turn into ruts.

The Internet provides an endless stream of novelty—new sex acts to watch and, more important, new women to ogle. The male brain sees a porn actress as a new potential sex partner to impregnate, and it will reward the viewer accordingly, with dopamine surges encouraging him to get the girl, chase her down. Porn stimulates the brain much as sex with a real woman would. The same dopamine reward and pleasure circuits light up in anticipation of sex; the same norepinephrine and phenylethylamine (PEA) get released as the viewer gets visually aroused, just as in love at first sight. And the same endorphin burst accompanies orgasm. Most concerning is that oxytocin, which in nature would be triggered by hugging and kissing, is still released by sex with a computer.

A Web site like Pornhub will provide a parade of more hot babes in ten minutes than the average man would be exposed to in the real world in a lifetime. It is unnatural, to say the least. Like rats with unlimited access to junk food who inevitably become obese, men given these extreme versions of rewarding images end up with dopamine levels so high their brains have to turn them down. The pleasure response gets numbed, and cycles of bingeing and craving result. The brain gets rewired to this cornucopia of potential mates and becomes picky. Men who get addicted to Internet porn find that they need ever more specific, intense visual images in order to climax. They are building up a tolerance to the hardcore stimulation. The biggest problem is erectile dysfunction. Sometimes men are surprised to discover that their flesh-and-blood girlfriends no longer do it for them the way hardcore videos do. Neuroplasticity expert Doidge recommends going cold turkey as the best way to remedy porn addiction and its ensuing relationship damage. His patients stopped using their computers for a time in order to weaken their neural networks, and, according to him, "their appetite for porn withered away." My advice to the porn junkies is two-fold: turn off your computer and turn toward your partner (or just leave your house, at least). Adding intimacy into the mix of your sexual repertoire will help to augment your pleasure.

Sex learned from a computer screen is visual; it's about how it looks to the camera or to someone watching you. That's very different from how sex feels, smells, and tastes, and the senses of connection, attachment, and intimacy. My complaints with porn are many, but first and foremost, it's creating a new normal for all of us. Women learn that we're supposed to be grunting and squealing with delight throughout sex and then climaxing repeatedly with minimal clitoral stimulation. Men learn that sex is mostly about pumping their penis like a piston into any orifice they choose. The women are nearly always shaved and many have breast implants. The men are often shaved, rock hard, and taking longer to ejaculate because they're pumped full of Viagra. Scenarios of sadistic, degrading, and humiliating sex abound online.

It's normal and common to have these fantasies inside your head (see the section below), but not many women enjoy being treated like this in real life. It's up to each of us to honestly educate our partners about what turns us on. Be specific about where the lines are. We must stand up for ourselves and stop acquiescing to sex based on hardcore pornography if it's not what we want. In the past ten years or so, I have seen a deeply concerning trend among my female patients. They are now engaging in sexual acts that they never thought they would try and, most important, that they don't enjoy. They are accommodating the desires of their partners without advocating for themselves. Please don't do this. If you don't want to have anal sex or aggressive oral sex, then you have to let him know immediately. This is one of those situations where you need to turn down your natural inclination to accommodate others. It will be better for both of you.

Communication is key during all sex play. Being forced to subjugate your desires and your power in favor of what he wants, whether it's playing a part in his fantasy or even having sex when you don't really want to, is never okay. Maybe it's too early in the relationship and you don't feel ready, or you've been married for years and just don't feel like it tonight. You need to speak up for your desires and needs, especially when the desire is "not now." Otherwise, your resentment will end up smoldering inside you, causing stress and depression and angry behaviors of acting out. Capitulation breeds contempt, which is decidedly unsexy.

A BODY BUILT FOR PLEASURE

As you may have noticed, men have all their stuff easily visible and accessible on the outside of their bodies. Women, sly creatures that we are, hide our erectile tissue inside our bodies. Let me be clear: the primary sex organ of a woman is the clitoris, not the vagina, which is the birth canal. The word *phallus* refers to both the external portion of the clitoris and the penis. During the arousal stage, when stimulated, a woman's erectile tissue fills with blood just like the tissue of the penis. We get erections, too, but, inevitably, wetness is how our arousal is measured and described in research and in porn.

The glans of the clitoris, replete with eight thousand nerve endings, is the most intensely innervated and sensitive part of a woman's body. Unlike the penis, used for expelling waste as well as DNA, the clitoris is used only for one thing: sexual pleasure. How's that for intelligent design? As for gender equality, our erectile tissue is nearly the same size as a man's. That little nub of the clitoris called the glans, visible under its protective hood, is just the tip of the iceberg. There is a large area of sensitive tissue right behind the glans called the clitoral body, or root, and there are extensions (called vestibular bulbs and legs) that course outward and down, like a fishbone, to circle the vagina and urethra inside the body, measuring between nine and eleven centimeters in total. To fully appreciate your sexual potential, you need to familiarize yourself with your clitoris. You need to become clitorate. I'd love us all to educate one another about the relatively new discovery of the 3-D anatomy of the clitoris. Spread clitoracy! (Thanks to artist Sophia Wallace for this great word.)

For sex to be good, we need to tackle the shame and discomfort we have with our bodies. We worry that our inner labial lips are too large or lopsided, that our clitoris is too small or hard to find, and that we smell bad or taste funny. Fully seeing and accepting your unique genitals as beautiful and perfect in their imperfection is crucial to relaxing and receiving sexual pleasure. Many sex therapists recommend you sit in a well-lit place with a hands-free mirror to examine and learn to appreciate all the beauty that is you down there. And if your partner isn't complimentary and verbally appreciative of your glory, tell him (or her) to get with the program. Not only should he put you at ease about your taste, smell, and appearance, but he also should assure you that he is in no hurry and will do everything it takes, and wait as long as required, for you to fully experience waves of intensifying sexual pleasure that crescendo in sublime spasms of release. This is your birthright, and I want you to exercise it.

Being fully present in your body and breathing deeply through your nose will go a long way toward helping you reach orgasm. Focus on your bodily sensations and what feels good to you instead of worrying about how you look, whether you're taking too long, and what your partner is thinking. Many women have a hard time receiving pleasure. When it comes to sex, we need to fight the urge to give. Sometimes being a little bit selfish is just what sex requires. Consider adopting the practice of orgasmic meditation, which cultivates attention to sensation and gives you permission only to receive.

OMNISEXUAL WOMEN

Each sexual and romantic experience further refines our idea of whom we should seek out for the next one. Gay males typically stay put, and true bisexuals males are rare, but women are more fluid about their orientation. Women are much more likely than men to vacillate between male and female partners. Some women see themselves as attracted to specific people rather than to their gender. Of self-identified straight women, more than one-third have had a same-sex experience or arousal. It may be that evolution has favored women with the capacity to bond with either sex, expanding options for child care (called alloparenting) if men are not available.

Our desire is adaptable, especially in service of attachment and maintaining committed relationships. Take your parents, for example. They started out looking and behaving fresh and flirty but grew grayer and more wrinkled down the line, and yet, as much as you're cringing right now, they got it on over the years. Their desires and libidos were fine-tuned to sustain their attachment. So it is with all long-term relationships. We find things that still arouse us, and they can change over time.

That's the story when it comes to committed relationships. We're particular and selective initially, but then we learn to adapt to maintain our attachment. When it comes to lust and sex, it's different. The criteria are much looser. And so are we. Women are omnisexual creatures, aroused by nearly anything. Women gaze just as long at porn as men do; we are no less fascinated. In studies measuring vaginal blood flow in women watching porn, everything turned them on: straight porn, gay porn, men masturbating, and our primate cousins the bonobos having sex. It all worked for them. Even gay women liked the gay men porn. (The gay men studied were the most category-specific, picky watchers.) Whether you know it or not, you respond to all sorts of sexy stimulus. And contrary to popular belief, sexual desire (lust) is not necessarily "sparked or sustained by emotional intimacy and safety."

Women are, by and large, not honest about what turns them on or about how much sex they're having. In studies measuring women's lubrication and engorgement, the physiological readings do not match self-reports of arousal. The women in these studies don't admit to what's turning them on nearly as much as the men do, suggesting more discord between what's happening in their bodies and in their minds. But, then, the erect penis is a strong signal. Women may be less aware of what turns them on due to the covert nature of their genitals and sexual response. They also may be giving the answers they think the experimenters want to hear. Women who are hooked up to what they're told is a lie detector report more frequent masturbation than the women who aren't, and they report more sexual partners than the men do. What's going on here? Instead of being in touch with our own bodies, we're in touch with society and what we *think* is supposed to turn us on. Once again, we're not living for ourselves and we're not in tune with the messages from our bodies. To have good sex, we need to do just that.

FANTASIES: FREE YOUR MIND TO TURN ON YOUR BODY

Your head can get in the way of sex, but it can also help you get in the game and stay there. Honoring your own fantasies is an important way to improve your lovemaking. Whatever arouses you, please know that it is all okay. Fantasizing about gangbangs, bondage, incest... They are all normal and common. If gay male porn turns you on, you are not alone. If girl-on-girl action titillates you and you don't identify as a lesbian, that is still normal. It is completely natural and very common to have sexual fantasies involving submission, humiliation, and even nonconsensual sex. The number of women who admit during interviews that this is the stuff that turns them on is between 30 and 60 percent. The actual number (due to shame about reporting it) is likely even higher.

Women (and men) who control every aspect of their lives, who are masters of the universe at the office and at home, are often the ones with sexual fantasies involving losing control. Everyone knows that the biggest spenders at the dominatrix's dungeon are the CEOs. It's not a mystery why *Fifty Shades of Grey* sold a bazillion copies. It turned on female readers everywhere with acts of surrender and subordination. For many women this is guaranteed to arouse. Part of the appeal is that there's no guilt if you didn't initiate the act, so there's less shame. Another part of it is basic narcissism. There is pleasure and gratification in feeling so wanted that your partner can't control his animal instincts. Being desired and desirable is a common theme in what turns women on. But there's something else that almost always works.

At a pharmaceutical dinner, I sat across from the presenter, a specialist on treating pregnant women with psychiatric complaints. She finished her talk, and it was time for us to ask questions. We dug into our entrées, and I picked her brain as she picked at her popover. "What do you do about low libido?" I asked her. "Try a new partner!" she answered immediately. "No . . . not you personally. I mean, what do you tell your patients?"

A new sex partner does wonders for a sagging libido. In truth, novelty is a more reliable stoker of lust than most other factors. Novelty is possible in the context of commitment, but it takes more work. (See chapter 4 for more on this.) You may feel guilty about fantasizing about someone other than your partner, but the truth is, you may be surprised to find that you actually have this in common with your partner. Men having cuckolding fantasies (watching their women with another man) is quite common. So are women having gangbang fantasies. The reason: they have a biological basis in reality. We are aroused by these scenarios because women and men are designed for sperm competition: may the best man win. The evidence for this theory can be found in the shape of a man's penis, the size of his testicles, and the makeup of his semen.

Did you ever wonder why after he finishes, you feel like you're just getting warmed up and could happily start all over again but he's fallen asleep? From an evolutionary standpoint, at least, women were designed for serial partners and sperm competition, an artifact from our days on the savanna, when we lived in egalitarian multipartner groups, sharing everything, not just food and shelter. So please don't feel bad about your fantasies of sequential partners; it is natural, in the truest sense of that word.

The crucial point of fantasies is that you don't actually have to want them to happen in real life. Make it clear to your partner that you want to talk about it and have fun with it, but you don't necessarily want to act on it. Often, the things that arouse us are forbidden and taboo. That's what gets us off. The adrenaline charge associated with feelings of fear or humiliation can stoke the circuits in the brain and body that help to bring about climax. Where we get into trouble is if our fantasies create shame in us, so we're second-guessing what turns us on. We wish it wouldn't because we think it shouldn't.

Arousal and plateau is the time to allow yourself any and every thought that makes you horny. And keep in mind that just as the characters in your dreams are often various parts of yourself, you play all the diverse roles in your sexual fantasies, too. Part of you gets off on the idea of being tied up, and another part of you is aroused by being the knot maker.

No one has to know what goes on in your head during sex and masturbation, and many times you have absolutely no intention of ever acting on these fantasies, especially if they'd be painful in reality. However, if you do end up sharing your fantasies with a lover and try to incorporate some of those themes into your sex play, be prepared for fireworks. Within the safety and intimacy of shared fantasy, what we most fear in real life is imbued with amazing erotic energy.

Some of us are more comfortable being the sexual aggressor and others prefer to be more passive. I have a patient who considers herself to be a bottom and is less comfortable with initiating sex acts. But she inadvertently married a bottom as well. She joked with me, "Foreplay for him is when he lies on his back." We had a good laugh but then agreed there's a real problem there. She wants him to lavish attention on her and make her feel desired, but he's more comfortable in the receiving role. Sexual relationships require negotiations, and sometimes you will need to take turns. But nothing will change if you can't talk about it. The same goes for technique. Your partner, whether man or woman, doesn't know exactly how you like it to be done. It is up to you to teach the "sex ed" class.

Masturbation is our first experience with sexual pleasure and a primary form of self-expression. It is one way we learn to love ourselves. Wilhelm Reich, a Viennese psychiatrist in the 1920s, said that how you feel about masturbation is really how you feel about sex in general. To improve your sexual response, you need to create a sexual relationship with yourself. Your body is built for pleasure. You can't wear it out. And let's be clear: orgasms beget more orgasms. You do not have a limited libido that will get depleted if you masturbate. Getting comfortable masturbating will make sex better and make it easier for you to climax with a partner. You are entitled to sexual ecstasy, whether alone or with a mate. Betty Dodson, a venerated sex therapist and orgasm whisperer, teaches that masturbation is the cornerstone of women's liberation.

Whether you want to use your fingers, a vibrator, a steady stream of water, or a pillow to grind on, experiment with a variety of stimulation until you get a sense of what works for you. You might need to be stroked a certain way initially, and then another way when you are more sexually stimulated, and then perhaps a different way to bring you to the finish line. Also, some people back off when they're getting close to orgasm out of fear of the unknown, or anxiety about pleasure or losing control. You need to power through that impulse to retreat. For my patients who've never climaxed or who have tremendous difficulty doing so, I often recommend they use the combination of a vibrator and any fantasies or visual stimulation they find titillating in an aggressive attempt to circumvent that hesitation. And yes, this sometimes includes female-friendly Internet porn.

Clitoral stimulation is what leads to orgasm for most women. If you want to climax, you are obligated to get in touch, literally, with your own clitoris and see what works for you. Mechanically, a penis thrusting in and out of a vagina is not what triggers orgasm for the vast majority of women. (Some sex researchers put that number as high as 80 percent.) Betty Dodson says, "my success rate in teaching women how to have an orgasm from intercourse alone has been zero," and she's worked with thousands of women.

Penile penetration does not stimulate the clitoris, unless you're one of the very few lucky women who have their clitoris unusually close to the entrance of their vagina. (Less than one inch seems to be the magic number.) Also, according to Alfred Kinsey, the average amount of time spent thrusting is two and a half minutes; precious few women can achieve anything in that amount of time, except maybe emptying the dishwasher. Masters and Johnson estimated the average time it takes men to climax is four minutes, but women required ten to twenty minutes—if they were with a partner. Interestingly, if women masturbated alone, the average time was again four minutes. That's important. Women are much quicker to climax alone than when they're paired up. Is this because we're taught from such a young age to hide our pleasure and sexual activity, whether alone or with a partner? Are we self-conscious about our sexuality and response, or maybe our orgasm face? Are we all brainwashed to believe we should be able to climax from penetration alone? I think the answer is yes to all three.

GETTING IN THE MOOD

With a partner, your sexual buildup to orgasm can take four times longer than his, and that's even if you're relaxed and horny. The women's magazines have one thing right when it comes to sex advice. Taking time to pamper yourself, lighting candles, putting on oils or lotions, and setting aside a few minutes to breathe, center, and destress are important first steps for sex. A hot bath or shower can help to get your blood flowing. Mothers will need even more time to switch gears from parent to partner. You'll likely need to fantasize. A lot. Start early, getting your mind in the game before your body follows. Allow yourself to conjure up any scenario that gets you hot. No judgments.

It's fine to masturbate before your partner joins in, especially if he is quick on the draw. Most men are completely turned on watching a woman touch herself, so don't be shy. Plus, it's a great way to teach him what works for you. And if you enjoy multiple erogenous zones being stimulated, as many women do, you can always ask him to lend a hand. For instance, while you stroke your clitoris, try one or two of his fingers in your vagina stroking the front wall, or have him suck your nipples.

Exercise is nature's Viagra. Just getting home from working out is a great time to have sex. Enhanced blood flow is exactly what you need to get started. Women shown porn after exercise have much more genital engorgement than those who don't exercise before watching. Frequent exercise is one strategy to enhance libido in women experiencing sexual side effects from their antidepressants. And then there's the ever-elusive (and efficient—two birds with one stone!) exercise-induced orgasm. This is rare, and most often associated with abdominal exercises, climbing, and lifting weights.

What else can get you going? How about how hot your guy is? Turns out, it does matter. Women reported more frequent and earlier-timed orgasms when matched with men who were rated as more masculine, dominant, and attractive. I know this is intuitive, but now you have a study to back it up.

VAGINAL BARBELLS, ANYONE?

You've probably heard about Kegel exercises, a great idea for every woman. They contract the pubococcygeus (PC) muscles, which compose most of the pelvic floor. These muscles need to be strengthened in many women, but especially after childbirth, during perimenopause, and after menopause. Locating your PC muscles is most easily done by trying to stop the flow of urine. Pilates exercises often encourage you to "pull up on the pelvic floor." In yoga, this is called *mula bandha*. Pilates and yoga can help keep your vaginal floor strong, enhancing the quality and ease of your orgasms. Now you know why those yogis look so blissful.

Once you've figured out where your PC muscle is, try squeezing and holding it for two or three seconds and then relaxing. Do this ten times. The goal is to do five sets of ten Kegels spaced throughout the day. Gradually extend the amount of time you can hold a contraction for up to eight or ten seconds. During intercourse, you can squeeze and hold your PC muscles to give both of you an extra thrill. Betty Dodson sells a special barbell called a Kegelcizer, a one-pound metal dildo that can help you strengthen your vaginal muscles. Dodson advises doing Kegels throughout sex or masturbation to enhance your pleasure and ease of climax. The healthier and stronger the PC muscles, the more powerful your orgasm will be. So get to work!

VIBRATORS

Vibrators started out as medical devices to induce "hysterical paroxysms" in women who were chronically sexually frustrated. A condition of irritability, fatigue, aches, pains, and general malaise was often diagnosed as hysteria, and the term wasn't officially removed from the diagnostic manual until 1952. Remember that this malady was treated by a doctor doing what women wouldn't or couldn't do for themselves—masturbate. In 1873, 75 percent of American women were in need of these treatments, making up the single largest market for therapeutic services. Many doctors were bringing off their patients with their hands to relieve their "symptoms," but in the 1880s, the vibrator came into vogue in doctors' offices to make this process more efficient. By 1917, vibrators outnumbered toasters in American homes.

Vibrators help some of my patients to achieve orgasm more easily and quickly than manual stimulation or even oral stimulation. For others, the buzzing feels too strong, or just wrong. Before you decide you're not a vibrator gal, wrap the head in a washcloth to minimize the vibrations, or try it on a lower setting, or put the head against your mons or vulva (outer vaginal lips) to cushion the stimulation the clitoris receives. Remember, especially when you're first getting warmed up, the clitoris is very sensitive and it doesn't take much to rub it the wrong way. Too much pressure will turn you off like a switch. The clitoris can get numb easily. Let your partner know this as gently as you can. The male ego can get bruised easily, too. As you get more aroused, during the plateau phase, the clitoris starts to pull back under the hood and protect itself from overstimulation. This may be a time when you can remove the washcloth or enjoy a stronger setting.

Starting off slowly and lightly is better than diving right in with intensity and pressure. Building up gradually is important, but the key is to not speed up when you think you're getting close, or to add too much pressure. It's great to mix it up in the beginning, but as you near the finish line, consistency is key.

Each pinnacle is unique. There is no one way or right way to have an orgasm. The key is being fully present. Stay in your body and put all of your attention and concentration on sensation. Keep your breathing deep, and clench and unclench your PC muscle.

IMPROVED TECHNIQUE

Proper foreplay is important for best results in sex. So read on and share this information with your partner if you'd like.

When touching the breasts, it's better to start with the sides and bottom of the breast before zeroing in on the nipple. Once the blood starts flowing to this area, the nipples have been primed for attention. Too early in the game, and they may be a bit numb. Some women go wild for having their nipples licked or sucked, but this is heavily influenced by hormonal factors. Nursing women are often much less sexually aroused by nipple play and are less horny in general. Perimenopausal or premenstrual women may not want you anywhere near their nipples if they're too sensitive at certain times of their cycle, likely the second half.

It's the same story with the genitals; diving headfirst into the clitoris is not the way to go. Attention should first be paid to the inner thighs and the outer and inner labia and vagina, before stimulating the clitoris. Start with indirect touching, perhaps through the outer labia or at least through the hood of the clitoris, before stimulating the glans of the clitoris under the hood, which should wait till much later. Many women are extremely sensitive in this area, so less is more. A very light and lubricated touch will work better than using more pressure, speed, or intensity, especially at first.

For oral stimulation, keep it very wet, and occasionally exhale heat onto the area. Kiss, lick, and suck all around the inner labia and clitoris, changing the speed, pressure, and type of stimulation you use. Combine oral and manual stimulation by putting one or two fingers inside the vagina, especially massaging the G-spot, the area directly behind the clitoris. Try to push the clitoris forward, toward your mouth, from behind. Try the flat part of your tongue around the area at the bottom of the clitoris, and then much later, after it is engorged, the tip of your tongue under the hood. Don't forget, pressure is best saved for later, if used at all. A lighter touch is almost always better. That goes for speed as well: slower at first, and faster later, if at all.

For intercourse, it's worth considering some new positions. Missionary is most common, and for many women, most intimate, but it's not great for clitoral stimulation. By making a few adjustments to the missionary position, more clitoral contact can be achieved with the *coital alignment technique*, increasing the likelihood of climax. He shifts his body a few inches northward toward your nose, so that either his pubic bone or the base of his penis never loses contact with your clitoris. The rhythmic motion is north-south. It is a down-and-up motion requiring coordination between both partners to accomplish. In the words of its creator, Edward Eichel, "less in and out and more rock and roll." The reduced focus on thrusting also helps the guy last longer.

Another modification to missionary position is using a pillow or two placed under your bottom or lower back, and bending his legs to go underneath yours. He lifts your hips up onto his thighs and your feet are firmly planted on the bed, knees bent. The more you can angle your pelvis for improved clitoral stimulation (using your feet for leverage), the better. Instead of his leaning on his forearms, he's on his hands, arms extended. You can also try to vary the angle by moving your knees to your chest. Experiment with what feels best.

When you're on top, have your guy sit up instead of lying down flat, so that his belly or pubic bone is rubbing against your clitoris. See what the best angle is for you, but aim for nearly vertical, with his leaning against the wall or headboard with a couple of pillows. Armless chairs are also great for a woman on top to be able to have a lot more clitoral pressure and control.

All sorts of positions are good for incorporating a vibrator or manual stimulation into your sex play: reverse cowgirl (you on top, facing away from him), rear entry, or the lazy position (man lies on his side to your left, you lie on your back with your left leg slung over his hip) all leave plenty of room for direct clitoral manipulation.

DIFFERENT KINDS OF ORGASMS

So what is an orgasm, exactly? Muscle tension and pelvic engorgement build to a release of between five and fifteen rhythmic involuntary contractions of the uterus, outer third of the vagina, PC muscle, and

anal sphincter. The first few contractions are stronger and closer together, becoming further apart, shorter, and weaker as the orgasm
peters out.

The pleasure of an orgasm can stay localized to the genital area,
which is more typical, or it can spread through your entire body. (Tantric
sex practices focus on whole-body orgasms by taking much more time to
build up, incorporating deep breathing, relaxation, and focus.) Arousal
creates blood pooling in the genitals, and an orgasm expels blood and
tension from all the pelvic organs, which returns the body to its original,
nonaroused state, called resolution.

The cigar- and cocaine-loving psychiatrist Sigmund Freud had the
idea that orgasms arising in the clitoris were immature and that a better-
adjusted woman would climax from vaginal stimulation alone. Thus
the idea of the vaginal orgasm was born. But Freud was a thirty-year-old
virgin with a complete lack of intercourse experience when he came up
with this theory. Masters and Johnson determined that all orgasms result from clitoral stimulation, and Betty Dodson agrees. However, there
are still those sex researchers who believe in different types of orgasms
arising from different forms of stimulation. Dr. Berman refers to a "pelvic floor" orgasm arising from stimulation of the G-spot, for example.

All sorts of stimulation can lead to an orgasm. There are women who
can reach orgasm without clitoral involvement. There are reports of people climaxing from stimulating just about every erogenous zone imagin-
able; even toe sucking can bring some women over the edge. Certain
paralyzed women can orgasm even after their spinal cord has been severed. Some women can climax from nipple stimulation alone, and other
women can orgasm simply from thinking about their breasts or genitals
being touched. Masters and Johnson found no subjects who could fantasize themselves to orgasm, but the Kinsey study put the rate of spontaneous orgasms (with no physical stimulation) at 2 percent in women. Did
you ever wake up in the middle of a dream and realize you just came?

Plenty of women have these "wet dreams." Two researchers put the number at exactly 37 percent. Nocturnal orgasms are related to "neurosis" or anxiety, meaning if you're really stressed out, your brain might be trying to do what it can to give you a short, calming orgasmic vacation.

Multiple orgasms are more accurately called serial orgasms. For many of us, after climax the clitoris is extremely sensitive and "off limits." This is the refractory period and is more definitive in men than in women. But if your partner continues to stimulate other erogenous zones and works his or her way back to the clitoris before things settle down too much, there are more aftershocks to be had. By contracting and relaxing the PC muscle, focusing on deep breathing, and rocking the pelvis back and forth, it is possible to move your way toward another set of sexual spasms.

DOC, I'M SEEING SPOTS

There are many places to stimulate inside your vagina. The G-spot (the Grafenberg spot, named after its "discoverer") is basically the backside of the root of the clitoris, a sensitive patch located on the front wall of the vagina about two to three inches in. Most of the vaginal wall feels fairly bumpy and rough, but there's a bean-sized area that feels smoother and, if massaged, at first makes you feel like you want to pee but then starts to feel good. The G-spot is more like a zone, an area that becomes swollen and easier to find once the other erectile tissue has become stimulated.

If your partner continues to stroke this area with a "come here" crooked finger, and is patient, an orgasm may result. My patients who do have G-spot orgasms say they are harder to achieve than clitoral ones and qualitatively different. Supporting this idea are studies out of Rutgers where women masturbate while in an MRI, keeping completely still, if you can imagine that. The MRI data comparing clitoral versus G-spot stroking suggests that different areas of the brain correspond to processing these different types of stimulation. G-spot orgasms do differ from direct clitoral orgasms because sometimes fluid is "ejaculated" through the urethra (where urine exits the body). This fluid is created in the Skene's glands, also called the paraurethral glands, which run internally alongside the urethra, homologous to a man's prostate gland. Whether some or all women can ejaculate, and what the fluid consists of, is disputed among sex researchers.

There's also the A-spot, or anterior fornix erogenous zone (AFE), a deep pocket of the vagina located between the cervix and the front wall, which requires a different angle entirely. A trick to remember is that stimulating the AFE can induce extra vaginal lubrication if you're a bit dry. Posterior fornix stimulation (also known as the cul-de-sac, the pocket between the cervix and the back wall of the vagina) can be best achieved with rear entry. Many women don't like to have their cervix stimulated, but some do. There is a phenomenon called cervical tapping that can lead to intense pleasure or orgasm in older women who have cultivated this sensation. See what feels good to you, and then communicate it to your partner. For those who like dildos, there are all sorts of width and shape options, designed in the hopes that these separate spots will be adequately massaged.

There are plenty of erogenous zones away from the genital area. Try behind the ear, the sides of the neck, the sides of the breasts, behind the knees, and especially the lowest part of the lower back. Most people have a special spot that does it for them, so don't be shy about sharing that information with your lover.

Maybe you're embarrassed by this, but you shouldn't be. The brain's wiring for genital stimulation is right next to the area that processes anal stimulation, so it is perfectly normal to be sexually aroused by anal play. Some women like oral or manual attention to the external area only, and others are comfortable with penetration. Lots of lubrication, going very slowly initially, and having the receiver dictate the pace and rhythm are crucial. The anus does not create its own lubrication as the vagina does, so lube is imperative. But extra care is needed because the bacteria in the rectum can cause vaginal infections, so change condoms when going from anal to vaginal, or wash the dildo or penis involved. Lie on your back instead of your front, so that any lube that drips down from the rectum avoids your vagina. Also, the tissue of the rectum can tear more easily than the ever-accommodating vagina, so the risk of HIV transfer is much greater in anal sex than in vaginal intercourse. Lubricated condoms are safest.

I wish it went without saying, but I have to remind my patients frequently: If you don't want to do something, say no clearly and without equivocation. No means no, whether it be a particular type of sex, or sex in general. A man is perfectly capable of finishing himself off if you don't want to participate any further. They do it nearly every day.

AND NOW, A WORD ABOUT SEMEN

So it turns out that semen has got a lot going for it besides that baby-making thing. Some components of semen show up in your bloodstream within a few hours of being deposited in the vagina. Semen contains testosterone and estrogen, both of which can make you feel more aroused, helping to enable orgasm. Now you know one reason why you get horny *after* he comes. Semen also has some dopamine, norepinephrine, and tyrosine, an amino acid used to make dopamine, which might help to explain why you're more awake after sex. Also, sperm can help to regulate the menstrual cycle due to its content of follicle-stimulating and luteinizing hormones. Weekly sex can help women keep their menstrual cycles regular.

Semen may even act as a natural antidepressant. It contains endorphins, and one study found that college women's condom use (or lack thereof) had effects on their mood, showing that females who were exposed to semen had lower scales on a depression inventory and fewer depressive symptoms and suicide attempts, all in proportion to their forgoing condom use. However, we all know condoms provide vital services, like protecting from STDs and decreasing the likelihood of pregnancy, so I don't recommend semen as an antidepressant unless you're with a steady partner and are postmenopausal or are using some other form of birth control.

Sex is a natural antidepressant, too, and the reasons why good sex makes us feel good are emotional just as much as they are physical. Being unified with your lover, enjoying space and time as one, can be a powerful spiritual experience. Chemistry is great for starters and may even carry you for the long haul of a committed relationship, but the depths of intimacy are endless. The path of creating closeness and safety has a big payoff. Receiving the loving attention of another helps you to love and accept yourself.

Eleven

Your Body: Love It
or Leave It

Any time you separate the mind from the body you're asking for trouble. One of the keys to getting healthy is to get in your body and stay there. Stay present, stay mindful, and stay connected to your breathing. Embodiment is the pathway to health. Walk, dance, swim, stretch. Your body is a temple, truly. Do anything that allows you to go inside and worship.

Physical inactivity is the single most important risk to your health and a grave public health problem. Our increasingly sedentary lifestyles are the fourth leading cause of death worldwide, racking up more global fatalities than cigarettes. Inactivity taxes the body as much as obesity does, increasing the risk of heart disease, diabetes, and many cancers, and shortening life expectancy. Currently, two-thirds of Americans are either overweight or obese, with one out of five considered morbidly obese. Seatbelts on airplanes are being lengthened and hospital CAT scan tables widened to accommodate our expanding girth. Just in the past decade, childhood fitness declined by 10 percent. Part of the reason for our obesity is that we sit. And sit. In our cars, at our desks, on our couches. And that level of inertia takes its toll. Keep in mind, if your head is buried in a screen, your body is immobile. (Or it had better be. Text and cross the street in Manhattan and you're putting your life in your hands, literally.)

The Centers for Disease Control recommends that adults get at least two and a half hours a week of moderate-intensity aerobic exercise (cardio), and seventy-five minutes of vigorous-intensity aerobic exercise. The CDC also encourages resistance training, like lifting weights, at least twice a week. No big surprise: nearly 80 percent of us don't get this recommended amount of exercise.

Exercise strengthens the heart muscle and improves blood supply to the entire body. It lowers cholesterol levels, prevents fatty buildup inside arteries, and assists in maintaining a normal weight. Exercise helps to prevent high blood pressure and heart disease, strokes, diabetes, and osteoporosis. Cardiorespiratory fitness is as important a health predictor as obesity is, and, in fact, physically active but overweight people have lower morbidity and mortality than normal-weight sedentary folks.

Women have a tendency to think about their bodies in aesthetic terms, setting up harmful comparisons with idealized models. As you engage your body, your sense of its worth changes. I bug my patients about doing cardio. A lot. Because it's not just good for your body; it's good for your head. Exercising gives you a sense of agency and autonomy and will help your mood. Then there are the chemical effects of exercise. We've all heard about how cardio can release endorphins, your body's internal morphine machine, making you feel happy and relaxed. Well, it turns out that's just a part of the story. It also improves levels of serotonin, dopamine, and norepinephrine, neurotransmitters implicated in depression and anxiety.

Moderate aerobic exercise reduces stress, eases anxiety, and lightens depression. It improves cognition, focuses attention, and enhances well-being. It can help to reverse or forestall aging effects on the brain and help to manage many of the effects of hormonal fluctuations in women, including libido. When it comes to sex, the more comfortable you are in your body, the better. Also, the more you get it moving and your blood flowing, the more horny you're going to be. Exercising immediately before sex significantly improves desire, sexual response, and orgasm, especially in those women who have sexual dysfunction. Scheduling regular exercise before sex may be a good way to combat the sexual side effects of antidepressants.

So it's good for your heart, good for your head, and good for your sex life. Are you at the gym yet? Well, wait. There's more. It turns out that exercise grows your brain, and obesity can cause the kind of inflammation that interferes with learning, making you stupid. So keep moving to stay smart.

BRAIN FERTILIZER

When my patients ask me how they can get off their antidepressant medications, the first thing I begin to talk about is exercise and, in particular, cardio. The brain responds to stimulation and prodding a bit like muscles do. It grows with use and shrinks with disuse. Exercise causes branches of nerve cells to grow new buds and new connections, binding with one another. The brain is constantly being rewired, growing and changing, and exercise fosters this plasticity.

Think of your brain as a lush forest of connected branches. From infancy to early adulthood, the brain becomes bushier with sprouts and shoots. Pathways become wider and faster when they're more often utilized. Neuroplasticity, the mechanism that enables behavior change, occurs primarily in the brain's memory center, the hippocampus. Since physical activity creates new brain cell connections in the hippocampus, cardio actually has beneficial effects on memory.

With regular cardio, the brain starts to show the same changes seen in people receiving antidepressants, namely, more BDNF, the chemical that precedes new nerve growth. BDNF allows neurons to sprout new branches, improving their function and protecting them against cell death. Part of the reason for a delay in antidepressants starting to work may have to do with waiting for neuroplasticity to kick in. People who respond to antidepressants often show elevated levels of the growth factor BDNF and new neuronal connections. BDNF itself may well act as an antidepressant. If you really want to grow your brain, combine exercise with antidepressants.

Another reason to stay chill: chronic stress not only tanks your mood but also disrupts neuroplasticity and BDNF. Fighting the effects of stress, the endocannabinoid system is a major influencer on how brain cells sprout and synapses connect in the hippocampus. As you'll read below, cardio can jump-start the endocannabinoid system.

THIS IS YOUR BRAIN ON OBESITY

One reason I encourage my depressed patients to lose weight is to reduce inflammation. Fat cells release cytokines, creating inflammation, and fatter patients have a lamer response to antidepressants. Obese individuals have the bad combo of higher kynurenine and lower tryptophan levels. This means more inflammation and less serotonin. When the weight is taken off, the ratio normalizes and their inflammatory status and mood improve.

Being obese (abdominal fat in particular) increases the risk for depression, and being depressed increases the likelihood of subsequent obesity. Obesity also is associated with anxiety disorders such as panic

attacks, generalized anxiety, and specific phobias. People with severe depression or anxiety sometimes get fatter over time regardless of whether
their mood symptoms improve or worsen. The stress and inflammation
fuel the obesity. And it gets worse.

Lab rats have been telling us for years that being overweight does the
brain no good. Obese laboratory animals show slower learning curves
and poorer memory than normal-weight animals. This may have to do
with inflammation interfering with neuroplasticity. Fat cells create a
proinflammatory cytokine called IL-1beta that can squeeze through the
blood-brain barrier into the hippocampus, the memory center crucial for
learning. Fat mice do a miserable job on measures of memory thanks to
this cytokine. If you give them liposuction, their cytokine levels plummet, and they ace their IQ tests. If the chubby rodents don't undergo surgery but instead adopt a cardio regimen of running on a treadmill, they
improve on their cognitive tests and show less inflammation and more
neuroplasticity in their hippocampi. Here's the freaky part: when researchers inserted the surgically removed fat pads into thinner mice,
their cognitive performance dropped. Talk about fatheads.

DO WHAT YOU LOVE

At first, I encourage my patients to stay on their medicines and get moving, but over time, once the cardio regimen is firmly in place, we can
start to slowly taper off their medicines and see how they feel. What's
crucial here is to find something you truly enjoy doing. Life is too short to
be resentful and groaning on the way to the gym. If you don't like the
gym environment, then don't go there! Just put on your sneakers and
head outside. Walking a few miles most days will do wonders not only for
your waistline but also for your mood. The most efficient thing you can
do, if you're pressed for time, is to run. Running will create new neuronal

growth more quickly and reliably than most other forms of exercise. When my patients tell me they have absolutely no time for exercise, I recommend they do daily seven-minute workouts. No matter what exercise you choose, what matters most is that you do it regularly, dare I say religiously?

When I was working weekends at Bellevue, I used to go to a ballet studio every Monday morning for a Pilates mat class. I was fried from working two nights in a row, and I had seen some things I really wanted to flush out of my brain. When I lumbered in and saw all those little girls in pink tights and leotards, I made a ritual of turning off my cell phone and pager as if I were entering my church. I saw the studio as a sacred space where I could devote my attention fully to my body and get out of my rattling head. These days I go to a Bikram yoga studio and see the same sweating people week in, week out, my church community. I have come to see yoga, dance, and any exercise as being as important as psychotherapy in healing my psyche.

So find something that puts a smile on your face. It can be Zumba, a hip-hop aerobics class, jumping rope, or kayaking. What really matters is simply that you do it, that you get your heart rate up and speed up your breathing and engage in it regularly. When your brain is fully oxygenated, when you're taking deep breaths and filling your lungs, bloodstream, and brain cells with oxygen, you are absolutely guaranteed to feel better. This is especially true if you have an anxiety disorder or suffer from panic attacks. The brain is much less likely to go into panic mode if you have plenty of oxygen on board. Never underestimate the power of oxygen.

Any exercise done out in nature earns extra points from me. You're crossing a few things off your list as you bathe in the sunlight, breathe some fresh air, and expose yourself to nature and its therapeutic effects. Another option for integrating exercise into your life is to live like a pioneer. Chop wood, carry water, hang your laundry out to dry, and do things the old-fashioned way. Take the stairs instead of the elevator. Walk or bike everywhere you need to go. If you naturally integrate vigorous physical activities into your day, then you don't necessarily have to take time out to "exercise."

When I asked one of my patients whether she does yoga, she replied, "It's all yoga to me. I go to the gym, I put on my favorite music, and I clear my mind." She, like many others, finds exercise to be meditative. When blood is required by the sensory and motor centers in the brain, it has to come from somewhere. The thinking and planning parts of your brain can go off-line while you move. During exercise there is a transient hypofrontality; blood is shunted away from the frontal lobes and toward these other structures. This may explain the "mindlessness" some of us experience while running or the "flow" we enter with more complicated movements like dance. I use my yoga time to practice a moving meditation, and back when I used to run, I would completely zone out and feel ultrarelaxed.

THE RUNNER'S HIGH

Most of us think of endorphins as the explanation for the runner's high, but that may not be where the full joy of cardio comes from. Exercise gets you stoned. It activates the endocannabinoid system, which plays a major role in rewarding effects both during and after exercise.

Your muscles have CB receptors on them, just as your fat cells do, in nearly equal numbers. The endocannabinoid system in the muscles decreases pain perception and reduces inflammation. In lab rats, even a single session of exercise can activate this system, reducing pain perception. We know that exercise releases anti-inflammatory cytokines from skeletal muscle just by movement. Myofascial manipulation, a type of deep massage, can enhance endocannabinoid activity in the muscles, getting you blissed out and relaxed. It may also be that simply moving your muscles helps to activate the endocannabinoid system and release these psychoactive substances.

You can also thank the endocannabinoid system for the fact that cardio makes you smarter. The positive effects of exercise on memory mediated by BDNF are dependent on the endocannabinoid system. The more you exercise, the more CB1 receptors and BDNF you have in the hippocampus. If the CB1 receptor is blocked in mice that run on a treadmill, it prevents exercise-induced memory enhancement and BDNF expression. But if the breakdown of anadamide, an endocannabinoid, is blocked, exercise-induced memory formation improves.

EXERCISE REORGANIZES THE BRAIN TO BE MORE RESILIENT AGAINST STRESS

Regular exercise quells the brain's response to stress and regulates the sympathetic nervous system. The two parts of the brain that help to chill out fight-or-flight reactions are the hippocampus and the frontal lobes. As exercise causes neurogenesis (brain cell growth) in the hippocampus and improves executive function (frontal-lobe inhibition of lower, emotionally reactive structures like the amygdala), it gives you two ways to improve your resilience to stress. Mice allowed to run obsessively on their treadmills showed new brain cell growth in the hippocampus, a brain region that can shut down overexcitement. The brains of inactive mice overreact to a stressor, while the exercisers stay calmer. This not only lowers anxiety but also helps to lower high blood pressure and normalize inflammation. Exercise also helps to improve the top-down control from your prefrontal cortex to the rest of your brain. Motor skills training and exercise facilitate and enhance executive function and may have a place in treating dementia and stroke.

Physical activity helps us learn. Our ancestors needed to track down food and remember where it was. If you're not moving, your brain assumes you have all the food you need and don't need to learn anything. Inactivity physically shrinks your brain and its connections, while exercise massively increases neurogenesis. Inactivity causes abnormal sprouting and neuron growth, which makes nerve cells more sensitive and more "apt to zap scattershot messages into the nervous system." This can sometimes lead to overstimulation of the sympathetic nervous system, potentially contributing to high blood pressure, heart disease, anxiety, and stress.

BDNF helps to promote serotonin neuron growth, and SSRIs help to enhance BDNF gene expression. This is one reason why it's a good idea to combine SSRIs with cardio. Serotonin helps to keep impulsivity, anger, and aggression down and your mood up. While chronic stress and depression can erode connections between neurons, shrinking the hippocampus, exercise creates a cascade of neurotransmitters and growth factors that can reverse this, bolstering the brain's infrastructure. Exercise gives you the triple threat of neurotransmitter enhancement, boosting levels of norepinephrine (arousal and attention), dopamine (reward and motivation), and serotonin (happiness and relaxation). One author likens going for a run to popping a Prozac and a Ritalin.

EXERCISE AND INFLAMMATION

Exercise has anti-inflammatory properties. It increases circulating anti-inflammatory cytokines from skeletal muscle and decreases body fat, which produces proinflammatory cytokines. One reason that exercise helps to protect against cardiovascular disease, diabetes, arthritis, and depression is that these are all diseases that progress in a setting of chronic low-grade inflammation. Decrease inflammation and you lower your risk of these illnesses.

In people with depression who don't respond well to medications, those with higher inflammatory markers have a greater response to exercise. When their depression improves via exercise, some of these markers fall.

WHITE FAT, BROWN FAT, AND IRISIN

There are two kinds of fat cells in the body, white and brown. Brown is the more metabolically active fat, generating heat, which means it can burn more calories. Brown fat cells also help to keep the body more sensitive to glucose, which is what you want; glucose insensitivity is a setup for diabetes and escalating fat stores. Irisin is a newly identified hormone that helps to turn white fat into brown fat. Exercise increases irisin levels in laboratory animals and in people, helping to explain why it can help you lose weight. Mice fed a high-fat diet but also given irisin had less weight gain and insulin resistance than controls, even without exercise. If you're thinking we may all be taking irisin pills in the future instead of hitting the gym, you may be right, but for now, please get your body off the bench and into the game.

TELL YOURSELF YOU LIKE TO EXERCISE AND TELL YOUR PHONE, TOO

My college friend Alex joined a group that goes on early morning runs in the park across the street from her house. She sent me a funny e-mail saying the whole time she's moving, there's a voice in her head saying, *I hate this. I hate this.* It got me interested in whether there was any evidence for inner monologues affecting your experience of exercise. There is. Motivational self-talk can have a significant effect not only on exercise endurance but also on perceived exertion. After gathering input from the muscles, the brain is the ultimate decider in exercise-related fatigue. Study participants pedal longer and report that it feels easier if their "voices" tell them they are doing well and feeling well. So try this, Alex: "I am a strong mama jama!" "I am up at six A.M. kicking ass!"

Try to reframe your thinking about exercise from "I have to" to "I get to." Consider it a privilege to spend time in your body, caring for yourself. And put your exercise schedule on your calendar in your phone. Make it a date you don't cancel, like a dentist's appointment, and add some helpful, healthful hints into your date book, too. Use your smartphone as the angel on your shoulder, whispering intelligent, competent advice into your ear. Reminders from FitBit and now the Apple Watch encourage people not only to exercise but also just to stand up and walk around more to avoid being too sedentary. My patients who are using these fitness technologies report they're moving their bodies more due to their obsession with their new toys.

PRETTY UGLY

How's this for unattractive? "I say that inner beauty doesn't exist. That's something that unpretty women invented to justify themselves." So says Osmel Sousa, the woman in charge of the Miss Venezuela pageant, when discussing the popularity of plastic surgery in her country. Unfortunately, girls learn from the time they're very young that they will be judged on their looks, and specifically on how sexy they are, rather than on the content of their character or what they have achieved. "For women... demands are made upon them to contour their bodies in order to please the eyes of others."

Many times, haute couture moves women further away from what's natural for them. Christian Dior once said, "My dream is to save women from nature." Plucked eyebrows, collagen-enhanced lips, or stilettos that arch our backs unnaturally are just a few examples. Even crossing our legs, a posture taught to young girls to communicate chastity, isn't good for us, increasing blood pressure and causing varicose veins.

In today's culture, we tend to assess ourselves and other women primarily by appearance. Our self-image is unduly influenced by how we think we look: we love ourselves when we decide that we look beautiful, but we can just as easily devolve into self-hatred when we have a pimple or a bad hair day or wear the wrong sweater. We compare ourselves with airbrushed and Photoshopped models designed to look like pubescent boys, long and lean. We want "extra body" in our shampoos and conditioners, we want sleek curves in our cars, but when it comes to our bodies, women seem to want neither. Rather than making peace with our own curvaceous hips and thighs, we are constantly at war. We want straight lines with no bulges or creases. We want thigh gaps to match the cropped and chopped pictures we see in magazines. It is unhealthy, unnatural, and, for the majority of us, unachievable.

Women need at least 17 percent body fat for their periods to begin in puberty, and 22 percent for regular menstrual cycles. Mannequins have become thinner over the decades, and their body proportions are quite different from those of normally menstruating young women. The skinny plastic forms that model clothing in department stores, if magically transformed into flesh, would not bleed. Models have also gotten progressively thinner over the decades, as have Playboy centerfolds. Barbie, the doll many of us grew up dressing and undressing, has body proportions naturally found in 1 out of 100,000 women. Ken's body shape is found in 1 in 50 men.

Girls get a lot of messages about what a "normal" body weight or shape is, when it actually isn't natural or achievable for them. Our consumer culture continually convinces us that what we have isn't good enough. More than half of the women surveyed in *Glamour* magazine were dissatisfied with their bodies, and 40 percent spent more than one-third of their time dieting. One-third said that feeling fat prevented them from having sex and that verbal compliments felt better to them than sex. Women who don't feel good about themselves need the affirmation of others, making them vulnerable not just to flattery but also to manipulation.

LOVE THAT BODY: HIPS, BOOBS, AND PUBES

The hips and thighs of swimsuit models and celebrities are unattainable for the average woman on the average American diet, without a personal trainer, personal chef, plastic surgeon, and, most crucial, Photoshop. Upper arms and thighs are planed down, and all wrinkles and blemishes are removed, on a computer screen. But our daughters look at these images as if they were reality, and it is making them miserable. Girls who look at fashion magazines end up feeling more depressed, both acutely and chronically. There is a large body of literature linking the "thin-ideal" focused media images with body dissatisfaction, shame, depressed mood, and disordered eating. Please don't fall for the "seduction of inadequacy."

Jeremy's old girlfriend Kate used to model. She is naturally thin, always has been, and eats like a lumberjack. She apologetically explained to me early in our friendship, "I just have those kinds of genes." Most models are statistical outliers; to some degree, you may even call them genetic mutants (sorry, Katie). Something else to keep in mind: many fashion designers, art directors, and stylists are absolute queens who hold in highest regard the lithe, limber shape of a prepubescent boy. So what's a Reubenesque gal to do? How about revel in your natural beauty, confident that heterosexual men will be aroused by your shape more than you could imagine.

The hospital police at Bellevue taught me to finally love my own ass. Wide hips signal the ability to carry and deliver a baby, and that shape has been ingrained in men for millennia. Neuroimaging studies show that men are hardwired to respond to a woman's curves the way a junkie responds to his next fix. Their reward centers light up, and no pile of fashion magazines will be able to surmount that animal instinct. Have you ever noticed that models in men's magazines are more curvaceous than models in women's magazines? Men who aren't gay happen to be turned on by a woman's round bottom. Curvaceousness is all about hips and breasts, with the waist creating an hourglass shape. The much-ballyhooed waist-hip ratio is controlled by sex hormones and influences the perception of attractiveness.

Men are genetically programmed to respond to wide hips and full breasts because they signify sexual maturity, the perfect vehicle for incubating their genetic material. A woman must have a certain amount of body fat in order to menstruate, conceive, and carry a child. So voluptuous curves indicate fertility. The waist-to-hip ratio is a "reliable and honest indicator of a woman's reproductive potential." You can diet yourself into the ground, but you're meant to have those hips and thighs.

BREAST AUGMENTATION

Agog, I stared at my nubile patient, who was turning just twenty-one in a few days. Jaw slack, I had no response to her exciting news. "Guess what my dad's getting me for my birthday.... A boob job!"

Face-lifts, liposuction, and nose jobs can't hold a candle to breast augmentation, America's most popular plastic surgery. The problem with fake breasts is that they create a new normal. Like steroids in baseball, or doping in biking, if everyone starts doing it, then the players who don't are at a disadvantage. We see actresses who are stacked; our boyfriends watch porn populated with perfectly round, firm tits, and pretty soon whatever Mother Nature bestowed upon us doesn't seem like enough. Boys growing up today are different from their fathers in two ways. They masturbate with their nondominant hand as the other roams the Internet for images, and they're exposed, at least visually, to many more factory-made breasts than natural ones.

Mammals are named for the female's mammary glands, used to nurse their young. In other primates, larger breasts exist only while actively lactating, giving the nipple some movement away from the ribs. In humans, breasts exist whether or not they're providing milk, helping us to stand upright and balancing out the weight from our hips and buttocks. There is more variability of women's breasts than any other body part, between a 300 and 500 percent difference in size. The breast constructs and deconstructs not only with each pregnancy but also, to a lesser extent, with each ovulation, just in case an egg should be fertilized. Over the course of our monthly cycle, the volume of the breast varies by more than 13 percent, due to water retention and cell growth. Also, one breast is usually one-fifth of a cup size bigger than the other, around 40 cubic centimeters, so please don't fret if you're uneven. We all are.

As a woman ages, especially with successive pregnancies, her breasts change, letting a man know about her youth and fertility and potential reproductive output. Women who've never given birth and nursed tend to have smaller nipples and lighter areolas. Many men are aroused by darker areolas, perhaps because it signals prior successful pregnancy and nursing.

In the 1970s and 1980s, breast augmentation surgery grew in popularity. A 1982 letter from the American Society of Plastic Surgeons to the FDA referred to small breasts (micromastia) as follows: "These deformities are really a disease which in most patients result in feelings of inadequacy, lack of self-confidence, distortion of body image, and a total lack of well-being, and of self-perceived femininity. The enlargement of the female breast is often very necessary to insure an improved quality of life for the patient."

Small breasts are not a medical problem, and they certainly aren't a disease, fellas. Nearly always, what nature gives you is just fine. To be functional for nursing an infant, the mammary gland needs to fill only half an eggshell; the breast will grow during pregnancy in order to adequately get the job done. Breast implants will often make it extremely challenging or impossible to nurse a baby. Lactation insufficiency occurs in between 28 and 64 percent of cases. Also, reduced nipple sensation is common. For many women, because the nipple is richly innervated, its stimulation is a key component of sexual pleasure. More than 80 percent of women surveyed listed nipple stimulation as a way to initiate or enhance their sexual arousal.

Other downsides to breast augmentation: In the 1990s, the largest-ever class-action settlement at that time, $3.2 billion, was paid out to 170,000 women by Dow Corning, maker of silicone implants. Women with ruptured implants were reporting fatigue, joint pain and swelling, numbness in the hands, and lupus-like or fibromyalgia-like symptoms. As implants age, their shape changes, with 25 to 70 percent of recipients experiencing something referred to as the "doorknob effect," an immune response where collagen accumulates, along with fibrous scar tissue, around the implants. A rare cancer can grow in this scar tissue, called anaplastic large cell lymphoma. This is not breast cancer per se, though implants can make it harder for mammograms to detect early breast cancer.

So here's the deal. The natural function of breasts is at least two-fold: sensation and lactation. They arouse us and they feed our babies. Putting bags of chemicals into our breasts risks interrupting these crucial functions. When we consider breasts sexy only to look at, but not to touch, and not whether they can function properly, we end up potentially deforming ourselves.

AU NATUREL

Exercise researcher Jean Denis Rouillon studied more than three hundred women for fifteen years to arrive at a surprising conclusion. Breasts get saggier with a bra than without one. Cooper's ligaments support the breasts. Jokingly referred to as Cooper's droopers, these ligaments atrophy when denied the benefits of gravity. In the women studied who didn't wear bras, their nipples lifted 7 millimeters a year toward their shoulders, their breasts became firmer, stretch marks faded more, and their back pain decreased.

Wearing a bra 24/7 cuts off your lymphatic drainage and may increase your risk of breast cancer. Premenopausal women who don't wear bras have half the risk of breast cancer compared with bra wearers. Sleeping without a bra can lower your risk of breast cancer by 60 percent.

If you'd like something stronger to link to breast cancer, try bisphenol-A (BPA), an artificial estrogen developed in the 1930s to prevent miscarriages, which didn't work. A by-product of refining petroleum, BPA is cheap to make and ended up being used to make plastics instead, a $6 billion business. BPA found its way into everything from CDs to cell phones, canned food linings, bike helmets, cash register receipts, and plane tickets. The problem is, BPA looks like estrogen to the breast cell, activating the estrogen receptors, causing cancer cells to replicate and grow invasively. BPA basically turns on and off the genes that form breast cancer. When young rats are fed BPA, they become more susceptible to getting breast cancer later on when they're exposed to other carcinogens. Breasts do most of their growing long after birth, during puberty, and the structures necessary for lactation don't grow until later in a pregnancy—two opportunities for incorporating carcinogens into the machinery.

Then there's atrazine, a pesticide often found in drinking water that increases activity of the enzyme aromatase, which converts testosterone and other hormones into estrogens. When developing mice are exposed to atrazine, they can't adequately nurse their young after they deliver. There are at least two hundred chemicals known to cause mammary gland tumors in animal studies. Hundreds of new chemicals come to market every year, joining thousands more, many of which affect our endocrine systems, acting as estrogens, antiandrogens, or thyroid hormone impersonators. Our mammary glands are the most sensitive organs to endocrine disrupters like atrazine, DDT (another pesticide), and BPA, yet when our government tests chemicals for their effects on our health, surveying kidneys, brains, and genitals, they leave out looking at breasts, perhaps the only time that men do.

SOMEONE SHAVED MY WIFE TONIGHT

Pubic hair is important. It is nature's way of letting men know that a woman is sexually mature and able to conceive. Making your pelvis look like an eight-year-old girl's is not natural, and it sends confusing signals to men's brains. Hairless girls are those who are not yet menstruating and shouldn't be engaging in sex just yet. Shaving/waxing away all of our pubic hair is one example of women completely going against nature. Anytime you do this, it helps to induce a little twinge of self-hatred, a feeling of needing to alter your natural body and that your body isn't good enough the way it is.

I had dinner with an old med school friend who was recently divorced and is back on the prowl. He was mortified to learn that there was nary a hair among the various women he'd been bedding. The fad took hold quickly; a whole generation of women is growing up with a completely different look from their mothers and his ex-wife. "When did this happen?" he asked me, baffled. "I didn't get the memo!"

What has me particularly worried is women permanently removing their pubic hair via laser treatment. Pulses of light are used to destroy hair follicles; this can result in complications, particularly when someone is not adequately trained in how to use lasers. The percentage of laser surgery lawsuits involving nonphysician operators has risen in recent years. Laser hair removal, when it works, is permanent. The follicle is incapacitated. The current trend toward a completely bare mons is just that. A trend. Fashions change. Pendulums swing. Please, if you must remove your pubes, at least don't do it forever.

I understand that it may have started with bikinis getting smaller and underwear getting thongier, but mostly, I don't blame clothing. I blame porn. Internet porn has made not only fake breasts but also a bare mons the new aesthetic norm. Sex has become much more visual than tactile, due to the Internet. On the computer, we look but don't touch, so fake boobs seem okay. Shaved pubic hair may look fine, as long as we're not rubbing up against the stubble. Looking but not touching is not real sex. Porn is like the junk food of sex. If you fill up on garbage, you'll end up malnourished. Porn has lowered our sense of how sexy we truly are, and now women everywhere are feeling like they need to ratchet it up to compete with the synthetic professionals. Like boys choosing Froot Loops over fruit, men are drowning in silicone and missing out on the sensuality of a natural body. In the process, real women are devalued.

Pubic hair removal, whether by shaving or waxing, causes inflammation and irritation at the hair follicle. Folliculitis is a common problem with shaving. Because a recently shaved hair can curl back around to irritate the skin, the hair follicle becomes infected with bacteria and sometimes fungus. Staph and strep infections thrive in the moist, warm atmosphere of your nether regions. Shaving and waxing cause repeated microtrauma to the skin, which can cause other skin infections, like cellulitis, abscesses, boils, and increased vulnerability to the viruses molluscum contagiosum and herpes. Then there's the contaminated wax or strips of cloth that can be colonized with bacteria, causing infections.

Instead of trying to eradicate an important indicator of your adult sexual status, consider the purpose of pubic hair. It cushions the skin and sensitive genitals from too much friction. Hair helps to reduce heat loss. It protects the skin and your vagina from dust, bacteria, and other particles that shouldn't enter your body. It helps to convey your natural scent, full of pheromones and information that your mate requires and that will turn him on. How someone smells affects us on a very deep, unconscious level, fortifying sexual attraction and solidifying attachment. Don't deny yourself and your lover that enhancement.

As long as we're in the area, there's one more thing to address. There is tremendous variability in the way our genitalia look, and, unfortunately, the demand for plastic surgery (called vulvoplasty) in this area is increasing. I would ask that you please not pay a plastic surgeon to alter your inner labia unless you are the victim of genital mutilation or are having physical pain during sex. The last thing we need is another "new normal."

Accepting yourself, your *natural* self, in all its splendor, is key to being happy and healthy. We all have an innate sense of what is natural for us, what feels right, like biting into a ripe, juicy peach. It is genuine: the real deal, no artifice. We demand all-natural ingredients when we shop for baby food or shampoo, yet somehow we don't demand it of our own bodies or our innate animalistic behavior. We all bristle at the obvious fakery of a saccharine smile, but we inject synthetic dermal fillers into our faces and inflate silicone balloons behind our nipples. This dichotomy fuels our discontent. Beauty is truth. If we can live in a way that is more aligned to what is natural and genuine for us, we will be calmer, more at peace, and more fulfilled.

Nature abounds with examples of beautiful imperfection. Take a walk on the beach sometime and examine the seashells. Each one is perfect in its individuality; it is naturally pleasing, but also irregular. Being dissatisfied with your natural self, feeling that it needs to be aggressively altered, leads to self-hatred that can spill over into self-abuse. We end up out of touch with our bodies: overeating, drinking, and taking drugs or medications to soothe the pain of this separation. In my practice, I see this time and time again. Women are feeling disconnected from their bodies and their natural selves, and they are miserable.

The solution is embodiment. Be inside your body; be in touch with your body. Women are taught to disregard their inner voice, their hunger, and their libido. We're led to believe that we can't trust our appetites, that they need to be tamed, or at least ignored. And so we suppress our innermost desires and intuitions: to eat, and screw, and throw off our bras, and let our hair grow. Body awareness and acceptance is what's best for your peace of mind. Good nutrition, proper exercise, sensual desire, and sexual response—it all comes back to being embodied and reveling in your body. Loving your body, trusting its signals, and inhabiting it fully... This is the way back to health.

Twelve

You. Need. Downtime.

W omen are constantly under pressure to do more. The day begins with chauffeuring kids to school and slips seamlessly into a jam-packed workday. When you clock out, the second shift begins: dinner, homework, housework, and maybe also caring for aging parents. And increasingly we lead a third life online—checking e-mail, browsing Facebook posts. Even the things we value and know will make us happy begin to feel like chores.

And so it may come as a relief to know that some of the most meaningful work you can do for yourself includes doing very little at all. Meditation and mindfulness studies tell us that just breathing (and paying attention to it) can do a world of good for our bodies and our brains. Even better if you move your practice outside. Nature has its own restorative properties and helps to quiet and calm the body and mind in a way that's likely to amplify your efforts. Whenever possible, be out in the sun and wind, bare feet on the ground, dirt under your fingernails, birdsong in your ears, surrounded by ocean, trees, mountain trails . . . anything to connect you to the earth.

Mindfulness sounds simple, but it's hard to be alone with your self and your feelings. Most people will expend all kinds of energy keeping busy in ten different directions to avoid it. One study showed that people prefer to give themselves an electric shock if it means they can be doing something instead of being left alone with their thoughts, doing nothing.

We need to develop sanctified downtime, a protected haven for recharging our batteries where we are not giving to others. The key here is creating *healthy* boundaries of unavailability instead of using alcohol, food, or drugs to incapacitate yourself.

I had a patient, the mother of two young girls, who worked a demanding job as the managing editor at a newspaper. We'd been working on her cigarette smoking, trying to taper it down, and she came into my office one evening proudly reporting that she'd managed to get her recent five-cigarettes-a-day habit down to exactly one last cigarette, but she couldn't quit that no matter how hard she tried: the one between work and home.

My patient was desperately trying to draw a line in the sand between her work life and her home life or, as some women say, her first job and her second. Boundaries help us to feel safe. We need a way to demarcate that part of the day that can feel like it's just ours. Instead of coming home and relaxing, like the stereotypical man in the La-Z-Boy with a beer, women tend to come home from work wiped out but continue to focus on others. For many of the women in my practice, "Miller time" is when the kids are in bed and they head for the fridge, mindlessly eating anything they can find to induce an altered state as reliably as a swami playing the flute for a cobra. If it's not that, then it's heading to the TV, computer, or phone, all portals to *elsewhere.*

We all find ways to forget ourselves, to get away from it all. We try to catapult out of our ruts and into a state of bliss. This is one of the reasons why we use drugs, alcohol, food, and screens. They readily induce a dissociated state, helping us to forget ourselves. We use them because we want things to be different. We're rejecting reality. The problem is, for most people, the drug (or other substance) makes them feel different, but not necessarily better. Yet they keep trying, hoping they can get what they were looking for. This is another example of scratching around an itch but never really satisfying the angst. Mindfulness teaches you to refrain from scratching. You notice the itch, but you don't react. And over time, the reflexive scratching, and then the deep-seated itch, both disappear. You learn to just be.

Sanctified, healthy rituals are vital to repleting our energy stores. A cup of herbal tea by the window during sunset, a warm bath with a candle, stretching, chanting, dancing, or meditating will all work to help center you. And if you can't do these things at home, then pack your bag and head to the gym or a yoga class. Even a quick down dog and child's pose while slowing down your breathing can be enough to lower your stress level. Demarcate work time from me time with something ritualized and reliable, and consider meditation and time outdoors as powerful options for the restorative downtime we all need.

LET NATURE TEACH YOU STILLNESS

When we are fully present in nature, we use all our senses simultaneously, the optimal state for learning. A nature walk can lead to greater mental acuity, restoring attention and decreasing mental fatigue. Directed-attention fatigue results from staring at a screen and causes irritability, diminished impulse control, and distractibility, all ADHD symptoms. Technology-aggravated attention deficits may be driving the ADHD overdiagnosis that is sweeping America (but don't let the drug companies off the hook). When kids with ADHD played outside, their

symptoms improved more than with indoor activities; they had significantly better concentration after walking in a park versus an urban
setting.

Adult subjects in an outdoor immersion program report a sense of
peace and an ability to think more clearly by being in nature, as well as a
reduction in anxiety and helplessness and improved cognitive reasoning
and creativity. Attention restoration is available to all of us, but we need
to peel away from our screens.

Being outside in nature at once calms and focuses us. It encourages
introspection, but at the same time, our senses blossom, welcomed by a
sense of awe, which expands time perception and enhances well-being.
Being enveloped in nature can help you become realigned with the
wholeness of life, a perfect way to feel a sense of belonging and connection that is critical and beneficial to the soul and the psyche.

SUNLIGHT, AIR, AND HOW WEATHER CAN AFFECT US

We have become a nation of vitamin D–depleted patients due to our diminishing time spent outside in the sunshine; three-quarters of us are
deficient in vitamin D. Exposure to sunlight can boost those levels and is
a great energizer. Vitamin D is made by your skin, as long as you get
twenty minutes of sunshine three times a week. But we don't get nearly
enough sunshine. We were meant to be outside in the fresh air and the
sun's glare. Instead, we spend the bulk of our days indoors under fluores-
cent lighting.

Low vitamin D levels correlate with depression, and giving patients
adequate doses of vitamin D improves their depressive symptoms. Vitamin D is essential for muscle health and bone growth. One study of people in an ER with complaints of bone pain and muscle aches found that
93 percent of them had a vitamin D deficiency. Just as important, many

of these patients also had a variety of psychiatric diagnoses, including fibromyalgia, chronic fatigue syndrome, and depression.

All of my Manhattan patients who bother to have their levels checked are surprised to find out they're low in vitamin D. I'm not surprised at all. Barely anyone in New York City is outside enough to keep those levels up. What did surprise me is that their internists gave them prescriptions for high-dose vitamin D instead of telling them to get outside, which is the natural solution. I tell my patients who are stuck in a cubicle in their offices all day, "You can at least leave your desk during lunchtime to get a few minutes of sun on your face." One tip: take those fashionable sunglasses off for a few minutes. Although any skin will do to make vitamin D, the sunlight needs to hit your retinas to exert its direct antidepressant effect, though of course you must never look directly at the sun, in case your mama never told you.

Nature affects us more than we realize. Human beings are just as light sensitive as other animals. The length of daylight dictates our energy level and behaviors. In the fall and winter, my private practice is busy, with many new patients coming in and old patients returning to restart their medications. They notice a darkening of their moods as the days shorten, and they're bothered by lower levels of energy, motivation, and concentration. In the spring and summer, most of my patients are feeling well and barely need to check in with me at all. They are outside in the sunshine and are more physically active, and consequently many of them lower their medication dosages or go off them completely. When the days lengthen and sunlight exposure increases, my bipolar patients are more likely to experience manic episodes. (When I worked at Bellevue, April and May composed what I used to call mania season.) But as soon as the clocks change in the fall, my phone starts ringing off the hook with people who can feel their depression coming on again.

Phototherapy is an excellent way to treat seasonal affective disorder or just the winter blues with no side effects like weight gain or libido loss.

Phototherapy lamps and visors are available online. The light should be placed above your head if at all possible, about a foot away from your eyes, and should emit 10,000 lux of full-spectrum light. I tell my patients to sit in front of the light for thirty minutes as early in the day as they can manage.

Many of us feel sluggish and blue on low-pressure days when it is cloudy, overcast, or raining. We are sensitive to weather in general, and to barometric pressure in particular. Depression is aggravated in lab animals when the barometric pressure is lowered. A survey of thousands of suicides in Finland shows a correlation between low pressure and suicide attempts.

Our moods often improve during high-pressure, good-weather days. These are often sunny days as well, so it's hard to tease apart the sun's effects, but barometric pressure does affect the fluid in our joints, causing pain in many people with arthritis or migraines in others. It's not unusual for pain to affect mood states. At Bellevue, I would often chat with NYPD officers about the weather affecting the city's inhabitants. Everyone had their theories, from temperature and humidity to the barometer's rise and fall, but there is no doubt that there is something there to explore.

Certain natural phenomena have the capacity to make us feel unusually good. Have you ever walked beside a waterfall or along the seashore as the waves crashed rhythmically at your feet? How about the way the air feels after it rains? Or even in the shower—how's your mood in there? Pounding water creates negative ions, which can improve our energy, mood, and stress levels. Fresh mountain air also has significantly higher amounts of negative ions than what you breathe in at your home or office. The cells in our bodies carry a negative charge, which means we attract positively charged ions toward us, such as dust, pet dander, and various microbes. Computers and cell phones generate positive ions, while air conditioners deplete negative ions; both are bad news for your head.

Studies using negative ion generators have demonstrated that exposure to negative ions can diminish symptoms of depression, lower stress and inflammatory markers, and increase alertness and mental energy.

Negative ion generators create a protective shield around you, deflecting positive ions. They can be purchased at reasonable prices and placed by your bedside for exposure while you sleep, but you know my advice, I'm sure. Go outside. Find a trail with a waterfall or stream, get to a beach or a mountain retreat, and, by all means, head out the door right after a spring shower to take in clean, negatively charged air. If you can't get outside, just take a shower. Call it hydrotherapy.

NATURE THERAPY

Being outside in nature enhances the body's ability to cope with stress and recover from injury or illness. Green exercise boosts resilience and immune function by enhancing the activity of natural killer cells. In a study comparing city folk and country folk, the former have greater fMRI activity in their fear centers (amygdalae) than the latter. The city folk also have greater anterior cingulate activity after stressful tasks than the country folk. The anterior cingulate is a part of the brain widely implicated in depressive symptoms. Take urban dwellers out into nature and they'll show a more positive outlook on life and higher life satisfaction. That translates into improved physical health, as genuinely happy people recover from illness more quickly and have been shown to seek out and act on health information, leading to longer lives.

In an American study, 22 percent of people felt more depressed after walking in a mall, while 92 percent felt less depressed after an outdoor walk. The outdoor walkers also felt less tense, angry, confused, and fatigued. The medical mile along the Arkansas River is a downtown walking path along the wetlands. Santa Fe, New Mexico, has a "prescription trails program," and a pilot program in Portland, Oregon, is pairing physicians with park professionals, who give feedback on whether their "outdoor prescriptions" are being filled by their patients. Many people, including doctors, are beginning to recognize the transformative power of nature.

Even looking at nature can be therapeutic. Patients who have a view of a tree outside their hospital window recover more quickly, take fewer pain meds, and have better nursing chart comments than those who don't. Canadian studies report that children with larger classroom windows showing views of nature have better test scores and graduation rates, and also that their teachers enjoy teaching more, with fewer discipline issues. Likewise, people in indoor workspaces with a window looking out onto natural views show better rates of heart-rate recovery from stress than those with an HDTV display of nature, who have better levels than those with a blank wall.

The research of Frances Kuo shows that play spaces in urban areas with more grass and trees generate fewer incidences of violence; crime rates are lower for those residences that have more green spaces. In Chicago public-housing projects, the presence of trees or greenery immediately outside the property correlates with improved concentration, less mental fatigue, and fewer incidences of domestic violence carried out by women against their partners. Yes, women. And here's another example of going green reducing violence. Couples in which both partners use cannabis have the lowest rates of domestic violence.

Immersion in nature helps us to feel connected to one another, valuing community and our relationships. Walking in a forest can provide a deep sense of homecoming. Research shows nature actually makes us more caring and generous. In a study of people looking at images of nature or man-made settings and being in a room with or without plants, the subjects who focused on the artificial elements rated wealth and fame more highly. Those exposed to the natural environment valued community and were more generous with their money. The natural world helps to connect people to their authentic selves. The hunter-gatherers we used to be depended on one another for survival. They were fiercely egalitarian and communal. When people get together to restore their communities or to improve or protect the environment, social capital increases, and they end up healing themselves. If we feel disconnected from nature, our sense of community can suffer, helping to fuel our hunger for drugs and other substitutes for that sense of belonging and unity we need. Going green is not only good for the environment; it is good for our own psyches.

BACTERIA FOR HEALTH

Americans have become obsessed with cleanliness and a sterile environment, but that is unnatural and potentially unhealthy. Dirt is natural; techno-clean is not. Antibacterial soaps and overprescribed antibiotics create "superbugs" that are resistant to typical chemicals and medications, causing more harm than other bacteria, and they create a sterile environment where we don't get to use our immune systems adequately, a setup for autoimmune disorders, asthma, and allergies.

Exposure to weaker pathogens (bacteria and viruses that cause illness) can stimulate our immune systems, dictating what kind of tolerance we have to pathogens that are potentially more hostile or deadly. Think of the immune system as a border crossing. If no outsiders enter, it's a lot harder to tell who's native and who's foreign because everyone looks the same. With no diversity, the body fails to recognize self versus other; it may end up going after its own tissues, as is seen in autoimmune disorders.

Having a large diversity of bacteria in the gut is healthier for our immunities and digestive functioning. Babies born by Caesarean section, not allowed to pass through the bacteria-filled vagina, have higher rates of asthma, allergies, and autoimmune symptoms. Also, children born by C-section are more likely to be obese later in life, because a wider array of gut bacteria improves metabolism. The solution could be as simple as swiping a swab from the mother's vagina into the newborn's mouth.

Farmers are putting antibiotics in their animals' feed to make them grow fatter in less time. The problem is, we're eating those antibiotics. When you combine high-calorie foods with antibiotics in mice, the males gain muscle and fat, but the females just gain fat.

Antibacterial soaps are another problem. There are concerns that triclosan and triclocarban might be disrupting thyroid function, amplifying hormone levels, and promoting drug-resistant infections. These antibacterial chemicals are found in our urine, our breast milk and our wastewater.

If you garden, forgo the gloves. Getting dirt under your nails might allow an "antidepressant bacteria" to do its job. Allowing exposure to bacteria in nature can make us smarter, happier, and calmer. *Mycobacterium vaccae* improves levels of serotonin and norepinephrine in the brain after exposure, and it stimulates growth of some brain cells, resulting in decreased levels of anxiety. Mice given live *M. vaccae* navigate a maze in half the time and with fewer anxiety behaviors than control mice. Bacteria also play a role in regulating the stress response. In laboratory animals and healthy human subjects, administering *Lactobacillus helveticus* and *Bifidobacterium longum* for two weeks significantly reduces anxiety-like behavior and negative emotionality. Some studies have found that certain bacteria are essential for normal social development in mice, whose autistic-like behavior improves when given the bacteria *Bacteroides fragilis*.

The take-home message is best summed up by Michael Pollan in his *New York Times Magazine* piece "Some of My Best Friends Are Germs":

"Minimize unnecessary antibiotics and hand sanitizers and let your kids play in the dirt and with animals." I tell my patients and friends to take probiotics to improve bacterial diversity (see the food chapter, page 182, for more on this).

SOILING THE NEST: POLLUTION AND PESTICIDES

We are indeed soiling our nest. The earth is being deforested, which directly leads to loss of species diversity and climate change. We are polluting our air and water in countless ways. Hormones are found in our water supply in record numbers. The millions of women who are on the Pill have higher levels of hormones in their urine, which, when recycled at wastewater-treatment facilities, are returned back to the environment. Hormones in the drinking water translate into elevated estrogen levels in our bloodstreams, increasing men's risk of prostate cancer and women's risk of breast cancer.

The estrogen receptor is the ultimate accommodator, and it is promiscuous. It isn't picky about what turns it on. Lots of other compounds trick the receptor into thinking it's occupied with estrogen, including synthetic chemicals, which are called xenoestrogens. In the bloodstream, estrogen often gets bound up by proteins, so lower levels actually reach the estrogen receptors. Chemicals with estrogenic activity remain unbound and go directly to the receptor and are therefore more estrogenic than estrogen itself. Most of the plastics that we're exposed to every day are estrogenic. When plastics are heated in a microwave they release even more of these chemicals. BPA, the chemical added to plastics to make them more flexible, is found in older sippy cups and baby bottles, in the linings of many aluminum cans, and on cash register receipts. BPA is highly estrogenic; chronic exposure brings on puberty earlier in girls and creates abnormal genitalia in boys. Research has tied BPA not just to infertility, genital deformities, and low sperm count but also to asthma, heart and liver ailments, ADHD, and cancer. BPA can switch off genes that suppress tumor growth, hence the increased risk for breast cancer discussed earlier.

Here's where it gets a bit like science fiction. The genetic changes can be passed down through generations. "A poison kills you. A chemical like BPA reprograms your cells and ends up causing disease in your grand-child that kills him." No industry-funded studies have reported signifi-cant effects of low doses of BPA, though more than 90 percent of government-funded studies have. The good news is that many manufac-turers have removed BPA from their products. The bad news: it's been replaced by other chemicals that still show estrogenic activity, in some cases more than that of BPA. The billion-dollar plastics industry is snow-ing us and strong-arming the government, just as Big Tobacco did, to minimize testing, public education, and product recall.

Phthalates are also used to make plastics flexible; they're also found in cosmetics and detergents to make them slippery. They've been corre-lated with cancers and birth defects, decreased sperm quality, and ab-normal testes development. They interfere with testosterone production, affect a woman's egg production, cause lower fertility, and should be con-sidered reproductive toxins. Exposure to phthalates brings on puberty earlier and is linked with breast cancer, diabetes, and obesity.

Since learning more about BPA and phthalates, I have tossed all the plastic containers in my house and replaced them with glass. Yes, it is crazy making, because plastic is everywhere. Please avoid wrapping your food in plastic, and above all, don't heat plastics, especially in the microwave, as the phthalates in them will be transferred to your food. Pregnant women, developing fetuses, and growing children are those most at risk.

ECOPSYCHOLOGY

The standard monotheistic narrative is one of mind over body; man separates from nature and dominates it. We transcend by spiraling up, and spirit is to be found in the heavens, out of the fray of nature, animals, and primal urges. But for indigenous cultures, nature is where the spirit is. Heaven is here on earth, not later but now. The forests and jungles are sacred; what flows from this is a desire to sustain them. Environmental damage hurts our psyches. The earth is suffering at our hands, and we, at least unconsciously, are in mourning.

We have a responsibility to take care of the earth and our natural surroundings, and doing so can make us feel better. As long as we feel separated from nature, we will not tend to the environment, and we may not feel unified. Having a sense of community is good for you. Being a part of something big and permanent, that needs your tending, is good for your soul. Becoming ecoconscious is, in and of itself, effective antidepressant behavior. Because we live here, being good to the environment is the same as being good to ourselves. Respect for the planet translates to self-respect. Helping the earth to survive and prosper, to stay green and healthy, allows you not only to live a healthier lifestyle but ensures that your children will as well.

We are all living in the same home. If some of us are polluters, we all lose. Luckily, what is healthiest for us as individuals is often what is best for the planet. Eating plants, being in sync with circadian rhythms and nature, and even using cannabis-based medicines as anti-inflammatories to increase our resilience to stress are all environmentally friendly behaviors. Hemp and cannabis are drought-resistant weeds that don't require pesticides that can make us sick. These crops put nutrients back into the soil, clean more carbon out of the air than trees do, and provide not just medicine but also fiber, fuel, and food. For many of us who do smoke, cannabis can help us to get into our bodies and appreciate fully the experience of being in nature. That makes it an apt medicine for moody bitches.

Paradise is not lost or forbidden to us, and there is no pill that will substitute for nature. The way to save yourself and the planet is to go out and find beauty in the world, whether it be the stream in your own back-yard woods or a national park, and revel in your right to be here. Then take care of the environment the way you'd take care of a loved one. Do unto others. Heal the earth, and you heal yourself.

When I walk on the beach in summer, I often find myself uncon-sciously gathering garbage that's tangled into the seaweed on the sand. The synthetic materials, mostly plastic, don't blend in with nature and are easy to spot. I've always hated plastic, a reminder of our insatiable need to buy and discard things. But since researching this book, know-ing it can actually disrupt our endocrine system and cause cancer, I'm looking at it in a new way. Mostly, I can't wait until we manufacture com-postable packaging made out of hemp.

There is a "plastic vortex" the size of Texas floating in the Pacific Ocean. Here at home, we have our own cancer of plastic. Synthetic fill-ers in our breasts and faces, fake sex partners on our computers, and artificial rationality from SSRIs are all choking the nature right out of us. We've gone too far toward technology and synthetics and away from fur and pheromones, and our bodies are suffering for it. Left over from our days of hunting and foraging for survival, we're still programmed to acquire. We are compulsively consuming this fakery without satiation or satisfaction.

We eat artificial sweeteners but our pancreas squirts out insulin as if it were sugar. Men ogle plastic breasts on their computer screens and their brains stimulate the same wiring as if they were having real sex. Chemicals in plastics act as if they're hormones, tickling our estrogen

receptors and disrupting our endocrine function and ability to reproduce. Exposure to others' traumas via mass media still triggers a stress
response in our bodies as if it were happening to us.

SCREENS ARE UNHEALTHY

When drugs are more plentiful, there are more cases of addiction. So it
goes with screens. America now has more Internet-connected devices
than it has people—311.5 million Americans own more than 425 million
personal computers, tablets, smartphones, and gaming consoles. You can
see it on the streets of Manhattan. Everyone is gazing into their iPhones
while they attempt to navigate the crowded sidewalks or, worse yet, cross
the street. While waiting on the subway platform, people are checking
their e-mail one last time or writing a text. When sitting in the subway
cars, they're playing mindless video games. All in an attempt to be elsewhere, anywhere but here. Technology, take me away. Paying attention to
a number of electronic sources at a superficial level, "continuous partial
attention," a term coined by Linda Stone, drains our ability to focus attention, think clearly, and be productive and creative.

We are so neurally invested in our smartphones that our brains fire
like crazy when they beckon to us, much as a junkie will release dopamine when looking at a needle and spoon. When a research subject hears
his phone ring, his insular cortex, an emotional center associated with
feelings of love and compassion, lights up as it would in the presence of a
loved one. It is insidious, our connection to our phones. A new term, *nomophobia,* has been coined to explain the unease many of us feel if we
can't find our cell phones or are losing battery power or a strong signal.

As social primates, it is imperative that we feel part of the troop. Our
status in the tribe affects how we feel about ourselves and our clan. We
groom one another verbally instead of eating bugs off fur, but it's groom-

ing nonetheless. Facebook has its own rules about how this is done, but it resonates with age-old primate behaviors of dominance hierarchies and displays of fertility, aggression, or tribal affiliation. We have an innate desire to be held, and we immerse ourselves in social media hoping to slake our thirst. But it is impossible to get enough of something that almost works. Social networking sites like Facebook and Instagram are pure fakery, as no one posts images of arguments with spouses, losing it with kids, or quaking in a meeting with the boss. And just as when we fill up on junk food, after bingeing on unsatisfying social interactions, we're less hungry for the real thing afterward.

One pseudoreligious ritual I'd like to recommend is to "keep the Sabbath holy." Be an honorary Jew and turn off your electronics for twenty-four hours, from sundown to sundown, Friday to Saturday. No e-mail, no texting, no television, no computers. Think you can try that for just one weekend to see how relaxing it is? Wait till you see how much more free time and energy you have when you do this. It's like a mini spa vacation.

YOUR LUNGS ARE A GATEWAY TO NIRVANA

Letting go isn't just good for your head; it's good for your whole body. And the quickest, easiest way to decompress is through the breath. It's hard for your brain to panic when it's fully oxygenated, and many of us are shallow breathers. When we're tense or fearful, we often take in even less air. One reason I stress cardio and yoga with my patients is that it fosters the ability to take in deeper, fuller breaths.

Breathing happens unconsciously, whether we think about it or not, but it can also be controlled consciously, as a voluntary function. When you focus on your breathing, you are doing spiritual work, helping to connect the mind and the body, consciousness and unconsciousness. Try these four different breathing techniques (appropriated from Andrew Weil's lectures on breath work) and see how each one feels to you.

1. Just follow your breath, using a slow in and out, with no influence on depth or speed. Notice how the air feels in your nose, your throat, your chest, your belly; notice your abdomen rise and fall. Just stay with your breath for as long as you can, and when you start to notice yourself thinking, just return to your breath, perhaps just saying to yourself, *Thinking,* as your attention falls back on your breathing.

2. Exaggerated exhales. Try to wring your lungs clean of all air before you take a new breath. Make each exhale slower, longer, and more complete than the last.

3. Breathe in for four counts, hold for seven, exhale for eight. Repeat ten times. This can help reduce anxiety and allow you to "come back to yourself."

4. Bellows breathing: take shallow breaths, in and out, as fast as you can go, through the nose. This breathing exercise is good for giving you more energy and focus, helping to wake you up and increase adrenaline.

Try to fit these breathing exercises into your daily schedule. When you're waiting in line, stuck in traffic, even at your computer waiting for something to download... Breathe. This allows you to "check in," to reinhabit your body and become grounded in your surroundings. Breathing resets you back to the now. Every breath can serve as a reminder, an opportunity to start over, to become conscious again, awakened, enlightened, and embodied.

Besides these four breathing exercises, I'd like to offer a few more suggestions. Just think of them as Dr. Julie's helpful hints for living calmly.

1. Choose peace. You've probably heard the phrase "Happiness is a decision." So is serenity. Whenever possible, make tranquillity a priority. Eliminate noise from televisions and radios. (You don't need them to "keep you company.") Have a zero-tolerance policy on yelling in the household.

2. Embrace the present moment. We spend a lot of energy fighting reality. Most of our suffering comes from wanting things to be different from how they are, from a denial of the now. Accept what is. Recognize and allow whatever is happening. You don't have to like it, but you do need to make a space for it to exist. This is a part of choosing peace.

3. Spend time in nature whenever you can. Getting outside where you can admire natural surroundings, whether a park, garden, forest, seaside, or mountain, will improve your mood.

4. In communicating with others, remember: people want to be heard and understood, so make sure you mirror what you're hearing and empathize with their feelings. People also want to feel that they belong. If someone is complaining to you about something, see if there isn't an element of her feeling left out or overlooked, and try to address her need for inclusion.

5. Find time to meditate or be mindful every day. Train your brain on one thing only, whether it's your breath, a mantra, or whatever you're doing at that moment. When you wash the dishes or cook dinner, focus intently on only that. Flip your switch from "transmit" to "receive" as you try not to generate any thoughts. Make a point of actively integrating relaxation into your day. Schedule it in your calendar if that's what needs to happen.

THIS IS YOUR BRAIN ON MINDFULNESS

Meditation can decrease stress, cortisol levels, blood pressure, and the risk of heart attack. It helps to improve resilience and tamp down inflammation, benefitting genes that control energy metabolism, insulin secretion, and telomere maintenance, important in slowing cell aging and death. Meditation practices are associated with neuroplastic changes in all the places that matter for stress, resilience, anxiety, and depression, such as the insula, the anterior cingulate cortex, and the connections between the frontal cortex and the limbic system. These changes in functional connectivity reflect improved sensory processing, awareness of sensory experience, and more consistent attentional focus. Most important, strengthening these connections improves self-regulation, one way to supplant your SSRI.

The longer people have an established meditation practice, the more brain folds they have. More folding (gyrification) means more brain connections. Perhaps because of this enhanced connectivity, people who meditate learn to regulate their emotions and their reactivity. Meditation not only helps you chill out while you sit, but you're calmer and less reactive "off the cushion" as well.

Meditation can help you be more resilient to stress. One part of the brain that can tamp down the amygdala's fear or rage response is the prefrontal cortex (PFC). The PFC helps to inhibit your anxiety. If you can strengthen or activate the PFC input (meditation is the best way to do this), you can inhibit the duration of the amygdala's response to stress and shorten the time it takes to recover from trauma, thereby enhancing resilience. This is top-down control in action. The PFC, amygdala, and hippocampus are all involved in resilience. Imaging studies of people who have survived a trauma but did not develop PTSD show stronger connections between the PFC and the hippocampus, implying that their higher cognitive functions were able to calm their emotional reactivity.

Advanced meditators are better at inhibiting pain signals and reactions to threats, one theory as to why they have reduced occurrences of depression and anxiety. Even after just eight weeks of mindfulness training, cell density increases in the hippocampus and decreases in the amygdala, a reflection of the dominance of the rational over the emotional. People who meditate are not only more psychologically healthy but are also generally more physically healthy than others. This is why I tell my patients not to strengthen just their PC muscles with Kegels but also to strengthen their PFC "muscle" with meditation and mindfulness. It is a pathway to living without antidepressants.

Meditation is not a belief system; it's a new way of paying attention. You don't need a fancy pillow or lessons from a shaman in order to slow down and breathe. The next time you're feeling like a moody bitch, you might consider closing your computer, putting down your phone, and focusing on your breath. Your only job is to be there, fully present. When you fixate your mind on the one thing you're doing, whether chores or sports, you will be in that blissful state known as flow.

As often as you can, create sanctified downtime. Use mindfulness to help you get a handle on reactive behavior, to modulate your emotionality. These days, busy is an addictive drug, and exhaustion is a status symbol. But chasing material possessions, acquisitions, and accomplishments will not fill the hole. Instead, sit motionless in that hole and realize it is a place of peace and stillness. Be happy with Less, with Empty, with Now. Be welcoming of uncertainty. Practice moderation in emotion and in consumption. Staying present and fully conscious, not checking out or becoming distracted, will ensure that this modulation can occur. Take time to fully feel and examine your feelings prior to expressing them. Let your higher, cortical brain, which plans, analyzes, and decides, be the master of your lower reptilian brain, which is reactive and sometimes even aggressive.

If sitting and meditating just isn't for you, then head to a patch of green instead. Realign with nature. Go into the woods. It is not hectic there; it is calm and still, and it can help you to be the same. Nature is a sustainable source of wonder. Having a sense of awe, of immenseness, can create feelings of abundance and satiety. If you feel you have more time available, you're less likely to feel impatient and more willing to volunteer your time to help others. You're even more likely to prefer experiences over material products. Feeling boundless and powerful, connected to the universe and all its inhabitants, is strong stuff that feeds your soul. Sublimating your smaller self into the larger picture, resting in the arms of an immense mother earth, is comforting for many and transcendent for others. The natural world of flora and fauna is the most learned paradigm available and the most potent force. This place of primordial perfection is sacred. Nature has given us all the answers we need for how to live fully and healthfully; we just have to pay attention, watch, and listen.

Being in sync with the rhythms of the earth is what's healthiest. Let the cycles of light and dark dictate your sleep. Let the seasons drive your caloric intake and energy expenditure. Let your ovulatory cycles influence your sexual priorities. Dualities and cyclical rhythms predominate in nature for a reason. Consistency and stability are not natural; homogenization is not natural. We thrive on diversity. There is strength in the synthesis of two opposites; hybrids are always hardier than purebreds. Learn to harmonize the yin and yang inherent in you, in your relationships, and in your community. This balance will bring you peace.

Conclusion:
Staying Sane in an
Insane World

Too many of us are out of sync with our bodies and our environment, and that disconnect is making us sick, fat, tired, wired, and miserable. We ignore or medicate away our body's own amazing feedback system, our *moods*. We take oral contraceptives that trick our bodies into not ovulating and then wonder why we're not horny. We spend our days indoors, yet are amazed when the doctor reports a vitamin D deficiency. We text and e-mail but can't understand why, as social primates who starve and even die from lack of physical touch, we feel so lonely. To plug these holes, we've become compulsive consumers of everything from food and clothing to pills and sex partners, always looking for a bargain in our rummaging but never fully satiated.

Our lives are big and messy and go in directions we would never expect, and the world often tells us that we should handle it all without breaking a sweat. We've been sold that bill of goods over and over again. Women are asked to do it all. We are raising our families and competing with men in the workplace. We are busier and more hassled and harried than ever and paying the price in pounds and pills. Modern women are suffering from our own energy crisis, and we're using anything we can to duct-tape our lives and ourselves together. We reach for comfort foods, lattes, alcohol, and an expanding array of neuromodulators like antidepressants, painkillers, energy drinks, and amphetamines in an effort to maintain our unnatural pace. Throughout the day, we're repeatedly traumatized by terrifying news reports and horrific images of suffering, and so we medicate away our unease. We take pills to quiet our anxieties, especially to help us get to sleep at night when the fears threaten to take center stage.

Our bodies and our lives are compromised in more ways than we'd like to admit, but we also have more power to reclaim them than we realize. All of us have the capacity to influence our emotional lives. This does not mean constant happiness of the kind we have come to expect and that the pharmaceutical companies promise to deliver. Our lives are not straight lines, and our moods aren't either. The oscillations of our changing hormones are a reflection of the endless permutations of our experiences in the world. Women know change—we live it every day—and it's an asset, not a hindrance. Our fluidity makes us adaptable. It makes us more resilient. To be optimally engineered means perfecting the balance between stability and flexibility. Being locked into one way of thinking, or having constantly artificially elevated levels of serotonin or estrogen, may be stable, but it is not natural or flexible, and very likely it is not adaptive.

We need a course correction so that we can live lives that truly honor how we feel. But in order to do that, we must be able to feel. We must be able to be our moody selves. Acknowledging our bodies in all of their complexity is the first step to wellness, and to wholeness.

If you are truly psychiatrically ill, then it's crucial that you take medication to manage your symptoms, but most people on antidepressants today are not genuinely ill. Granted, they are miserable, and it's true that enhancing serotonin can ease the misery, but it also mutes the sensitivity. SSRIs might lengthen your short fuse, but they also help to numb you, dulling your sensibilities. Masking the symptoms won't fix the problem. Change can come only from the discomfort and awareness that something is wrong. Not feeling the pain makes it impossible to address its causes. A nation hooked on psychic painkillers is not going to pull itself up by the bootstraps and fix what's broken. If medicated ends up meaning complacent, it helps no one.

Taking a medicine that makes it harder to cry and be sensitive, to be irritated and reactive, and to be motivated to make changes is not a decision that should be taken lightly. For more of us, the better solution is to slow down, to get into our bodies and out into the natural world, away from screens, shopping, and psychiatric medication. Listening to your intuition, and knowing what's right, will help to right your course. Tune in to your body to tune in to your knowing. Hear that faint voice tell you where you're sick and need healing or which behaviors or foods are the problems, not the solutions. Particularly in times of despair, or during PMS or perimenopause, if we tune in to our bodies and our intuition, if we hear that voice and follow its message, there's no telling how powerful we could become or how much good we could unleash on the world. It is during these times that the gloves come off. When we allow ourselves to feel more critical, less accommodating, and less accepting of the status quo, we can really clean house.

We need to modulate our moods, not dull them entirely. I hear my medicated patients marvel at how they no longer get upset or tearful at what used to make them flustered or snippy. But it would be healthier, and less extreme, to achieve top-down control, to help our rational brain tame our "lower" emotional centers. Mindfulness, meditation, and physical activity all help us to stay present and gain control over our emotional responses so that we can moderate our reactivity without needing a daily dose of meds. Mastery of mood need not require a pharmaceutical cocktail every day for the rest of your life.

Best for our bodies are those things that limit inflammation: a colorful whole-food diet, moderate exercise, and stress reduction. Our immune systems need to be tamed to not attack the self, just as our emotional brains need to be tamed to not lash out at loved ones. Pay attention to what your body is telling you about your own wants and needs. Find the rhythms in your cycles. There is wisdom in our biology. Above all, do what feels best. Making healthy choices feels good. This is not deprivation. It is nourishment, on all levels; it is the opposite of neglect. Being in your body will allow you to experience the most gratification, whether from sex or food or exercise. You will stay fit as you enjoy not only the pleasures of movement but also the feelings that healthy foods impart.

Remember when you make those hard decisions about what to eat, when to exercise or go to sleep, that you are caring for yourself; you are *taking* care. There is a time to be sensitive to the needs of others, and there is a time for nurturing ourselves. Like a mama lion protecting her cubs, be aggressive in demarcating time that is just for you. Women are often givers and sometimes martyrs. Life doesn't always have to be about pleasing other people. Resist being a pathological accommodator. Practice saying no. Finding ways to replete your energy is crucial to your functioning; you can't pour from an empty pitcher.

Being a moody bitch means being a warrior, and your first point of defense should be yourself. Be your own best advocate. You deserve downtime and pleasure, and your needs matter. Honor your hearty appetites for food, sex, and sleep. Stop beating yourself up with "shoulds." Find the healthiest thing that soothes your aching heart and give it to yourself without shame. If at all possible, avoid the cycle of impulsive gratification followed by self-flagellation. Nothing healthy develops in a medium of self-hatred, rejection, and resentment.

We are all beautiful and imperfect. You can't postpone self-acceptance until after you've lost fifty pounds or switched jobs or found a partner. Start where you are. You need to call a piece of earth a garden before it can bear flowers. You have to cordon off a square of weeds and rocks before you work the soil and plant the seeds in order to cultivate anything. This is a case of "act as if." If loving care is not applied first, there will be no forward movement. You can't care for something you don't care about.

Often, behaviors can change brain chemistry. Smiling can improve your mood, and breathing deeply can immediately calm you. Feeling the stillness and the calm inherent in nature can help you to be the same. Green psychiatry, as I see it, is using nature to heal your psyche. Being outside in the grass and trees, bathed in sunlight, eating plants, honoring your appetites, and accepting your natural body (less perfume, shaving, and silicone parts) are the building blocks for decreasing stress and improving mood. *Be natural* to be healthier and happier.

Many of the solutions in *Moody Bitches* involve not only embracing nature and what is natural for us as human animals but also integrating the many forces that pull us in opposite directions. These opposing demands exist in all parts of our lives. They are part of what makes marriage so hard and transitions between work and home life so awkward. It is difficult to find a balance between living in your mind, on your computer, and getting back into your body so you can move it and not lose it. It is challenging to walk the line between millennia of cultural dictates that demonize female sexual pleasure while battling our evolutionary design for joy and promiscuity. It is a struggle to slake our thirst for the luxury of unscripted time amid the regimented schedules of our lives.

We can't avoid these opposites in our lives, and we shouldn't try to. Finding balance between two poles is what health and wholeness are all about. Learn to cultivate a healthy interplay between work and play, between movement and stillness, between rational and emotional. Becoming mentally healthy involves integrating and harmonizing disparate parts of our selves. For a woman, this means accepting the boy inside of her who wants to compete, to score, to lead. But it also means getting reacquainted with the girl who's vulnerable and open.

People resonate with authenticity, so go ahead and be yourself, speak your mind, and follow your gut. *Act naturally*. We all have the capacity to be more powerful in our lives. Stop playing small, rationalizing that it helps others to feel more comfortable. It helps no one. Better to shine. It encourages all who see your light to burn more brightly. Lead by example. If you learn to use your moods, they will become your most powerful resource—personally and professionally, physically and spiritually.

As I have found in my office, no one prescription for better living is going to work for everyone. Our lives and our needs are complex and unique. Your individual genetics affect how you process everything from food to trauma. Some of my patients are making it out in the world unmedicated, while others require steady doses of antidepressants or mood stabilizers. Some of the women take SSRIs only when their incapacitating premenstrual symptoms come around, while others take them only in winter. But no matter what you decide, you can improve how you feel by learning more about how your body was made to function. My hope is that you will take in the advice I've offered in *Moody Bitches* and then let your own body be your master teacher.

Remember that the solutions you create for yourself as a single thirtysomething woman might not work when you're a forty-year-old new mom or when caring for aging parents while combating hot flashes. Jettison what is not serving you. Your body changes, your mind changes, your life changes, and the way you care for yourself will, too. Women are made to be in tune with the earth, cycling with the moon. In honoring the seasons and the tides, we learn to honor our own cycles. From the springtime of puberty through perimenopause, the autumn, we must attend to our bodies and all the changes they undergo. This includes making a sacred space for aging and death, an integral part of nature.

And if we attune ourselves to these cycles that are within and around us, we will feel that direct connection with something bigger than ourselves, and we will be more at peace. Be a wise woman, a healer, and a warrior for peace—yours and others'.

Acknowledgments

First, I'd like to thank the talented deep thinker Jeremy Wolff, for marrying me, fathering our children, and coming up with great ideas for *Moody Bitches* thereafter. I couldn't have done this without him. Deep gratitude goes to the wise women who shepherded this project from the beginning, Suzanne Gluck, my agent at William Morris Endeavor, and Ann Godoff at Penguin Press. To my two editor doulas who helped me to deliver this manuscript, shoulders and all, Ginny Smith Younce and Lindsay Whalen, I offer you large golden medals for bravery and perseverance in helping me to shape, mold, and otherwise extrude this book out of my brain. A huge thank-you goes to the meticulous genius copyeditor Randee Marullo, to Jane Cavolina, who wrangled the notes and citations, and to Noirin Lucas, associate director of copyediting at Penguin Random House. And Claire Vaccaro art directed a beautiful book.

Thank you Kathie Russo, who finished what Spalding had started long ago, which was to hook me up with the great and powerful Suzanne.

I'd also like to thank Erin Conroy, Eve Atterman, and Clio Seraphim at WME. I look forward to many happy years in your care.

There were two literary agents early on who helped me hone my pitch, Richard Pine and Jim Rutman, and I'm grateful for their time and advice. I hope they understand that, in the end, this book simply needed to be created by women.

Writer Michael Pollan fed me general wisdom on writing and publishing. For specific tidbits, I'd like to thank the following authors and researchers. For food: Orsha Magyar (neurotrition.ca). For pheromones and cycles: Winnifred Cutler. For sex: Daniel Bergner, Maryanne Fisher, Justin Garcia, Jim Pfaus, and Martie Haselton. For all things hormonal: Chris Creatura, C. Neill Epperson, Ellen Freeman, Irwin Goldstein, Tierney Lorenz, Lila Nachtigall, Jennifer Payne, and Sari van Anders. For sleep: Paul Glovinsky. For mind/body and addiction: Gábor Maté. For neurotransmitters and receptors: Charles Nichols. For inflammation: Elissa Epel, Vladimir Maletic, Charles Nemeroff, and Charles Raison. For evolution: Chris Ryan. For crying: my childhood friend Eileen Murphy. For neural circuitry: Zoran Josipovic. For the endocannabinoid system: Paul Bregman, Greg Gerdeman, Matt Hill, and Ethan Russo. For bacteria: Martin Blaser and Larry Forney. For herbal advice: Paulina Nelega.

Michael Hogan's grin when I secured MoodyBitches.com back in 2007 told me I was on the right track, and I appreciate his reading and supporting this project throughout. The same goes to the wise and lovely Alex McKay. Jessica Wolff, yet again, was a tremendous help with editing and talking. There are several women whose books and lectures helped to ground and nourish me through many years: Pema Chodron, Tara Brach, and Geneen Roth. I also feel compelled to thank my main writing environments, the Metro-North trains and the Hudson Valley and CLAMS libraries. My local librarians assured me this was a necessary book for women, and I know they're eager for their copies!

To my parents, Clare and Richard, and my sisters Ellen and Debbie, I thank you for your belief in me from the very beginning, and for your love. To my children, Molly and Joe, I owe you one summer vacation. Thank you for understanding how preoccupied I got. That goes for you, too, Jer. I love growing up with you.

Appendix

> ## Naming Names:
> ## A Guide to Selected Drugs

ANTIDEPRESSANTS

SSRIs (Prozac, Zoloft, Paxil, Celexa, Lexapro, Luvox, and Others)

Specific serotonin reuptake inhibitors do just that. They specifically block the reuptake of serotonin. They don't affect any other neurotransmitters, hence the term *specific*. Blocking reuptake means that more serotonin is available to get across the synapse to the next nerve cell, or neuron. Think of it this way: There is a pitcher neuron and a catcher neuron. The balls are the serotonin. The pitcher can scoop up any balls that aren't caught immediately with its mitt and throw them again, or just hold on to them. If you block the pitcher's mitt, there are more serotonin balls available to eventually be scooped up by the catcher's mitt. This blockage results in enhanced serotonin getting across to the catcher. This is referred to as increased serotonergic tone. Now, why this translates into feeling happy and relaxed is complicated and not well understood. There are changes that occur long term in the number of catcher's mitts produced; the postsynaptic neuron learns to accommodate the extra serotonin in the synapse by adjusting how many receptors there are. This is called downregulation. (If there were less serotonin in the synapse, the number of receptors would increase, called upregulation.) This up- and downregulation is the neurologic basis for tolerance to a drug. If you keep on taking a drug that increases a neurotransmitter level, you will eventually develop fewer receptors for that transmitter. So there are two stages to adapting to a new antidepressant: an immediate response to having more neurotransmitter available and then a delayed, more chronic response that involves the up- or downregulation of the receptors. There may also be a lag because of neuroplasticity and BDNF needing time to do its job. The bottom line is that these are the medications used to treat depression and anxiety, and they work slightly better than placebos in many patient groups and significantly better than placebos in other patient groups.

Not everyone who is depressed, anxious, or obsessive has measurably low levels of serotonin when you look at them in research settings, so very likely there are other things going on chemically that we have yet to fully understand. SSRIs, sometimes called serotonergic medications, are good for decreasing depression, anxiety, and obsessiveness. Obsessive-compulsive disorder is treated with SSRIs exclusively. The other types of antidepressants that affect other brain chemicals really don't work that well in OCD.

Unfortunately, increasing serotonin in your brain often translates into feeling less horny and making it harder to climax. Some SSRIs can make your pelvis feel numb, with decreased sensitivity of the genitals. Zoloft is well known for causing this problem. Most of the SSRIs make it take longer to climax, and sometimes the quality of the orgasm is reduced. This side effect is worse upon initiating the medicine and gets better over time, though for some people it is a lasting problem. In my experience prescribing these medicines, the SSRI with the fewest sexual side effects is Lexapro, but there can still be decreased libido and increased time to orgasm at higher doses. Other psychiatrists prefer Prozac, the original SSRI, which they feel is less likely to cause weight gain and sexual side effects. My issue with Prozac is that it has the longest half-life of any of the SSRIs. This means that even if you stop using the medicine, it stays in your system for days or weeks. One of the main advantages to using Lexapro, because it has a shorter half-life, is that you can stop it for a day or two and markedly decrease its blood level and therefore its side effects.

Celexa was my SSRI of choice until Lexapro came along. They are chemical sisters, more alike than different. Celexa works fine for many of my patients, but Lexapro seemed to be a bit "cleaner," leaving my patients less foggy and more mentally sharp. When I give my patients a prescription for Lexapro, I tell them to break the tablet in half to start. I usually start with the 10-milligram tablets, but sometimes I'll start with 5-milligram tablets in people who are very sensitive to medicine or have absolutely no history of taking anything that alters their brain chemistry. I recommend the half tablet for a few days (three to five) before going up to the full tablet. Also, it's better to take SSRIs on a full stomach or with food and not on an empty stomach, as nausea becomes much more likely. The presence of food protecting the stomach lining helps to diminish this side effect. (This is true for many medicines. In general, if a pill makes you feel nauseated, you should take it with food unless the bottle specifically states that you need an empty stomach for it to work, as is the case with Synthroid and some antibiotics.)

A big issue with many SSRIs is timing—when to take the pill. With Lexapro, many people find the best time to be late afternoon, three or four P.M. Sometimes taking Lexapro first thing in the morning will make you very sleepy after lunch (I call it the exaggerated siesta response), so taking it in the late afternoon will delay that sleepiness until closer to bedtime. Others get a lift from it and take it first thing in the morning after breakfast. Still others, though fewer, take it right before bed and it helps them to sleep. The only problem with taking it before bed is that it can enhance the vividness of your dreams. It doesn't cause nightmares but may give you very intense and memorable dreams that seem quite real. Also, I occasionally hear about people feeling a bit hungover in the morning if they take it before bed. It's harder to get out from under your warm blanket. So I tend to recommend "tea time" as the best time to take Lexapro; the only problem with that is remembering to take it, which is crucial in order for it to work! The bottom line with the timing issue is that you really have to experiment and figure out which of those three types of people you are. And if late afternoon works best for you, set an alarm on your cell phone or anchor it to something you do regularly that time of day, like picking up the kids from school or hiding from your boss.

As for the other SSRIs, there are a slew of them, and they all have different side-effect profiles. As there are serotonin receptors in the stomach, many of these medicines can cause nausea or stomach upset. I don't prescribe Zoloft much because when it first came out, we referred to it as "the puke drug." Nausea, vomiting, diarrhea, and stomachaches were big problems in my patients. I have a colleague I respect tremendously who uses Zoloft preferentially, though, and it is widely prescribed by many other physicians, so obviously not everyone feels the way I do. (I have a theory on how Zoloft became so popular with internists. They saw drug reps from Pfizer who gave them samples of medicines for blood pressure and threw in some Zoloft for their depressed patients.)

Paxil is another SSRI I don't typically prescribe. It tends to be sedating and makes people feel hungover the next morning when they take it at night. It has actions similar to Benadryl, an antihistamine, and can also cause increased appetite and weight gain more often than some of the other meds. Also, it is tricky to discontinue due to its short half-life.

In my experience, Paxil is the SSRI that is hardest to stop, with the most significant withdrawal syndrome. There is an extended-release version, Paxil CR, that is easier to taper off.

So let's talk about that whole withdrawal issue. While it isn't as much of an issue with SSRIs as it is with the SNRIs (see the section below), it can be a bit uncomfortable to come off these medicines. It is important to slowly taper the dose over several weeks so that you can avoid the headaches, spacey feelings, and disorientation that can come from abruptly discontinuing the medicine. I have a number of patients who notice that if they miss a day or two of their SSRI they are irritable, grumpy, or angry. They have a shorter fuse than usual. Other people feel acutely depressed when they miss a few doses of their medicine.

There is some literature that shows that if someone is in the bipolar spectrum, SSRIs can aggravate rather than ameliorate some symptoms, so it is an important distinction. People with a history of manic episodes shouldn't take SSRIs, and even sometimes people with bipolar relatives would be better off with a different medication choice. (I often choose Lamictal for these folks. See below.)

SNRIs (Effexor, Effexor XR, Cymbalta, and Pristiq)

This second group of antidepressants blocks the reuptake of serotonin and norepinephrine (similar to the brain's adrenaline). These antidepressants are particularly good for anxiety and panic disorder, and they work very quickly, often relieving depressive symptoms within a week. Effexor was a popular choice at Bellevue when I was working there, because we would start to see the antidepressant effects kick in within three or four days. Like the SSRIs, they also make it difficult to achieve orgasm and can cause weight gain in some people.

Unfortunately, this group of antidepressants has more of a discontinuation syndrome than the SSRIs. Effexor withdrawal is legendary.

Google it and you'll see. I have heard patients going through withdrawal complain of the following: nausea, dizziness, disorientation, extreme anxiety, agitation, electric shocks running from their head to their arms (sometimes called brain zaps), feeling their brain move inside their skull, feeling their vision lag behind their eyes, and feeling something like cold water running down their spine. I had one patient who obtained relief only by locking herself in her closet and screaming; this was a mild-mannered gal, not a screamer. When she got online, she was relieved to see that other people had taken this approach to dealing with their discomfort. I had another patient feel so out of it, disoriented, and ditsy that he almost got hit by a cab crossing the street. I have learned not to be too surprised when I hear about people's experiences trying to get off Effexor. Most important, I have been able to assist people in their attempts to get off it by starting them on an SSRI (either Lexapro or Prozac) prior to doing a slow taper of the Effexor. Cymbalta is another SNRI that is difficult to discontinue, but it isn't as legendary as Effexor in difficulty.

Cymbalta, which has received FDA approval to treat fibromyalgia, is touted as an antidepressant that also helps with pain syndromes. All the SSRIs and SNRIs can help with any types of pain, but especially neurogenic pain, the tingling that occurs from nerve pressure. Because SNRIs do things that SSRIs don't (mainly, they affect a second neurotransmitter system, norepinephrine, that the SSRIs don't affect), if you have a partial response to an SSRI, it makes sense to try an SNRI to see if you can have a more robust response.

Wellbutrin, Wellbutrin SR, Wellbutrin XL, and Zyban (Bupropion)

The makers of Wellbutrin don't give a lot of information about how it works, except to say it doesn't increase serotonin. As such, it doesn't do much for obsessiveness or anxiety, but it's great for certain types of depression. It seems to enhance dopamine function, so if you have a low-energy, foggy, can't-get-off-the-couch type of depression, Wellbutrin can be a great choice. It often increases energy, concentration, and motivation. What's even better, it reliably decreases appetite, helps with willpower (making it to the gym, sticking to your meal plan), and has no sexual side effects. Some women even find that it's easier to climax and that they have more libido on Wellbutrin.

The biggest downside with Wellbutrin is initiating the medicine. The first few days are tricky. Many people feel "speedy" when they start taking it, like they've had too much coffee. Also, it can cause difficulty falling asleep. Taking the pill after eating a meal first thing in the morning can help. Also, I have found that it helps to eat a little bit of protein throughout the day on the first few days, like a hard-boiled egg or some almonds. Eventually, the jitteriness smooths out, but it can be a tough ride in the beginning.

One caveat: if irritability and a short fuse are issues for you, Wellbutrin can make that worse, especially at the higher doses. Wellbutrin comes in immediate release, SR, and XL. In my experience, XL is the best, but it's also harder to get started on than SR because the lowest dose isn't all that low. Sometimes I'll start people on a lower dose of the SR formulation and then switch over to the XL.

Many people need only a half dose of Wellbutrin XL (150 milligrams) instead of the 300-milligram maintenance dose. If someone can't get by without the 300-milligram dose, I'll often add a small amount of Lexapro to counter the edginess. Adding a second medicine to counteract side effects of the first is never a good idea, except here. The combination of Wellbutrin and Lexapro does fabulous things. Between the two of them, they are like buckshot, knocking down every symptom of depression and anxiety. And their side effects cancel each other out, to some extent, so the low libido and potential weight gain with SSRIs can be countered by adding Wellbutrin. Also, the low motivation and lackadaisical side effects seen in higher doses of SSRIs can be countered by adding a bit of Wellbutrin. Many of my patients are on this combination, and I look forward to the day when some genius in the pharmaceutical industry realizes they should just make one pill with both these medicines bundled together.

Remeron (Mirtazapine)

Remeron is considered a tetracyclic, a medicine that effectively increases serotonin in multiple ways, but not by blocking the reuptake site as SSRIs do. It blocks certain serotonin receptors (5-HT2A, B, and C, and 5-HT3). It also increases norepinephrine transmission, as Effexor and Cymbalta do. It can help with anxiety and is quite sedating, making it a good choice for people with insomnia. It also can quell nausea, vomiting, and irritable bowel symptoms. The main drawback is that many people experience increased appetite and weight gain from Remeron, but in the right patient this can be a plus. (People who are chronically ill or anorectic, for instance.)

Tricyclics and MAOIs

These are older versions of antidepressants that are seldom used anymore. The tricyclics (Elavil, Anafranil, Tofranil, Pamelor, Vivactil, and many others) are quite effective at treating depression, as they raise levels of two neurotransmitters, serotonin and norepinephrine, by blocking their reuptake. The problem is the signal-to-noise ratio, or the positive effect to side-effect balance. Even though they block those two transporters, they also hit a lot of other neurotransmitter receptors, so you pay a pretty high price for efficacy with dry mouth, constipation, difficulty climaxing, and sedation. Also, they are dangerous in an overdose, as opposed to the SSRIs, which have a much wider margin of safety. There are still some psychiatrists who prescribe them, but not many. I am not among those who do. That goes for MAO inhibitors also. These medicines (Nardil, Marplan, Parnate) prevent the breakdown of many neurotransmitters, including serotonin, norepinephrine, and dopamine, thus increasing their levels, but you have to follow a strict diet and avoid many medications (including cough and cold preparations) or you risk having a marked rise in blood pressure. There are newer MAOIs that don't require much in the way of diet restrictions, including a patch called Emsam, but it's not a medication that I typically prescribe.

A word about antidepressants in general: while some increase serotonin and others enhance norepinephrine or dopamine, many have one underlying effect in common, called hippocampal neurogenesis. It turns out that the brain can grow new neurons, new connections, especially if brain-derived neurotrophic factor gets involved. BDNF is increased by many antidepressants and results in new brain cells being formed and new connections being made. But exercise does the same thing, people. Numerous studies have shown that regular cardio enhances BDNF and hippocampal neurogenesis. This is why when my patients ask me about getting off the meds, the first thing we start to talk about is an exercise regimen. Neurogenesis is a delayed effect of the antidepressants, taking weeks to fully kick in. Sometimes my patients start to feel better very quickly when we start certain medicines (Lexapro, Viibryd, and Effexor seem to kick in more quickly), but most meds need a good six to eight weeks to fully settle in and do their job.

The two medicine groups that are immediate acting, instead of taking weeks to kick in, are the stimulants and the antianxiety medicines. In some ways, it makes more sense to consider these to be drugs instead of medicines because of their near-immediate effect.

STIMULANTS

Amphetamines like Adderall and Dexedrine help to give energy, motivation, focus, and concentration. They work within an hour. The main side effects are that they are stimulating, make it hard to calm down or to sleep, and also cut appetite. These medications were used for treating depression in the 1960s, until it was discovered that they can cause tolerance and dependence and that the withdrawal can bring about a horribly depressed mood. These days they are used almost exclusively for attention-deficit disorder, though many people try them out as appetite suppressants. (The problem here is that this effect diminishes over time, so they need to be used sporadically, if at all, for that indication.)

There is no quick and easy way to diagnose ADHD. The gold standard is a battery of neuropsychological testing that takes many hours and costs around one thousand dollars at a minimum. Many people come to my office having read an article on ADHD and feel fairly sure they have the diagnosis. There is a sense that their concentration and attention are faltering, and maybe their impulse control isn't 100 percent. Sometimes people undergo a trial of stimulants to see if they have ADHD, but the truth is, anyone who takes these medicines will experience an increased focus and less distractibility. Many of my patients who are taking stimulants have been on them since grade school and demonstrate clear signs of hyperactivity and inattention. But some of my patients take stimulants because they're sitting at desks in front of computers for a dozen hours a day and find that the prescriptions help them stick with their work for long stretches.

With Adderall and Dexedrine, there are tablets and capsules. The tablets come on a bit more quickly and peak and "crash" to some extent. They last about three or four hours. The capsules come on a bit more slowly and have a longer plateau with much less of a crash, lasting about six to eight hours. I often prescribe both the capsules and the tablets to my patients so that they can experiment with each and see which they prefer, though many of my patients end up using both of them throughout the week, depending on the demands on their time. Many people take a capsule earlier in the day and a tablet later on if they need more medicated time.

I usually start with the lowest dose, 5 milligrams. The tablets can be broken in half, unlike the capsules. For people who've never had stimulants before, I start with the tablet and have them break it in half, just to make sure they're not too sensitive to it and don't have some unforeseen problems with it. But most people don't really get by on 2.5 milligrams. They need either 5 or 10 milligrams. So they can start with a half, go up to one tablet, and if they need two, it's fine.

The most common side effect of stimulants is feeling a bit revved up, like you've had too much coffee. Interestingly, the people who really do have ADHD don't feel so stimulated; they feel calm and focused. (This is also their response to cocaine and speed, which can help to diagnose someone. Also, these are the people who can have a cup of coffee right before bed. Stimulants don't seem to rev them up as they do other people.) One of the many downsides of stimulant use is a headache when the crash comes (when it wears off). Also, importantly, it cuts your appetite quite a bit.

One word of advice I usually provide: eat before you take the medicine, so you won't be too ravenous when it wears off. One reason people notice the crash is that they haven't had anything to eat or drink for six to eight hours and so their stomach hurts and they have a headache. I encourage them to eat something like a salad or fruit or at least a protein bar at some point during the day, so their blood sugar won't tank. Also, don't take them too late in the day or it will be difficult to fall asleep.

There is an extended-release amphetamine medicine that lasts longer than the Adderall or Dexedrine capsules called Vyvanse, which lasts twelve hours or more. Some of my patients who have been taking stimulants for years and work very long hours appreciate what Vyvanse can give them.

You may be wondering why I haven't mentioned Ritalin, or the long-acting forms of Ritalin called Concerta or Metadate. I don't prescribe these ADHD medicines, and I don't think the medicines in this class work nearly as well as the amphetamines. When it was first introduced, Ritalin supposedly had a lower abuse potential, and it also didn't have the baggage of the amphetamines because it had a new name and was a new compound (methylphenidate). However, it really doesn't work as well as Adderall or Dexedrine in my experience (and my patients' experiences), and many psychiatrists, including me, think it actually is more likely to be abused. If someone comes to me and has tried both and is absolutely sure he or she prefers Ritalin, then I will acquiesce and prescribe it, but so far that has been a rare occurrence. Most people who come to me on Ritalin and switch over to Adderall or Dexedrine appreciate the new medicine.

BENZODIAZEPINES

Antianxiety drugs like Valium, Xanax, Klonopin, and Ativan belong to the family of medicines called benzodiazepines, often called benzos. These medicines help to soothe and calm anxious feelings. I had a mentor once who called them psychic pain relievers. A smaller dose will "take the edge off" anxiety, while a larger dose will put you in a zone where you simply don't care or react much to the storm outside the window. But take too much and you are "shlogged" or just plain asleep. There's an old movie with Goldie Hawn and Burt Reynolds where Goldie takes one too many Valiums and ends up with her face in a plate of egg salad. The real danger is mixing benzos with alcohol, which can cause coma or death but more commonly causes falls down stairs or off curbs.

One big difference between the antidepressants and the benzos is how quickly they work. The SSRIs and SNRIs can quell anxiety, but they will take days or weeks to do so. The benzos are more like drugs than medicines in that they work very quickly. Once your stomach has absorbed them and they are processed by your liver (not all of them are, though; Ativan and Serax do not get broken down by the liver), they then make their way to your brain, where they increase the transmission of a neurotransmitter called GABA. This chemical is an inhibitory neurotransmitter, and higher levels result in a brain that is less excitable. In an emergency room, if a patient comes in having a seizure, the doctors will inject benzos into a muscle or vein to stop the brain from misfiring. Orally, most benzos work within twenty to forty minutes, depending on how much food is in the stomach. (One way to make them work faster is to put the pill under your tongue, thus bypassing the stomach and liver. The veins beneath your chin will drain the medicine directly to your heart which will pump it to your brain. This is particularly common to do with Ativan, called lorazepam as a generic.)

The main side effect of benzos is that they make people sleepy and unfocused. One shouldn't drive or operate machinery and should never mix them with alcohol. Another problem is interference with memory consolidation. At higher doses, benzos can turn your brain into Teflon, and things don't stick as well. New memories aren't formed appropriately and so become irretrievable. The workplace is not the best environment for these medicines, and I typically advise patients with chronic anxiety who need to stay sharp that they're better off taking an SSRI or SNRI instead. The other big caveat is addiction. These meds can cause tolerance, dependence, and withdrawal. It is possible (though rare) to have withdrawal seizures if a chronic high dose is abruptly discontinued. Also, the issue of rebound anxiety is worth mentioning. If you take benzos consistently, especially Xanax, your brain comes to expect them, and when they wear off, the anxiety you're trying to quell comes back like gangbusters, often earlier and earlier, necessitating more frequent dosing of benzos or higher doses of them. In my practice, whenever possible, I encourage only intermittent, sporadic use of benzos and stimulants, which is the key to using them. Don't get into any patterns of regular use where your brain starts to expect a certain medicine at a certain time.

The most commonly used benzodiazepines are Ativan (lorazepam), Xanax (alprazolam), Valium (diazepam), and Klonopin (clonazepam). For panic and anxiety, all these medications work, but they have different times of onset and levels of sedation, so it can be challenging to find the right medicine for the job. The sedation is a very big deal. Many of my patients can't tolerate taking a benzo at work, for instance, because they get too cloudy and spacey. The trick is to cut the anxiety without completely wiping you out so that you feel as if you have to head to bed. Some people find Ativan to be the least sedating, and others notice Klonopin is better for them. It's very hard to predict which patient will like which medicine, so sometimes there's a bit of trial and error. Also, many people notice that after they take Xanax they are depressed or otherwise feel "off" the next day.

Delayed onset is a drag when you're dealing with a fifteen-minute panic attack, so Klonopin isn't a great choice for this because it takes up to an hour to fully kick in. One nice thing about Ativan is that you can dissolve it under your tongue to work more quickly than any of the others. With Ativan, sometimes there's delayed sedation, sometimes not. The usual dose is either .5 or 1 milligram (though at Bellevue we would give either 2 or 4 milligrams, depending on how agitated the patient was, and we would give it as an intramuscular injection).

Many people use benzos for fear of flying, and, depending on the length of the flight, there are many options. Klonopin lasts the longest, with a half-life of roughly twenty-four hours, so it's too long acting for most plane rides. It's a good choice for chronic anxiety, though. Klonopin is also a good choice to take before bed if you wake up with anxiety in the morning, as there is a bit of a hangover effect due to its long half-life. Typical doses are .5 or 1 milligram.

Valium is the only benzo that also relaxes skeletal muscles, so it's particularly good if you have tension headaches or tight neck muscles, or if you have a back spasm. It's medium to long acting, with a half-life of thirty hours, but it has an active metabolite with an even longer half-life. Typical doses are 5 or 10 milligrams.

Xanax is medium length, moderate onset, but often pretty specific to the brain and less so to the body (unlike Valium). Its half-life is around eleven hours. Dosages range from .25 to 2 milligrams. Sometimes you can find a dose of Xanax that is good for planes, like .25 or .5 milligram. Taking a bit once you are at the gate and a bit more once you're settled in your seat is what I often advise. The trick is to not be so sedated that you can't carry your baggage once you get off the plane. Your balance might be affected, as well as your coordination, and remember: don't drink any alcohol if you're taking benzos. Not on a plane or anywhere else. They act synergistically and the chances of falling are markedly increased. Also, some people get disinhibited when they take benzos, the way some get when they drink alcohol. A little too loose and loopy. So it's not always the best choice to take benzos before that big presentation in the conference room just because you're nervous. (Beta blockers, like propranolol, are a much better choice in this situation.)

MOOD STABILIZERS

The usual treatments for bipolar disorders are mood stabilizers like lithium, Depakote, or Tegretol. Many of the mood stabilizers in the current psychiatric armamentarium come from the field of neurology and are actually medications used to control seizures, thus called AEDs, anti-epileptic drugs. Lithium is the exception. It is not an epilepsy medication but rather a mineral, with a long history of being used as a "tonic" to soothe the nerves. Lithium was even an ingredient, once upon a time, in 7UP.

Lithium continues to be the gold standard for treating classic manic symptoms, but many people don't like the way it stifles their creativity, causes salt/water balance issues of excessive thirst and urination, and also puts their thyroid at risk. (Chronic use of lithium can often lead to hypothyroidism, for which people need to add Synthroid to their medication regimen.) Also, you need to monitor blood levels and make sure the kidneys are functioning adequately, so being on lithium means going to a lab to get blood tests. Even given these downsides, I do prescribe lithium frequently for my bipolar patients because it works. Usually, though, I use it in combination with another mood stabilizer so that the dose can remain quite low.

Depakote and Tegretol also require blood draws to check levels and make sure the liver and bone marrow are still doing their job; doctors have to monitor white and red blood cell counts, platelet levels, and liver function. Depakote can cause hair loss, acne, and swollen gums, and Tegretol is no picnic either, with nausea, vomiting, and blurred vision as potential side effects. These two meds are not for the faint of heart, but if you need them, you take them.

Lately, the second-generation antipsychotics are gaining traction in being used as mood stabilizers, and many are FDA-approved to treat bipolar disorder. These are medicines like Risperdal, Seroquel, and Abilify. (The first generation of antipsychotics, like Haldol, Prolixin, and Thorazine, don't typically have the mood-stabilizing properties of the second generation.) No need for blood draws goes in the "pro" column. In the "con" column are weight gain, sedation, and the potential for irreversible diabetes and movement disorders (tardive dyskinesia). These medications, while effective, are in no way benign. The problem is that bipolar disorder is hardly benign either. Suicide rates are very high when people are in either the manic or the depressive phases of the illness. And I've seen people ruin their marriages, their credit rating, and their children's serenity while in manic phases. Bipolar illness takes a toll on patients and families, and it is very tricky to treat. Balancing the risks and benefits of each treatment and tailoring the options to the patient's particular symptoms gets complicated; it's important to see a psychiatrist and not an internist if you have bipolar disorder. If you can find someone who specializes in bipolar treatments, so much the better.

Abilify (Aripiperazole)

In 2007, Abilify, a medicine formulated to treat schizophrenia, was approved by the FDA to treat depression, as an add-on medication. So if someone is on an SSRI or Wellbutrin and isn't having a robust response, she can augment her medication regimen with a small dose of Abilify. Abilify is also used as a mood stabilizer. In schizophrenics and bipolars, the typical dose is in the 15- to 30-milligram range. For depression, the range is 2 to 5 milligrams, which should lighten the side-effect burden, one would think, but in truth, Abilify can be a bit tricky to initiate due to its side effects. The drug company calls it activation, but it can feel like agitation. I warn my patients that they may feel more energetic and "antsy," and it's not uncommon to have some insomnia when starting Abilify. It has a very long half-life, so even if it's taken in the morning, it may lead to difficulty initiating sleep. Many people are better off taking it before bed, so the peak blood level comes during the day. I usually start with a 2-milligram dose and ask my patients to break it in half for the first few days. The activated feeling usually passes by the end of the first week or clears up as the dose is increased over time. I have some patients who end up on 5 milligrams, but many more stay in the 1- to 2.5-milligram range.

I do have several people with schizophrenia in my practice who are doing well on Abilify and quite a few with treatment-resistant depression who require a combination of antidepressant and low-dose Abilify.

Lamictal (Lamotrigine)

Lamictal has become increasingly popular among psychopharma-cologists, but is rarely considered by internists trying to treat their depressed patients. A great medication for depression or anxiety with no sexual side effects and no weight gain, Lamictal is well tolerated with minimal side effects, if you can get past one big issue: a very serious rash that is often described as life threatening. Stevens-Johnson syndrome is a dangerous potential reaction to many medications, especially mood stabilizers, including Tegretol and Lamictal. To decrease its likelihood, you need to go up very slowly on the medication; this is called a slow titration. The Lamictal titration is typically prescribed over a six-week course: 25 milligrams for two weeks, 50 milligrams for two weeks, 100 milligrams for a week, then 125 milligrams for a week, finally stopping at 150 milligrams, which is when you might start seeing some results. Sometimes people don't turn a corner until a higher dose, and it takes time to find the right one. Given the six-week titration schedule and then fishing around for where the person will remain dosewise, Lamictal isn't for those patients who are in a hurry to feel better. It's a good medication to choose when someone comes to me already on another medicine but only getting a partial response, when we have the luxury of time. Also, it's a great choice if you've been on a bunch of antidepressants and they all work well at first but then "poop out" after a year or two, or if you've tried SSRIs, SNRIs, and Wellbutrin but nothing has worked. Lamictal often works when nothing else does, and it's very subtle. With many medicines you can feel side effects, or you can somehow sense when you've taken the medicine versus when you've missed it. You feel medicated. Most of my patients don't feel like they're taking any medicine when they're on Lamictal. They just notice an absence of symptoms.

PROSEXUAL MEDICINES

The short answer is that there are currently no FDA-accepted medications that can reliably induce sexual arousal in women, but, rest assured, Big Pharma is working on it. However, the FDA has already shot down several prosexual drugs for women. I often wonder if the FDA won't approve any proposed sex drug that works too well because they fear these pills will turn women into impulsive, uncontrollable sex fiends, and society as we know it will break down. Or perhaps they're worried about the drug falling into the wrong hands and being used as a date-rape drug. While I sympathize with the latter concern, it doesn't explain the holdup in this approval process. (See the perimenopause chapter for more on this.)

Prosexual Meds Currently Available by Prescription

Testosterone, the hormone most responsible for sexual interest, desire, and some part of sexual response in women, is FDA approved only for use in men. Some doctors will prescribe small doses of testosterone for women, but it is considered an off-label use. Desired effects include a boosting of sex drive, clitoral enlargement, and increased frequency of sexual activity and thoughts. Undesirable side effects include weight gain (mostly due to muscle mass), acne, increased facial (and upper thigh) hair, and possibly liver problems if administration is oral. If you use sublingual drops or spray or a transdermal cream or patch, you bypass the liver issues. Pregnant women should never take testosterone, as it will cross via the placenta and affect the baby's development.

Normal testosterone levels in women run between 14 and 76 nanograms per deciliter, with the most common range between 20 and 50 nanograms per deciliter. The ideal dose of testosterone is between .25 and 2 milligrams per day in the pill form. For creams, it's a 2 percent cream applied three times a week at bedtime or thirty minutes before sex if the sex falls on a night when you aren't taking your dose.

Testosterone may well make you horny, engorged, lubricated, and more able to climax. It may also make you hairy, pimply, and a bit aggressive. I do have some patients who are taking testosterone prescribed by their gynecologists. It seems to work reliably in many of them, but the desire it stokes is indiscriminate. A man on the subway, your boss, and the pizza delivery boy all seem like reasonable sex partners. Remember, testosterone is not the hormone of monogamy; it is the hormone of novelty. Also, it causes more masturbatory behavior.

In women who have a primarily physical basis for their sexual dysfunction, such as female sexual arousal disorder, Viagra significantly improves sexual functioning. When taken by women, Viagra, Levitra, and Cialis do make genitals engorged and lubricated. For some women this will assist in arousal and even climax, but they do very little in terms of stoking desire. The Berman sisters researched Viagra on 48 prescreened women. It significantly increased the blood flow to the vagina, clitoris, labia, and urethra in all of them. The ability to climax increased in 67 percent of them, and more than 70 percent said they felt more sensation in the genital area during stimulation. In another of their studies, out of 202 women, 82 percent were more pleased with lubrication and sensation. Also seen were improvements in ability to orgasm, enjoyment during intercourse, and overall sexual satisfaction. It's important to note that the Berman studies eliminated women with low desire and low testosterone as well as those who would have responded better to psychotherapy. Another study, this time by Basson, showed that Viagra was no better than a placebo among 577 women who weren't screened the way the Berman studies' women were.

For Viagra, you'll need a prescription from your doctor and your insurance is unlikely to pick up the bill, though it'll pay for it for men. The dosage is 50 to 100 milligrams an hour before sex, on an empty stomach and with no alcohol on board. If you're not sure about the timing of when sex will occur, ask your doctor for Cialis, which lasts much longer. Neither of these is FDA approved for use in women yet.

Side effects can include nasal congestion, facial flushing, indigestion (possible worsening of gastroesophageal reflux disease, or GERD), and a temporary blue tinge in vision. You should avoid mixing it with nitrate medications or a dangerously low blood pressure can result. Also important, Viagra has been known to delay orgasm in men and women.

Buspirone (brand name Buspar) is a prescription serotonin agonist (5HT1A receptor). In studies with animals, the experimental serotonin agonist that works at the 1A receptor site, 8-OH-DPAT, was consistently shown to lower the threshold for ejaculation. Buspirone, which works at the same receptor site, was also shown to be effective. Clinical studies of women on SSRIs with sexual dysfunction showed that more than half improved when buspirone was added. Lybridos contains buspirone as its second ingredient, after testosterone (see below).

Cyproheptadine is a prescription serotonin antagonist (5HT2 receptor) that can mute the sexual side effects of SSRIs if taken before sex, but it's incredibly sedating, so you have to work fast.

Experimental Medicines in the Pipeline or Recently Rejected by the FDA

Lorexys is a combination of buproprion (found in Wellbutrin) and trazodone (Desyrel). These are two common antidepressants, one activating and one sedating, that may boost libido via dopamine enhancement. Clinical trials performed by developer S1Biopharma are under way.

Lybrido is a pill with an outer coating of testosterone and an inner core of Viagra. The testosterone enhances desire, arousal, and response, as well as triggering dopamine production for more pleasure. Viagra enhances blood flow, creating genital swelling, which ramps up sensation. The manufacturer (Emotional Brain) hopes to have FDA approval and distribution by 2016.

Lybridos is a pill with an outer coating of testosterone and an inner core of buspirone that slows down serotonin release, leading to short-term serotonin suppression, which improves desire and sexual response. The manufacturer (Emotional Brain) hopes to have FDA approval and distribution by 2016. Lybrido is about a year or so ahead of Lybridos in terms of clinical trials.

Flibanserin modulates serotonin in prosexual ways, thus turning down the inhibition and turning up the juice on desire. It is a 5-HT1A receptor agonist and 5-HT2A receptor antagonist (sort of like combining buspirone and cyproheptadine). It was rejected by the FDA in 2010, ten to one, due to the drug reportedly not being much better than a placebo, the side effects of dizziness, fatigue, and nausea outweighing the benefits in a study of eleven thousand women. Studies of prosexual drugs for men with fewer participants and more significant side effects have garnered FDA approval in the past, so the manufacturer (Sprout Pharmaceuticals) is resubmitting to the FDA in 2014.

Intrinsa is a testosterone patch for women developed by Procter & Gamble and rejected by the FDA in 2004. Remember the "women don't need this" line in the perimenopause chapter? The official party line is that they were concerned about "off-label use."

Libigel is a testosterone ointment that failed to sufficiently separate from a placebo in clinical testing in 2011 (Biosante). Phase III clinical trials were being conducted anew, with more than three thousand post-menopausal women enrolled, but are now at a standstill.

Luramist is a transdermal spray testosterone (developed by Vivus, then sold to Acrux) withdrawn from consideration for FDA approval in 2004, reconsidered for submission as of 2012, and now MIA. Acrux makes Axiron, a transdermal testosterone gel approved for use in men, instead.

Estratest was a popularly prescribed pill containing estrogen and testosterone combined in dosages of either 1.25 mg estrogens/2.5 mg methyltestosterone or 0.625 mg estrogens/1.25 mg methyltestosterone. The brand was discontinued in 2009 for mysterious reasons. There is a generic available called EEMT HS (esterified estrogens and methyltestosterone.)

Apomorphine is an FDA-approved medicine for the treatment of Parkinson's disease. It is a subcutaneous injection that stimulates the release of dopamine, resulting in feelings of pleasure and erections. It was also an experimental prescription medicine in a sublingual form called Uprima, rejected by the FDA in 2000 over concerns of nausea, vomiting, and fainting. The company Nastech had a nasal-spray form of apomorphine in 2000, but the trail goes cold when trying to track down what ever became of it. E-mail me if you know.

Bremalanotide (Palatin Technologies) was the most promising medicine to enhance sexual desire ever. I even bought stock in the company when I heard about it, which I have only done one other time and that was with Pfizer's Viagra. Delivered via nasal spray and stimulating the medial preoptic area of the hypothalamus (the so-called ground zero of desire), it sent extra dopamine surging in all the right areas. The FDA shot it down, citing nausea, vomiting, decreased appetite, and increased blood pressure. An injectable version is in the works, with clinical trials proceeding nicely. Given the FDA's track record on approving drugs that actually work to enhance women's desire, don't hold your breath here.

Phentolamine is available as a prescription medicine called Vasomax (for men) or Vasotem (for women) that works faster than Viagra and is safer to take with nitrate medicines. It is a blood-flow-enhancing agent combined with an alpha-adrenergic receptor blocker. Side effects include low blood pressure, diarrhea, and nasal congestion (sound sexy?). The drug is not FDA approved in the United States but is available in other countries (Brazil and Mexico).

APPETITE SUPPRESSANTS

Please, start with eating whole, raw foods, more protein, and fewer carbs, and avoid flour and sugar as much as possible. If you have any sense that dairy is making you gassy, cut that out, too. Add probiotics and omega-3 fatty acids to your supplements. And move your body. If things still aren't going in the right direction, you can try the following things to boost your efforts.

Prescription Meds for Appetite Suppression

Topamax, Phentermine, and Qsymia

Topamax can reliably cut appetite and stimulate weight loss, but you need to be careful of side effects. We doctors often call it dopamax, because it can make you stupid if you push on the dose. Cognitive complaints are common with this medication, from memory lapses to word-finding difficulties, so I usually use lower doses, typically 25 to 50 milligrams once or twice a day. It can often help with depression and headaches as well.

Phentermine is the half of Fen-Phen that wasn't taken off the market. (Fenfluramine, the other half, is a potent serotonergic medicine that can cause brain changes in serotonin nerve cells and was shown to cause heart valve disease and pulmonary hypertension.) Phentermine comes in both tablets and capsules, which are short acting and long acting, respectively. The tablets can be broken, so I often recommend that people start with half a tablet in case they're sensitive to its effects. I have patients who like this better than Adderall for the combination of appetite suppression and concentration.

Some doctors are combining Topamax and phentermine in their obese patients who want to lose weight. There is a brand-name pill that combines these two generic medications, called Qsymia. (Your guess on how to pronounce this baby is as good as mine, but keep in mind that you can typically take two generics more cheaply than one brand-name medicine.)

Adderall, Dexedrine, and Other Amphetamines

Back in the fifties, using prescription speed was the way to lose weight. Amphetamines were widely prescribed to dieting women. They do cut appetite, but this effect typically wanes over time. And if you continue to take them and increase the dose to chase that initial reaction, you run the risk of becoming psychotic or paranoid, hallucinating or thinking bugs are crawling all over you. It's rare, but if it happens to you, you're going to be hospitalized for longer than you'd like. Amphetamine-induced psychosis is notorious for taking a long time to clear—weeks, not days, which is how long cocaine- or PCP-induced psychoses take to resolve. So the best way to take these stimulants, if you're going to try them, is sporadically, with no pattern of use that your brain will adjust to, to avoid tolerance. But really, my advice is not to use them at all, unless you need them for ADHD.

Acomplia (rimonabant) is a medicine designed and marketed by Sanofi-Aventis that I was excited about when I heard it was in the pipeline. It is a cannabinoid receptor antagonist, which means it's like a pill to stop the munchies. Because it induced a depressed mood, it's not available in the United States, but my assumption is that there will be some other, more refined cannabinoid antagonist coming down the pike at some point that will cut appetite without making you miserable.

Belviq (lorcaserin) is a selective 5-HT2C receptor agonist. Activation of these receptors in the hypothalamus activates proopiomelanocortin production and consequently promotes weight loss through satiety.

PRESCRIPTION SLEEP AIDS

Ambien (Zolpidem)

Ambien (zolpidem) is the most often prescribed and most requested sleep aid in my office and the most maligned in the press. It is a powerful sleeping pill with some pretty quirky side effects. Number one is Teflon brain. Once it kicks in, in twenty or thirty minutes, nothing sticks. You will not lay down new memories. This is why I tell my patients to take it IN BED once they're done with EVERYTHING. No more e-mails, texting, phone calls, or Internet purchases, unless you want to have absolutely no recollection of what was said or done. I have a patient who used to wake up in the morning and see his cell phone on his pillow. Scrolling through the list of recent calls was a waking nightmare. Numbers of his ex-girlfriends. What did he say to them? No clue. I have heard of "Ambien sex," in case you haven't. Some women find it easier to loosen their inhibitions with Ambien. If you don't mind having no memory whatsoever of the event or what was said, give it a try, but to me, that's all pretty risky. You might say things you wish you hadn't or do things you'd typically not do, with a patchy memory at best of what went down. This is best for established couples with few secrets, not for early in the relationship or with casual partners.

Then there's the sleepwalking and nighttime eating. I have a number of patients who won't take Ambien anymore because it makes them raid the fridge after it kicks in. One guy woke in the morning to find the kitchen a mess, pots and pans everywhere. He'd cooked himself a full meal and had no recollection of preparing it. Others awoke to find empty ice cream cartons and candy wrappers littering their bedsheets. And we've all heard about people sleepwalking or driving their cars in the middle of the night erratically (Patrick Kennedy, Tiger Woods), blaming Ambien for at least some of their bizarre actions.

Besides these memory-related side effects, there is the issue of Ambien's half-life. It is short. It puts you to sleep but does not keep you there. Many of my patients pop awake three to four hours later and then have trouble getting back to sleep. The joke I always make in my office is, "Ambien sings you a lullaby and rocks you to sleep, but then it slams the door on the way out." I often recommend that people take half a pill before bed and save the other half by their bedside for when they wake up. I call this the "poor man's Ambien CR." The controlled-release version of Ambien automatically gives you that second dose in the middle of the night, but the problem for many of my patients is that it's not sufficiently front-loaded to knock them out adequately in the beginning of the night. The upside is that after years on the market, they're both finally generic, and I do have some patients who combine a bit of immediate release with the long-acting version. But they need to be careful about the total dose. Ambien comes in 5 milligrams and 10 milligrams, but the 5s are usually right for most people. Older people should take even less. Ambien CR comes in 6.25 milligrams and 12.5 milligrams. If you break them, you lose the controlled release aspect of them, so it's not recommended.

Many of my patients notice that if they take Ambien nightly, sometimes it just doesn't seem to work. It's a bit unreliable. There may be a cumulative tolerance issue that develops, and so you need to take breaks in using it. Actually, it isn't recommended (or FDA approved) for chronic use but, unfortunately, many people are taking it that way. The other downside of Ambien is that it really doesn't work well on a full stomach, so if you're a late dinner eater, you're out of luck. There are some sublingual versions of zolpidem that you can put under your tongue. Remember, sublingual administration bypasses the stomach and the liver, so these meds will always work faster; what time you eat becomes irrelevant. The sublinguals Edluar (impossible to pronounce) and Intermezzo are both brand names and expensive for now, but they'll go generic eventually.

Lunesta (Eszopiclone)

Lunesta (eszopiclone) is like Ambien but better for many of my patients in that it works more reliably, especially on a full stomach. Lunesta lasts a bit longer, with less of the middle-of-the-night bouncing up, fully awake. And from my patients, at least, I have had no reports of night eating or "drunk dialing." One downside is its own quirky side effect. At least 10 percent of the people who take Lunesta (16 percent at 2 milligrams, 33 percent at 3 milligrams) get something called metal mouth, waking up with a horrible taste on their tongue, as if they'd slept with a few pennies in their mouth. Most things you drink or eat taste funny, and brushing your teeth makes no difference because there isn't a coating on your tongue. This is a neurological side effect, meaning it's mediated through your nervous system. It's harmless and it fades as the day progresses, but for the one out of ten who get this side effect, it's usually a deal breaker. Lunesta comes in 1-, 2-, and 3-milligram tablets. Don't break them; they taste horrible. For what it's worth, I don't get metal mouth and this is my favorite sleeping pill when I need something stronger than the herbal remedies.

Sonata (Zaleplon)

Even shorter acting than Ambien, Sonata (zaleplon) is great for people who have trouble falling asleep but not staying asleep. And it's even better for those who fall asleep fine but wake in the middle of the night and can't get back to sleep, because it clears your system in time for you to take it pretty late at night and still get up for work. It's been around long enough to be a cheap generic, and most of my patients like it. If you're a restless sleeper with insomnia that lasts all night long, it's not a good choice, but for most other people, it's worth a try. It comes in 5- and 10-milligram doses.

Benzodiazepines for Sleep

Restoril, Xanax, Klonopin, and Ativan are all potentially good sleeping pills in the benzodiazepine family. They each have a different half-life and, therefore, a different hangover potential. Klonopin lasts the longest and has a morning carryover effect, so it's particularly good if you have trouble not only falling asleep but are also waking up anxious. Typical doses are .5 to 1 milligram, but it takes awhile to kick in, so you may need to take it an hour before bedtime. Restoril is medium acting and is a good choice for most people. I usually prescribe 15 or 30 milligrams. Ativan is shorter acting and, for some, less sedating, but if all the other benzos leave you hungover, it's the one to try. A dosage of .5 or 1 milligram will help decrease nighttime anxiety to allow for sleep, but at Bellevue we would give 2 milligrams to really knock someone out. Xanax is its own special little complicated benzo. Medium to long acting, sedating for many, it's great for killing anxiety. If your insomnia is all about worrying, then this is the one for you. But I have many patients who feel that they're a bit depressed and "off" the day after they take Xanax for sleep, so it isn't for everybody. Doses range from .25 to 1 milligram.

I don't like to give benzos for sleep induction. People get used to their effects and need higher doses as tolerance becomes an issue. I limit their use to treating anxiety, but many other doctors prescribe them for insomnia. Also, benzos should never be combined with alcohol, and they have a higher potential for abuse, physical dependence, and withdrawal than other medicines, so you really need to watch your dosing and frequency. Being honest with your prescriber about how you're taking it is your first and best line of defense against misuse and addiction.

Trazodone

Trazodone is a medicine that's been around for a long time (and so is generic) and was originally used as an antidepressant. It has a low potential for abuse and there's no tolerance, so it's a good choice for people with addiction issues. The problem for many of my patients is that it makes them feel kind of crappy in the morning, headache-y and a bit hungover, but that typically goes away pretty quickly once they shower, have a cup of coffee, etc. Doses range from 50 to 150 milligrams to induce sleep. (Doses for treating depression are higher.)

One of the very rare side effects of trazodone, or so I was taught in medical school, is that it can induce an erection that doesn't go away, called priapism. When I was a fourth-year student at Temple, we had a brain-damaged patient who was given trazodone nightly so that he (and the nightshift) could have a quiet night. He never spoke to me, but every morning I had to go into his room and check his diaper to make sure he didn't have a hard-on. He never did. But still, I had to do my job, five days a week. One day I didn't get there until lunchtime, and when I came in to have a peek at his penis, he croaked out, "I've been waiting for you." I almost wet my pants. No one had ever heard him speak!

Rozerem (Ramelteon)

This is a prescription sleep aid that acts like melatonin, hitting the same receptor that melatonin hits (so it's a called a melatonin receptor agonist). The few times I prescribed it, my patients reported feeling strange and trippy, so I stopped. I e-mailed many of my colleagues to find out their experiences and received responses like "It doesn't work, so I stopped prescribing it" and "My patient got crazy high from it." The makers of Rozerem point out that it doesn't hit the benzodiazepine receptors and so has a low potential for abuse, but when you do a search on drug users' networks, it does come up as having a "weed-like high . . . especially if you've already had a good night's sleep and take it during the day." It comes in 8-milligram tablets, to be taken thirty minutes before bed.

Tricyclics

These are older antidepressants that have fallen out of favor for treating mood disorders due to side effects like sedation, dry mouth, trouble initiating urination, and constipation. But some of them are still used at nighttime to induce sleep, especially in people with pain syndromes, particularly neuropathy, or with depression or anxiety (and by older doctors who haven't learned new tricks). Elavil is a popular tricyclic used for sleep in doses that range from 10 to 100 milligrams, as are Sinequan (doxepin) and Pamelor (nortriptyline).

Remeron, Cymbalta, and Paxil

These are the more sedating antidepressants. If you're depressed, anxious, and have insomnia, these medicines might be good choices for your doctor to make for you. But all three of them can cause weight gain, so they're not too popular in my office!

Seroquel

This is an antipsychotic medicine initially formulated to treat schizophrenia and is also FDA approved to treat bipolar disorder or as an add-on in depression pharmacotherapy. Doses of 200 to 800 milligrams are used for these major psychiatric illnesses, but many doctors prescribe 25 or 50 milligrams to induce sleep. I personally don't prescribe antipsychotics unless someone is psychotic, due to serious side-effect possibilities (movement disorders, metabolic syndrome, or irreversible diabetes). But many doctors do reach for this prescription for their patients with insomnia. The most common issue with Seroquel is weight gain. I have one older gal with horrendous, debilitating insomnia who swears by her Seroquel as she pats her roll of belly fat, telling me it's the "cost of doing business," but as I want to stay in business, I don't typically prescribe this one.

NONPRESCRIPTION SLEEP AIDS

Benadryl

Used commonly by tons of people, this one doesn't require a doctor's prescription and is cheap and plentiful at every drugstore. For most people, 25 or 50 milligrams will knock them out for the night. Downside?

Dry mouth, hangover, and waking up foggy as all get-out. There are more significant cognitive complaints in some people, especially the elderly. It's definitely not good for anyone with Alzheimer's. It's great for people with allergies or a cold, as it dries you out as well as sedating you, though this can mean trouble for your sinuses, including pain and inflammation. Many over-the-counter sleeping pills, like Sominex, Unisom, Sleep Eze, and Nytol, have generic Benadryl (diphenhydramine) or doxylamine (another antihistamine) as their active ingredient.

PRESCRIPTION DRUG ABUSE: OPIATE PAINKILLERS AND ADHD MEDS

A small proportion of Americans are addicted to cocaine and heroin and an even smaller percentage of those are women. Where women *are* gaining ground is in the painkiller department. Sales of opiates (those medicines derived from the poppy flower) like oxycodone (Percocet), hydrocodone (Vicodin) and OxyContin (a long-acting oxycodone) have ballooned, and deaths from overdoses have tripled during the past decade. Between 1991 and 2010, prescriptions for these medications in America increased from 30 million to 180 million, a six-fold increase. The manufacturing of the drug oxycodone increased from 8.3 tons in 1997 to 105 tons in 2011, an increase of 1,200 percent.

In our nation of quick-fix answers, our medicine cabinets are full. We are 5 percent of the world's population, yet we account for about 80 percent of the world's pain medicines. We have enough painkillers to keep every American adult medicated around the clock for a month.

Too many opiates and you simply stop breathing. More people are killed by prescription opiates than by heroin and cocaine combined. Emergency room visits related to the abuse or misuse of pharmaceuticals are more common than those for illicit drugs, 435 versus 378 per

100,000. Motor vehicle accidents were always the number one cause of accidental death in the past. Now, in more states, it's overdose deaths that are number one. And according to the National Institute of Drug Abuse, women are more likely to be prescribed painkillers than men, and they're more likely to use these drugs nonmedically. A CDC report (2013) showed that the use of opiate painkillers by women has quintupled since 1999 and that overdose deaths are rising faster among women than among men. Younger women in their twenties and thirties tend to have the highest rates of opioid abuse, but the overdose death rate was highest among women ages forty-five to fifty-four, where the drugs were often prescribed for pain.

So why are women more vulnerable to opiate use, misuse, and addiction? One reason is that women naturally somaticize, or convert anxiety and psychic pain into physical aches and pains. Feeling tense, put-upon, and burdened translates into backaches, neckaches, and headaches. Fibromyalgia, a syndrome of achy muscles and joints typically treated with antidepressants, is a good example. (But please consider a diagnosis of Lyme disease if you live in a tick-infested area, before you assume it's fibromyalgia.)

Sometimes we say yes to everyone's requests, piling on more responsibilities for ourselves by accommodating and gratifying others, until our bodies finally say no. Also, women with a history of childhood sexual abuse are more likely to somaticize than others, and there's no question that these women are overrepresented among the ranks of addicts.

The truth is, opiates feel great—you feel warm all over and everything seems all right. They soothe many aches and pains and offer psychic pain relief as well. It is easier to suffer the slings and arrows of everyday life with an analgesic on board, and it's very easy to hide an addiction to pills. Pinpoint pupils can give you away, but if people don't know to look for that, there's really no other outward sign that you're high on painkillers, except an easily overlooked slackening of the facial muscles and droopy eyelids. Your breath doesn't give you away as it does in alcoholism or nicotine addiction, and you don't typically stumble around or slur your speech. And when it's easy to hide, it just adds to the adrenaline charge of the duping delight.

Many treatment options are available for opiate addiction, including buprenorphine (a replacement drug similar to methadone except that it blocks the brain from getting high on your drug of choice), acupuncture, supplements like DLPA (an amino acid that helps you make endorphins), and, of course, rehabs and twelve-step programs.

As always, the first step is admitting that you have a problem and you need help. No easy feat for anyone, but especially the working mother who does it all seamlessly. While painkillers may work for some, others opt for stimulants instead. Pills like Adderall, Ritalin, and Dexedrine are typically prescribed for children with ADHD, but they are also prescribed in growing numbers for adults.

Supermoms may take ADD medicines so they can do more and last longer, all while running on empty. Between 1991 and 2010, prescriptions for stimulants increased from 5 million to 45 million, a nine-fold increase. High school and college-aged kids are a huge black market for study pills like Adderall, Ritalin, and Dexedrine, but it turns out moms like prescription speed, too. Like cocaine and methamphetamine (speed), ADD meds increase the amount of dopamine available in the brain, enhancing concentration, cutting appetite, and making it easier to stay awake longer. The downsides are headaches and stomachaches when the pills wear off and the need for higher doses more frequently if the use becomes long term.

Many of my patients on ADD meds notice that although they become more efficient and productive, their social skills and empathy are sacrificed in the process. One of my patients only takes her ADD meds when she has paperwork to do, not when she has clients to meet, noticing that she is unable to engage in small talk or warm eye contact. "With the

Adderall, I turn into 'laser-brain,' wanting to cut through all required niceties to get to the knot and untangle it. I'm too intense and in too much of a hurry."

I have a patient with horrendous ADD. If she comes to my office in the morning before she's taken her medicine, it is nearly impossible for me to get a word in edgewise as she talks in circles, never quite arriving at her destination. She tells me her daughter starts many of her sentences with, "Mommy, focus!" For her, the Adderall isn't a luxury or a drug of abuse; it is truly the medicine her brain needs to function normally. What people need to understand is that everyone responds to stimulants in similar ways, with increased focus, concentration and impulse control, whether they have ADD or not. The difference between people who have ADD and those who don't is the stimulant effect. Unlike people without the diagnosis, who get jazzed and can't sleep, people with ADD can have caffeine, cocaine, speed, or Adderall and not feel very jacked up.

If you are prescribed stimulants for ADHD, stay conscious and mindful of your use; make sure you're honest with your physician about how often you're taking your medicine and under what conditions. I can help my patients who stay in touch with me about their patterns of use; it's the ones who keep the behavior hidden who miss out on my guidance. If you are abusing stimulants, it's important to seek help from a clinician who can help you wean yourself off. Abrupt cessation can cause a syndrome of very low energy and mood, not to mention a ravenous appetite bouncing back from being suppressed.

COCAETHYLENE

In New York City, people go out for a few drinks and end up in a bathroom stall snorting a line or two of cocaine. No big deal. Except it is.

Combining cocaine and alcohol actually creates a third drug in your system, cocaethylene, which is more toxic to your brain and heart than either drug alone. This is the only time ingesting two drugs creates a new one in your body. We know that alcohol kills brain cells and liver cells. Cocaine constricts blood vessels, which puts you at risk for heart attacks and strokes. Cocaethylene is even more likely to cause these two catastrophic medical situations.

Just say no to this combination.

MDMA (ECSTASY, MOLLY)

MDMA (methylene-dioxy-meth-amphetamine) used to be known as Ecstasy, but these days, it goes by the rebranded name Molly. MDMA is a potent serotonin releaser, causing most people to feel happy and relaxed. It is also a dopamine and norepinephrine enhancer, so people are awake, focused, and euphoric. What's unique about MDMA is that it also triggers oxytocin release, creating feelings of closeness and connection. Since the 1980s, this drug has been growing in popularity. Emergency room visits reporting Ecstasy use increased from roughly 4,500 to 10,000 between 2005 and 2011. (I do feel compelled to offer, for comparison, the emergency room visits related to misuse of prescription medications, which rose from 636,472 to 1,345,645 between 2004 and 2010.) I believe the rising popularity of this drug reflects our growing need for social cohesion in our digital age. We are more connected yet less. We are all communicating like never before, yet without touch, eye contact, or closeness. On the dance floor, you get all of the physical closeness you crave, plus the intense bonus of emergence. When a flock of birds turns all at once into a new direction, a slight ripple of delay detectable, you can see the phenomenon of group cohesion. Group mind is intoxicating, and universal consciousness is a common psychedelic-induced euphoria. Many people who make dance a regular part of their lives will tell you that the sensation is better than drugs.

Because of the increased demand for this unregulated drug, there has been rampant drug substitution. Counterfeit drugs that contain no MDMA are common. In the early 2000s, tablets sold as Ecstasy often contained combinations of chemicals, none of which were MDMA. In response to this, people started selling white powder and calling it Molly instead of ecstasy, with the understanding that Molly was pure MDMA powder, not like those adulterated tablets that were going around. Unfortunately, the truth is quite the opposite. In 2013, the DEA's Miami field office reported that out of 106 samples of seized Molly, 43 contained different substances: the most common substitutes are methylone and mephedrone, more commonly known as bath salts. Nineteen substances were so obscure they were unidentifiable.

Lesson number one: buying a white powder at a concert or nightclub is dangerous and unwise, even if it now carries the name of an innocent, freckle-faced little girl. There is no telling what chemicals you've just purchased, and pressed tablets are also no guarantee of purity. Lesson two: the behavior that accompanies Ecstasy use is often a bigger risk than the drug itself. With MDMA in a warm environment, there is an increased risk of heatstroke, so dancing for hours on end can lead to serious health risks. Also, MDMA causes water retention, especially in premenstrual women, so drinking too much water is also risky. MDMA, when used in medically supervised settings at a low dose, infrequently, without overheating or water intoxication, can provide therapeutic benefits. But in the recreational setting, where you don't know exactly what you're ingesting, dancing for hours without taking breaks, or drinking too much water, the risks outweigh any potential benefits.

CANNABIS

Cannabis is an ancient medicinal plant that has been used for thousands of years to decrease inflammation, nausea, muscle spasms, and chronic pain; induce sleep; and improve mood and appetite. Even if you don't smoke pot, your body uses its own cannabinoids to regulate nearly every bodily function.

Before it was rechristened marijuana, the scary Mexican slang specifically designed to conjure up frightening images of migrant workers made insane from loco weed, cannabis was known to doctors and patients alike as an incredibly useful medicine. Up until the late 1930s, it was a mainstay in the American pharmacopeia, used to treat ailments ranging from menstrual cramps to insomnia. Ignoring and even misrepresenting the AMA's request, Congress made cannabis illegal, mostly bowing to industrial interests against hemp, and renamed the well-known medicine using a smear campaign based on xenophobia. After the repeal of Prohibition, the federal machinery in place to enforce the ban on alcohol morphed into the one we have in place today, fighting the war on drugs.

America arrests and imprisons more people than any other nation on earth for nonviolent drug offenses, but it has done nothing to shrink the rates of drug abuse. We are the biggest consumers on the planet. Eighty-two percent of Americans believe we're losing the war on drugs and 78 percent believe cannabis should be legal, but our government spends more than fifty billion dollars every year invading our privacy, tearing apart families, targeting low-income communities, enriching drug cartels, and denying patients access to less toxic medicine.

In places with legal cannabis or medical dispensaries, fewer motor-vehicle fatalities and opiate overdoses are recorded. Every nineteen minutes in the United States someone else dies from an opiate overdose. Alcohol, which is associated with domestic violence, homicide, and suicide, causes 100,000 fatalities a year in the United States. Cannabis has no such associations. No one has ever died from an overdose, something you can't say about nearly any other prescription medicine or drug of abuse. Chronic pain patients can lower their use of opiates significantly and reduce their risk of overdose by adopting a regimen including cannabis, since they act synergistically. Curious about who's funding the war on medical marijuana? The makers of OxyContin and Vicodin, for starters.

If you are lucky enough to live in one of the growing number of states with medicinal cannabis laws, I encourage you to educate yourself about what this plant can do for you. (One place to start would be *The Pot Book*, a nonprofit book I edited, published in 2011.) What is most important with using cannabis or other drugs, or food for that matter, is if you are choosing to do it, honor the pleasure. If you are more conscious and conscientious, using drugs as a ritual sacrament imbued with meaning and inducing reverence, you will become less compulsive and destructive in your drug-taking behavior.

CIGARETTES AND HOW TO QUIT SMOKING

The percentages of people who try a drug and go on to become addicted are as follows: inhalants, 4 percent; psychedelics, 5 percent; sedative hypnotics (sleeping pills and antianxiety meds), 9 percent; cannabis, 9 percent; alcohol, 15 percent; sniffing cocaine, 17 percent; smoking cocaine (crack) and heroin, 23 percent; tobacco, 32 percent. Addiction to heroin and cocaine are distant seconds to the vicelike grip of nicotine dependence. Cigarettes are the most addictive drug known to modern science, and they kill half their users.

Here's how I get my patients to stop smoking cigarettes. First, we set up a taper schedule. This does two important things: it gives your brain time to adjust to receiving less nicotine, and it gives you time to say goodbye to your friend. If you smoke a pack a day, you make a timetable for cutting down to nineteen cigarettes a day, then eighteen, and so on. You can do this over twenty weeks, twenty days, or anything in between, as long as it's a consistent step-down schedule. Some of my patients slow down the schedule as they get to the last five cigarettes or so.

Next, you learn to substitute other behaviors when you're triggered to want a cigarette. Smoking consists of two things, sucking and breathing. Sucking releases endorphins and endocannabinoids, causing pleasure (if that weren't the case, babies would not suckle and survive), and deep breathing calms you down. Some people are helped in the process of quitting by sucking on spoons, their thumbs, or their tongue. But the most important thing is the breathing. Whenever you take that first drag of a cigarette, you take a deep breath, hold it in, and then let it out slowly. I tell my patients to go ahead and do the sucking and the breathing, but without the cigarette. Take a deep breath, hold it and let it out slowly, again and again (see the breathing exercises at the end of the downtime chapter). Whenever you're anxious, fidgety, or want to smoke, take a look at what is driving the behavior and write it down, and then get to work on regulating your breathing. As with regulating all drug use and abuse, the answer starts with consciousness. Be aware and in your body, not lost in a fog.

Quitting smoking is tough and often requires multiple attempts. It will be even harder if you're living with a smoker or if your lover or friends smoke. Acupuncture involving ear stimulation can help immensely, as can hypnosis. Nicotine replacement patches can be helpful if you'd rather step down that way instead of a cigarette taper, but I've seen too many people end up addicted to nicotine gum, so I don't typically recommend that to my patients.

An interesting side effect of the buproprion-containing antidepressants (Zyban, Wellbutrin) is that they seem to make cigarettes taste awful and not give you the same rewarding experience they used to, which is why Zyban is a popular prescription for smoking cessation.

The other medicine used for smoking cessation is Chantix (varenicline). It's not recommended for people who have any sort of psychiatric history, though. Every time I've prescribed it, my patients have gotten intolerable side effects, such as acutely depressed mood, suicidality, and crazy nightmares. It may work well in others without a psychiatric history, but I have no experience with this.

Glossary

Adrenaline—a chemical released from the adrenal glands that helps to raise heart rate and blood pressure, preparing the body to fight or flee; often accompanied by cortisol

Agonist—a chemical that activates a receptor in the brain or body

Amygdala—the fear center of the brain; associated also with aggression and anger (the plural is amygdalae)

Anandamide—the main internal cannabis molecule, or endocannabinoid, that enhances pleasure and appetite; helps to tamp down the stress response, and is metabolized by FAAH

Androgen—a classically "male" hormone like testosterone or DHEA (though these are present in women's bodies)

Antagonist—a chemical that antagonizes an agonist, competing for the receptor site or blocking it

Anterior cingulate cortex—a part of the brain where attention, emotion, and memory interact; responsible for emotional regulation and processing; felt to be overactive in depressive disorders

Antiandrogen—something that blocks production of an androgen, or its docking onto a receptor

BDNF—brain-derived neurotrophic factor, a chemical secreted by brain cells that fosters growth of neurons, driving neuroplasticity

BPA—bisphenol A, an artificial estrogen found in plastics that can cause breast cancer, among other illnesses and abnormalities

Cannabinoid—any cannabis-like molecule that stimulates the endocannabinoid system, often by binding to cannabinoid receptors

CB1—the cannabinoid receptor found in the brain

CB2—the cannabinoid receptor found everywhere else in the body, including the white blood cells, skeleton, muscles, liver, spleen, bladder, and uterus

Cortisol—a stress hormone released from the adrenal glands that acutely suppresses immune function and raises blood sugar levels; often released with adrenaline

CPAP machine—a medical device for sleep apnea that keeps the airway open via continuous partial airway pressure

Cytokine—small proteins important in cell signaling, often enhancing or dampening immune responses

DHEA—dehydroepiandrostenedione, an androgen found in men's and women's bodies; a precursor to testosterone

Dopamine—the neurotransmitter that underlies motivation and reward/pleasure

Dysthymia—chronic, low-level depression that lasts for years, not months

Endocannabinoid—internal cannabis-like molecules like anandamide and 2AG (2-Arachidonoylglycerol)

Endocannabinoid system—a bodywide system to fight inflammation, maintain metabolism, and enhance resilience (sometimes abbreviated ECB; the endocannabinoid system is often abbreviated ECS)

Endocrine system—the network of hormone-producing glands, including (but not limited to) pituitary, thyroid, adrenals, and ovaries

Endorphin—an internal opiatelike chemical that activates the opiate receptor, causing pain relief or pleasure

Executive function—the frontal cortex's role in planning, analyzing, paying attention, problem solving, and time management, among other things

Frontal cortex—the front part of the brain that helps to inhibit "lower" impulses from the emotional center (limbic system)

Ghrelin—the hormone that makes your stomach growl, stimulating hunger and feasting

Hippocampus—the brain's memory center; tamps down reactivity in the amygdala

Hypothalamus—the part of the brain involved in balancing temperature and appetite regulation, circadian rhythms, sexual desire, and other functions via hormone release

Kynurenine—a metabolite of serotonin; increased levels are associated with depression and inflammation

Leptin—the hormone that tamps down hunger, turning off the eating switch

Limbic system—a circuit of brain structures involved with motivation and emotion, among other things

Major depression—a mood disorder characterized by at least two weeks of low mood as well as changes in sleep, appetite, and energy level; a.k.a. chemical depression or clinical depression

Major histocompatibility complex (MHC)—molecules on the surface of cells that help to dictate immune responses and compatibility, as in organ transplants

Menarche—the very first menstrual period

Norepinephrine—an activating neurotransmitter involved in anxiety and vigilance

Neuroplasticity—the growth of brain cells; new connections being made

Neurotransmitter—a chemical in the brain that allows two neurons, or brain cells, to communicate

Parasympathetic—the nervous system responsible for eating, resting, and reproducing

Phenylethylamine (PEA)—an amphetamine-like neurotransmitter thought to be present during orgasm and love at first sight.

Polymorphism—different versions of inherited genes

Prefrontal cortex (PFC)—the higher-functioning part of the cortex that can inhibit activity in the amygdala, tamping down reactivity, providing top-down control

PTSD—posttraumatic stress disorder, a cluster of symptoms among survivors of trauma

Receptor—a site on a cell where a transmitter docks

Serotonergic—having to do with serotonin (e.g., serotonergic neurons are those that have receptors for serotonin)

SERT—the serotonin reuptake transporter protein, docking site of SSRIs; blocking this site stops recycling of released serotonin back into the neuron so that more gets across the synapse to the next neuron

SHBG—sex hormone binding globulin, a protein in the blood that binds up testosterone

SNRI—serotonin and norepinephrine reuptake inhibitor; antidepressant medicines that block the recycling of both serotonin and norepinephrine, so that less gets recycled into the "sending" neuron and more makes it across the synapse to the "receiving" neuron

SSRI—specific serotonin reuptake inhibitor; antidepressant medicines that block the recycling of serotonin into the "sending" neuron, allowing more serotonin to get across to the "receiving" neuron

Sympathetic—the nervous system responsible for the fight-or-flight response

Telomere—the tip of a gene, which shortens as cells replicate

Top-down control—when the frontal cortex "tames" the lower emotional centers, rationality inhibiting reactivity

Transcranial direct-current stimulation—an experimental treatment of depression and anxiety involving placing electrodes on the scalp to modulate neuronal activity

Xenoestrogens—synthetic chemicals (from plastics, soaps, pesticides, and more) that dock on the estrogen receptor

Notes

Introduction

2   **one in four American women:** Medco Health Solutions, "America's State of Mind Report," November 2011.

4   **By 2006 the antidepressant Zoloft:** Charles Barber, *Comfortably Numb: How Psychiatry Is Medicating a Nation* (New York: Random House, 2009).

4   **The latest news is particularly:** IMS National Prescription Audit, IMS Health 2013 (accessed at http://www.medscape.com/viewarticle/820011).

4   **Prescribing antipsychotics:** Daniel E. Casey, "Tardive Dyskinesia and Atypical Antipsychotic Drugs," *Schizophrenia Research* 35 (1999): S61–S66; Wildon R. Farwell et al., "Weight Gain and New Onset Diabetes Associated with Olanzapine and Risperidone," *Journal of General Internal Medicine* 19, no. 12 (2004): 1200–1205; Robert L. Dufresne, "Weighing In: Emergent Diabetes Mellitus and Second-Generation Antipsychotics," *Annals of Pharmacotherapy* 41, no. 10 (2007): 1725–27.

5   **we take 50 percent:** IMS Institute, "Medicine Use and Shifting Costs of Healthcare: A Review of the Use of Medicines in the U.S. in 2013," April 2014.

5   **Four out of five prescriptions:** Ramin Mojtabai, "Clinician-Identified Depression in Community Settings: Concordance with Structured-Interview Diagnoses," *Psychotherapy and Psychosomatics* 82, no. 3 (2013): 161–69.

5   **surveys of primary care doctors:** Christopher M. Callahan and German Elias Berrios, *Reinventing Depression: A History of the Treatment of Depression in Primary Care, 1940–2004* (USA: Oxford University Press, 2005).

Chapter One: Own Your Moods

14   **By evolutionary design:** J. O. Wolff and J. A. Peterson, "An Offspring-Defense Hypothesis for Territoriality in Female Mammals," *Ethology Ecology & Evolution* 10, no. 3 (1998): 227–39; Shelley E. Taylor, *The Tending Instinct: Women, Men, and the Biology of Relationships* (New York: Macmillan, 2003).

15   **Drug makers had found:** Jim Rosack, "Drug Makers Find Sept. 11 a Marketing Opportunity," *Psychiatric News*, March 11, 2002.

15   **Glaxo doubled its advertising:** Charles Barber, *Comfortably Numb*.

16   **As the *New York Times* explained:** Amy Harmon, "Young, Assured and Playing Pharmacist to Friends," *New York Times* 16 (2005).

16   **Numerous medical chart:** World Health Organization, Department of Mental Health and Substance Dependence, *Gender Disparities in Mental Health*, 2002.

17   **People who don't really need these meds:** Substance Abuse and Mental Health Services Administration, *Results from the 2012 National Survey on Drug Use and Health: Mental Health Findings*, NSDUH Series H-47, HHS Publication No. (SMA) 13-4805, 2013.

18   **it's more complicated:** Many concepts in this book have been simplified. There are three types of estrogen in the body (17-beta estradiol, estrone, and estriol), yet I use the word *estrogen* throughout

this book. I may talk about low levels of this or that hormone or neurotransmitter, but one molecule does not completely cause a behavior. Nothing happens in a vacuum in the human body, and every shift in one chemical is liable to set off a cascade of events in others. Small events can trigger larger countermeasures as the body and brain struggle to reach a new balance, or homeostasis. The brain adapts to new conditions as receptors upregulate or downregulate in response to the low or high functioning of a specific neurotransmitter. Also, nothing is one-size-fits-all because everyone's genes are different; individuals process drugs in idiosyncratic ways thanks to genetic variability, and many are more susceptible to psychiatric complaints because of their genetic predispositions.

18   **When serotonin levels are lower:** Khaled M. K. Ismail and P. M. S. O'Brien, "Premenstrual Syndrome," *Current Obstetrics & Gynecology* 11, no. 4 (2001): 251–55.

19   **Patients report having less:** W. J. Barnhart et al., "SSRI-Induced Apathy Syndrome: A Clinical Review," *Journal of Psychiatric Practice* 10 (2004): 196–99; R. Hoehn-Saric et al., "Apathy and Indifference in Patients on Fluvoxamine and Fluoxetine," *Journal of Clinical Psychopharmacology* 10 (1990): 343–46.

19   **Women's brains develop differently:** Louann Brizendine, *The Female Brain* (New York: Random House, 2007); Helen Fisher, *Why We Love: The Nature and Chemistry of Romantic Love* (New York: Macmillan, 2004).

20   **Even more brain changes occur:** Ibid.

20   **Our memory center:** Fisher, *Why We Love.*

20   **The hippocampus can calm:** Cora Hübner et al., "Ex Vivo Dissection of Optogenetically Activated mPFC and Hippocampal Inputs to Neurons in the Basolateral Amygdala: Implications for Fear and Emotional Memory," *Frontiers in Behavioral Neuroscience* 8, no. 64 (2014).

20   **are larger in men:** Jill M. Goldstein et al., "Normal Sexual Dimorphism of the Adult Human Brain Assessed by in Vivo Magnetic Resonance Imaging," *Cerebral Cortex* 11, no. 6 (2001): 490–97.

20   **have receptors for testosterone:** C. E. Roselli et al., "Quantitative Distribution of Nuclear Androgen Receptors in Microdissected Areas of the Rat Brain," *Neuroendocrinology* 49, no. 5 (1989): 449–53.

20   **When under acute stress:** Benno Roozendaal et al., "Stress, Memory and the Amygdala," *Nature Reviews Neuroscience* 10, no. 6 (2009): 423–33.

20   **The biggest problems:** Ajai Vyas et al., "Chronic Stress Induces Contrasting Patterns of Dendritic Remodeling in Hippocampal and Amygdaloid Neurons," *Journal of Neuroscience* 22, no. 15 (2002): 6810–18.

20   **It becomes atrophied:** Scott L. Rauch et al., "Neurocircuitry Models of Posttraumatic Stress Disorder and Extinction: Human Neuroimaging Research—Past, Present, and Future," *Biological Psychiatry* 60, no. 4 (2006): 376–82.

20   **seen in anyone undergoing chronic stress:** Bruce S. McEwen, "Plasticity of the Hippocampus: Adaptation to Chronic Stress and Allostatic Load," *Annals of the New York Academy of Sciences* 933, no. 1 (2001): 265–77; Lisa Eiland and Bruce S. McEwen, "Early Life Stress Followed by Subsequent Adult Chronic Stress Potentiates Anxiety and Blunts Hippocampal Structural Remodeling," *Hippocampus* 22, no. 1 (2012): 82–91.

20   **Intuiting the motives and feelings:** S. Baron-Cohen, *The Essential Difference* (New York: Basic Books, 2003).

21   **The better we are at sensing:** A. D. Craig, "Human Feelings: Why Are Some More Aware Than Others?" *Trends in Cognitive Sciences* 8, no. 6 (2004): 239–41; Beate M. Herbert et al., "Interoceptive Sensitivity and Emotion Processing: An EEG Study," *International Journal of Psychophysiology* 65, no. 3 (2007): 214–27.

21   **The insula:** Tania Singer et al., "A Common Role of Insula in Feelings, Empathy and Uncertainty," *Trends in Cognitive Sciences* 13, no. 8 (2009): 334–40.

21   **is noticeably bigger:** John S. Allen et al., "Sexual Dimorphism and Asymmetries in the Gray–White Composition of the Human Cerebrum," *Neuroimage* 18, no. 4 (2003): 880–94.

21   **The insula not only helps:** Kirsten G. Volz and D. Yves Von Cramon, "What Neuroscience Can Tell About Intuitive Processes in the Context of Perceptual Discovery," *Journal of Cognitive Neuroscience* 18, no. 12 (2006): 2077–87.

21   **Women have more brain circuitry:** Brizendine, *The Female Brain.*

21   **Testosterone impairs empathy:** Jack Van Honk et al., "Testosterone Administration Impairs Cognitive Empathy in Women Depending on Second-to-Fourth Digit Ratio," *Proceedings of the National Academy of Sciences (PNAS)* 108, no. 8 (2011): 3448–52; S. Lutchmaya et al., "Fetal Testosterone and Eye Contact in 12-Month-Old Human Infants," *Infant Behavior & Development* 25 (2002): 327–35; E. Chapman et al., "Fetal Testosterone and Empathy: Evidence from the Empathy Quotient (EQ) and the 'Reading the Mind in the Eyes' Test," *Social Neuroscience* 1 (2006): 135–48; Simon Baron-Cohen and Sally Wheelwright, "The Empathy Quotient: An Investigation of

Adults with Asperger Syndrome or High Functioning Autism, and Normal Sex Differences," *Journal of Autism and Developmental Disorders* 34, no. 2 (2004): 163–75.

22   **Oxytocin, the hormone:** Jorge A. Barraza and Paul J. Zak, "Empathy Toward Strangers Triggers Oxytocin Release and Subsequent Generosity," *Annals of the New York Academy of Sciences* 1167, no. 1 (2009): 182–89.

22   **It also helps us:** Carsten K. W. De Dreu et al., "The Neuropeptide Oxytocin Regulates Parochial Altruism in Intergroup Conflict Among Humans," *Science* 328, no. 5984 (2010): 1408–11.

22   **In hostile environments:** Shelley E. Taylor, *The Tending Instinct: Women, Men, and the Biology of Relationships* (New York: Macmillan, 2003).

22   **playing out as aggression:** Shelley E. Taylor, "Tend and Befriend Biobehavioral Bases of Affiliation Under Stress," *Current Directions in Psychological Science* 15, no. 6 (2006): 273–77.

22   **Protective mothers' maternal aggression:** Beth L. Mah et al., "Oxytocin Promotes Protective Behavior in Depressed Mothers: A Pilot Study with the Enthusiastic Stranger Paradigm," *Depression and Anxiety* (2014); Oliver J. Bosch, "Maternal Aggression in Rodents: Brain Oxytocin and Vasopressin Mediate Pup Defense," *Philosophical Transactions of the Royal Society B: Biological Sciences* 368, no. 1631 (2013): 20130085.

22   **Girls flock together:** Brizendine, *The Female Brain*.

22   **Estrogen triggers dopamine:** Ibid.

22   **Whereas women tend to discuss:** Deborah Tannen, *You Just Don't Understand: Women and Men in Conversation* (New York: HarperCollins, 2001).

22   **The connections between the areas:** Brizendine, *The Female Brain*.

22   **Women also have more bilateral processing:** Madhura Ingalhalikar et al., "Sex Differences in the Structural Connectome of the Human Brain," *Proceedings of The National Academy of Sciences* 111, no. 2 (2014): 823–28; Theodore D. Satterthwaite et al., "Linked Sex Differences in Cognition and Functional Connectivity in Youth," *Cerebral Cortex* (2014): bhu036.

23   **better at multitasking:** Gijsbert Stoet et al., "Are Women Better Than Men at Multi-Tasking?" *BMC Psychology* 1, no. 1 (2013): 18.

23   **Men's brains have more linkages:** Ingalhalikar et al., "Sex Differences."

23   **Men tend to outperform women:** Satterthwaite et al., "Linked Sex Differences," bhu036.

23   **outperform men on a "lost key":** Stoet et al., "Are Women Better Than Men," 18.

24   **In adulthood, women are twice as likely:** R. C. Kessler et al., "Sex and Depression in the National Comorbidity Survey. I: Lifetime Prevalence, Chronicity and Recurrence," *Journal of Affective Disorders* 29 (1993): 85–96; G. F. Placidi et al., "The Semi-Structured Affective Temperament Interview (TEMPS-I): Reliability and Psychometric Properties in 1010 14–26-Year-Old Students," *Journal of Affective Disorders* 47, no. 1–3 (1998): 1–10; Jules Angst et al., "Gender Differences in Depression," *European Archives of Psychiatry and Clinical Neuroscience* 252, no. 5 (2002): 201–9; C. Kuehner, "Gender Differences in Unipolar Depression: An Update of Epidemiological Findings and Possible Explanations," *Acta Psychiatrica Scandinavica* 108 (2003): 163–74.

24   **two to four times more likely:** Robin W. Simon and Leda E. Nath, "Gender and Emotion in the United States: Do Men and Women Differ in Self-Reports of Feelings and Expressive Behavior?" *American Journal of Sociology* 109, no. 5 (2004): 1137–76; Richard Gater et al., "Sex Differences in the Prevalence and Detection of Depressive and Anxiety Disorders in General Health Care Settings: Report from the World Health Organization Collaborative Study on Psychological Problems in General Health Care," *Archives of General Psychiatry* 55, no. 5 (1998): 405.

24   **The increased risk:** Marco Piccinelli and Greg Wilkinson, "Gender Differences in Depression: Critical Review," *British Journal of Psychiatry* 177, no. 6 (2000): 486–92.

24   **Although some of the increased incidence:** Janet Shibley Hyde et al., "The ABCs of Depression: Integrating Affective, Biological, and Cognitive Models to Explain the Emergence of the Gender Difference in Depression," *Psychological Review* 115, no. 2 (2008): 291.

24   **mood changes caused by variations:** E. W. Freeman et al., "Hormones and Menopausal Status as Predictors of Depression in Women in Transition to Menopause," *Archives of General Psychiatry* 61 (2004): 62–70; Jennifer L. Payne et al., "A Reproductive Subtype of Depression: Conceptualizing Models and Moving Toward Etiology," *Harvard Review of Psychiatry* 17, no. 2 (2009): 72–86.

24   **specific sensitivity:** P. J. Schmidt et al., "Differential Behavioral Effects of Gonadal Steroids in Women with and in Those without Premenstrual Syndrome," *New England Journal of Medicine* 338 (1998): 209–16.

24   **some lucky ones don't, possibly dictated by genes:** J. Guintivano et al., "Antenatal Prediction of Postpartum Depression with Blood DNA Methylation Biomarkers," *Molecular Psychiatry* (2013): 1-8.

24   **when your hormones aren't fluctuating:** Payne et al., "A Reproductive Subtype of Depression," 72–86.

24   **After menopause:** P. Bebbington et al., "The Influence of Age and Sex on the Prevalence of Depressive Conditions: Report from the National Survey of Psychiatric Morbidity," *Psychological Medicine* 15 (2003): 74–83.

24   **especially two years after:** Ellen W. Freeman et al., "Longitudinal Pattern of Depressive Symptoms Around Natural Menopause," *JAMA Psychiatry* 71, no. 1 (2014): 36–43.

25   **Progesterone is implicated:** J. H. Gold et al., "Late Luteal Phase Dysphoric Disorder: Literature Review," *DSM-IV Sourcebook* 2 (1996).

25   **postpartum depression:** Mohammed T. Abou-Saleh et al., "Hormonal Aspects of Postpartum Depression," *Psychoneuroendocrinology* 23, no 5 (1998): 465–75.

25   **dysthymia:** C. Neill Epperson et al., "Gonadal Steroids in the Treatment of Mood Disorders," *Psychosomatic Medicine* 61, no. 5 (1999): 676–97.

25   **The increased incidences of depression:** Barbara L. Parry, "Reproductive Factors Affecting the Course of Affective Illness in Women," *Psychiatric Clinics of North America* 12, no. 1 (1989): 207–20.

25   **If women develop these behaviors:** Randolph M. Nesse, "Is Depression an Adaptation?" *Archives of General Psychiatry* 57, no. 1 (2000): 14–20.

25   **When women feel under threat:** J. E. Y. Wei et al., "Estrogen Protects Against the Detrimental Effects of Repeated Stress on Glutamatergic Transmission and Cognition," *Molecular Psychiatry* (2013); R. E. Bowman et al., "Chronic Stress Effects on Memory: Sex Differences in Performance and Monoamines," *Hormones and Behavior* 43 (2003): 48–59; R. E. Bowman, "Stress-Induced Changes in Spatial Memory Are Sexually Differentiated and Vary Across the Lifespan," *Journal of Neuroendocrinology* 17 (2005): 526–35.

25   **One of the ways estrogen builds resilience:** David R. Rubinow et al., "Estrogen-Serotonin Interactions: Implications for Affective Regulation," *Biological Psychiatry* 44, no. 9 (1998): 839–50; Hadine Joffe and Lee S. Cohen, "Estrogen, Serotonin, and Mood Disturbance: Where Is the Therapeutic Bridge?" *Biological Psychiatry* 44, no. 9 (1998): 798–811.

25   **Serotonin activity is greater:** I. Hindberg and O. Naesh, "Serotonin Concentrations in Plasma and Variations During the Menstrual Cycle," *Clinical Chemistry* 38, no. 10 (1992): 2087–89.

25   **When estrogen surges:** C. L. Bethea et al., "Ovarian Steroids and Serotonin Neural Function," *Molecular Neurobiology* 18, no. 2 (1998): 87–123.

25   **causes serotonin receptors:** Barbara E. H. Sumner et al., "Effects of Tamoxifen on Serotonin Transporter and 5-Hydroxytryptamine 2A Receptor Binding Sites and Mrna Levels in the Brain of Ovariectomized Rats with or without Acute Estradiol Replacement," *Molecular Brain Research* 73, no. 1 (1999): 119–28. Zenab Amin et al., "Effect of Estrogen-Serotonin Interactions on Mood and Cognition," *Behavioral and Cognitive Neuroscience Reviews* 4, no. 1 (2005): 43–58.

25   **to be made:** 5HT2A.

26   **The natural process of stress:** Ibid.; Rubinow et al.; Sumner et al., "Effects of Tamoxifen," 119–28.

26   **normalizes our:** increased SERT production, the presynaptic reuptake inhibitor upon which SSRIs dock.

26   **sexual side effects:** There are gender differences in serotonin receptor numbers and sensitivity. Women have slightly different responses to the serotonin-enhancing drug MDMA (called Ecstasy or Molly) due to these receptor differences, for example. Researchers have shown sex differences in the serotonin transporter where the SSRIs dock, called SERT. If you have more SERT, you have more recycling of serotonin back into the pitching cell, so less is available for the catching cell. More SERT is the opposite of more antidepressants, which block the SERT site. The gene implicated in depression that helps to guide the manufacture of SERT, called SLC6A4, has a "switch" that is turned on by estrogen. Other subtypes of serotonin receptors have gender differences or estrogen responsiveness as well. The number of SERT docking sites decreases as depressed women age, but not depressed men. This may have to do with waning estrogen levels seen after menopause. Aging seems to affect women more than men when it comes to their serotonergic systems.

26   **People on SSRIs report less:** M. Oleshansky and L. Labbate, "Inability to Cry During SRI Treatment," *Journal of Clinical Psychiatry* 57 (1996): 593; Jonathan Price et al., "Emotional Side-Effects of Selective Serotonin Reuptake Inhibitors: Qualitative Study," *British Journal of Psychiatry* 195, no. 3 (2009): 211–17; Adam Opbroek et al., "Emotional Blunting Associated with SSRI-Induced Sexual Dysfunction. Do SSRIs Inhibit Emotional Responses?" *International Journal of Neuropsychopharmacology* 5, no. 2 (2002): 147–51.

27   **SSRIs affect emotional processing:** Price et al., "Emotional Side-Effects of Selective Serotonin Reuptake Inhibitors," 211–17.

27   **medications often can:** The exception here is if you've had more than one major depressive episode. Then the current recommendation is that you get on and stay on your antidepressant medication to avoid a likely relapse.

28   **A clear, visible sign:** Robert W. Levenson, "Blood, Sweat, and Fears," *Annals of the New York Academy of Sciences* 1000, no. 1 (2003): 348–66.

28   **In one study of medicated women:** Robert J. Gregory et al., "Ethical Dilemmas in Prescribing Antidepressants," *Archives of General Psychiatry* 58, no. 11 (2001): 1085.

29   **stuffing down your feelings:** Gabor Maté, *When the Body Says No: The Cost of Hidden Stress* (New York: Random House, 2011).

29   **The suppression of anger:** William T. Riley et al., "Anger and Hostility in Depression," *Journal of Nervous and Mental Disease* 177, no. 11 (1989): 668–74.

29   **People who've experienced depression:** Cindy L. Brody et al., "Experiences of Anger in People Who Have Recovered from Depression and Never-Depressed People," *Journal of Nervous and Mental Disease* 187, no. 7 (1999): 400–405.

29   **Depressed patients have higher levels:** M. Weissman et al., "Clinical Evaluation of Hostility in Depression," *American Journal of Psychiatry* (1971): 12841–46; Roger C. Bland and Helene Orn, "Family Violence and Psychiatric Disorder," *Canadian Journal of Psychiatry/La Revue canadienne de psychiatrie* 31, no. 2 (1986): 129–37.; K. B. Koh et al., "Predominance of Anger in Depressive Disorders Compared with Anxiety Disorders and Somatoform Disorders, *Journal of Clinical Psychiatry* (2002): 63486–92.

29   **the more anger, the more severe:** A. P. Schless et al., "Depression and Hostility," *Journal of Nervous and Mental Disease* 159, no. 2 (1974): 81–100.

29   **In an examination of women's employment reviews:** Keiran Snyder, "The Abrasiveness Trap: High-Achieving Men and Women Are Described Differently in Reviews," *Fortune*, August 26, 2014, http://fortune.com/2014/08/26/performance-review-gender-bias/.

29   **SSRIs reduce aggression:** Menahem Krakowski, "Violence and Serotonin: Influence of Impulse Control, Affect Regulation, and Social Functioning," *Journal of Neuropsychiatry and Clinical Neurosciences* 15, no. 3 (2003): 294–305.

30   **SSRIs augment social dominance:** S. Tse Wai and Alyson J. Bond, "Serotonergic Intervention Affects Both Social Dominance and Affiliative Behavior," *Psychopharmacology* 161, no. 3 (2002): 324–30.

30   **elevating an animal's status:** M. J. Raleigh et al., "Serotonergic Mechanisms Promotes Dominance Acquisition in Adult Male Vervet Monkeys," *Brain Research* 559 (1991): 181–90.

30   **girls who hold on to their assertiveness:** Maté, *When the Body Says No.*

30   **In the nineteenth century:** Pierre Janet, *The Major Symptoms of Hysteria* (New York: Macmillan, 1907).

30   **One treatment for hysteria:** Rachel Maines, *The Technology of Orgasm: "Hysteria," the Vibrator, and Women's Sexual Satisfaction* (Baltimore: Johns Hopkins University Press, 1999).

30–31 **removal of the clitoris:** Elizabeth Sheehan, "Victorian Clitoridectomy: Isaac Baker Brown and His Harmless Operative Procedure," *Medical Anthropology Newsletter* 12, no. 4 (1981): 9–15.

31   **Epidemiological studies show:** Linda LeResche, "Epidemiologic Perspectives on Sex Differences in Pain," in *Sex, Gender, and Pain*, ed. R. B. Fillingim (Seattle: IASP Press, 2000), 233–49; Linda LeResche, "Epidemiology of Pain Conditions with Higher Prevalence in Women," in May L. Chin et al., eds., *Pain in Women* (New York: Oxford Univeristy Press, 2013); M. Von Korff et al., "An Epidemiologic Comparison of Pain Complaints, *Pain* 32 (1988): 173–83.

31   **Men are less apt:** Ann Vincent et al., "Prevalence of Fibromyalgia: A Population-Based Study in Olmsted County, Minnesota, Utilizing the Rochester Epidemiology Project," *Arthritis Care & Research* 65, no. 5 (2013): 786–92.

31   **Women's sensitivities extend:** A. M. Unruh, "Gender Variations in Clinical Pain Experience," *Pain* 65 (1996): 123–67; Marieke Niesters et al., "Sex Differences in Analgesic Responses," in Chin et al., eds., *Pain in Women.*

32   **overwhelming laboratory evidence:** Mordechai Averbuch, and Meyer Katzper, "A Search for Sex Differences in Response to Analgesia," *Archives of Internal Medicine* 160, no. 22 (2000): 3424–28; R. B. Fillingim and W. Maixner, "Gender Differences in Response to Noxious Stimuli," *Pain Forum* 4 (1995): 209–21; R. B. Fillingim and T. J. Ness, "Sex-Related Hormonal Influences on Pain and Analgesic Responses," *Neuroscience & Biobehavioral Reviews* 24, no. 4 (2000): 485–501; Riley, "Anger and Hostility in Depression," 668–74.

32   **Women are also more apt:** Cosgrove et al., "Evolving Knowledge of Sex Differences," 847–55.

32   **our hormones:** M. B. Dawson-Basoa and A. R. Gintzler, "17-Beta-Estradiol and Progesterone Modulate an Intrinsic Opioid Analgesic System," *Brain Research* 601 (1993): 241–45; Yolanda R. Smith et al., "Pronociceptive and Antinociceptive Effects of Estradiol Through Endogenous Opioid Neurotransmission in Women," *Journal of Neuroscience* 26, no. 21 (2006): 5777–85.

32   **where we are in our menstrual cycle:** Zsuzsanna Wiesenfeld-Hallin, "Sex Differences in Pain Perception," *Gender Medicine* 2, no. 3 (2005): 137–45; Cristina Tassorelli et al., "Changes in

Nociceptive Flexion Reflex Threshold Across the Menstrual Cycle in Healthy Women," *Psychosomatic Medicine* 64, no. 4 (2002): 621–26.

32   **Our psyches are silently screaming:** Maté, *When the Body Says No.*

32   **In the journal *Pain*:** J. S. Mogil and M. L. Chanda, "The Case for the Inclusion of Female Subjects in Basic Science Studies of Pain," *Pain* 117 (2005): 1–5.

32   **reports of chest pain:** J. Ayanian and A. Epstein, "Differences in the Use of Procedures Between Women and Men Hospitalized for Coronary Heart Disease," *New England Journal of Medicine* 325 (1991): 221–25; M. Delborg and K. Swedberg, "Acute Myocardial Infarction: Difference in the Treatment Between Men and Women," *Quality Assurance in Health Care* 5 (1993): 261–65.

32   **lung cancer:** C. Wells and A. Feinstein, "Detection Bias in the Diagnostic Pursuit of Lung Cancer," *American Journal of Epidemiology* 128 (1988): 1016–26.

32   **in general complaints:** K. Armitage et al., "Responses of Physicians to Medical Complaints in Men and Women," *JAMA* 241 (1979): 2186–87; S. Colameco et al., "Sex Bias in the Assessment of Patient Complaints," *Journal of Family Practice* 16 (1983): 1117–21.

32   **psychiatric complaints:** Ann A. Hohmann, "Gender Bias in Psychotropic Drug Prescribing in Primary Care," *Medical Care* 27, no. 5 (1989): 478–90; Cynthia M. Hartung and Thomas A. Widiger, "Gender Differences in the Diagnosis of Mental Disorders: Conclusions and Controversies of the DSM–IV," *Psychological Bulletin* 123, no. 3 (1998): 260.

32   **Until recently, surgeons knew much less:** Jennifer Berman and Laura Berman, *For Women Only: A Revolutionary Guide to Reclaiming Your Sex Life* (New York: Macmillan, 2001), 127.

33   **Eight of ten drugs withdrawn:** J. Heinrich et al., "Drug Safety: Most Drugs Withdrawn in Recent Years Had Greater Health Risks for Women," United States General Accounting Office, Washington, D.C., 2001.

33   **After twenty years on the market:** David J. Greenblatt et al., "Gender Differences in Pharmacokinetics and Pharmacodynamics of Zolpidem Following Sublingual Administration," *The Journal of Clinical Pharmacology* 54, no. 3 (2014): 282–90.

Chapter Two: Feeling Bitchy Like Clockwork

36   **Somewhere between 3 and 8 percent:** Lorraine Dennerstein et al., "Epidemiology of Premenstrual Symptoms and Disorders," *Menopause International* 18, no. 2 (2012): 48–51.

37   **when you ovulate:** The feeling of ovulation is called *mittelschmerz*, German for "middle pain." It is a short, sharp pain usually felt in one corner of your lower pelvis. The side may alternate monthly, but not always.

37   **what to expect:** Google "Monthly Mood Cube" for a cute idea.

37   **The peak estrogen levels:** Elizabeth Hampson, "Estrogen-Related Variations in Human Spatial and Articulatory-Motor Skills," *Psychoneuroendocrinology* 15, no. 2 (1990): 97–111.

40   **there is some evidence:** Christiane Northrup, *Women's Bodies, Women's Wisdom: Creating Physical and Emotional Health and Healing* (New York: Bantam, 1994).

40   **Because of lower serotonin levels:** Eliza Reynolds, *Mothering and Daughtering: Keeping Your Bond Strong Through the Teen Years* (Sounds True, 2013).

41   **There are studies that claim:** Debra A. Zellner et al., "Chocolate Craving and the Menstrual Cycle" *Appetite* 42, no. 1 (2004): 119–21.

41   **your body requires more calories:** Roy F. Baumeister and John Tierney, *Willpower: Rediscovering the Greatest Human Strength* (New York: Penguin, 2011).

41   **your magnesium levels are low:** Kristen Bruinsma and Douglas L. Taren, "Chocolate: Food or Drug?" *Journal of the American Dietetic Association* 99, no. 10 (1999): 1249–56.

41   **In depression and in PMS:** Richard J. Wurtman and Judith J. Wurtman, "Carbohydrate Craving, Obesity and Brain Serotonin," *Appetite* 7 (1986): 99–103; Richard J. Wurtman and Judith J. Wurtman, "Do Carbohydrates Affect Food Intake Via Neurotransmitter Activity?" *Appetite* 11 (1988): 42–47.

42   **Cardio, in particular, can help:** Amanda Daley, "Exercise and Premenstrual Symptomatology: A Comprehensive Review," *Journal of Women's Health* 18, no. 6 (2009): 895–99.

43   **when you started having sex:** Winnifred B. Cutler et al., "Sexual Behavior Frequency and Menstrual Cycle Length in Mature Premenopausal Women," *Psychoneuroendocrinology* 4, no. 4 (1979): 297–309.

43   **If you started earlier:** Winnifred Berg Cutler et al., "Sporadic Sexual Behavior and Menstrual Cycle Length in Women," *Hormones and Behavior* 14, no. 2 (1980): 163–72; Winnifred Berg Cutler et al., "Sexual Behavior Frequency and Biphasic Ovulatory Type Menstrual Cycles," *Physiology & Behavior* 34, no. 5 (1985): 805–10.

43   **Weekly sex:** Cutler et al., "Sexual Behavior Frequency and Menstrual Cycle Length," 297–309;

Cutler et al., "Sexual Behavior Frequency and Biphasic Ovulatory Type Menstrual Cycles," 805–10.

43 **In a group of women:** W. B. Cutler et al., "Coitus and Menstruation in Perimenopausal Women," *Journal of Psychosomatic Obstetrics & Gynecology* 17, no. 3 (1996): 149–57.

43 **antidepressant withdrawal:** Junk food is addictive, our phones are addictive, cigarettes are addictive. Why would we think antidepressants are any different?

45 **In one study of women:** H. Joffe et al., "Impact of Oral Contraceptive Pill Use on Premenstrual Mood: Predictors of Improvement and Deterioration," *American Journal of Obstetrics & Gynecology* 189 (2003): 1523–30.

45 **estrogen causes the manufacture:** Barbara E. H. Sumner and George Fink, "Estrogen Increases the Density of 5-Hydroxytryptamine 2A Receptors in Cerebral Cortex and Nucleus Accumbens in the Female Rat," *Journal of Steroid Biochemistry and Molecular Biology* 54, no. 1 (1995): 15–20.

45 **About a third of women:** Merja Viikki et al., "Interaction Between Two HTR2A Polymorphisms and Gender Is Associated with Treatment Response in MDD," *Neuroscience Letters* 501, no. 1 (2011): 20–24.

45–46 **Synthetic progestin is horrible:** Lila Nachtigal, personal communication with author, June 4, 2014.

46 **The oral contraceptives Yaz and Yasmin:** Wolfgang Oelkers, "Drospirenone, a Progestogen with Antimineralocorticoid Properties: A Short Review," *Molecular and Cellular Endocrinology* 217, no. 1 (2004): 255–61.

46 **synthetic hormones seem to interfere:** P. W. Adams et al., "Effect of Pyridoxine Hydrochloride upon Depression Associated with Oral Contraception," *Lancet* 301, no. 7809 (1973): 897–904.

47 **Taking extra estrogen:** Peter R. Casson et al., "Effect of Postmenopausal Estrogen Replacement on Circulating Androgens," *Obstetrics & Gynecology* 90, no. 6 (1997): 995–98.

47 **It gets worse: a research study:** Panzer et al., "Impact of Oral Contraceptives on Sex Hormone-Binding Globulin and Androgen Levels: A Retrospective Study in Women with Sexual Dysfunction," *Journal of Sexual Medicine* 3 (2006): 104–13

47 **he told me it never returns:** Irwin Goldstein, personal communication with author, June 4, 2014.

47 **Part of every woman's monthly cycle:** Stephanie H. M. Van Goozen et al., "Psychoendocrinological Assessment of the Menstrual Cycle: The Relationship Between Hormones, Sexuality, and Mood," *Archives of Sexual Behavior* 26, no. 4 (1997): 359–82.

48 **a book called *Sexy Mamas*:** Cathy Winks and Anne Semans, *Sexy Mamas: Keeping Your Sex Life Alive While Raising Kids* (Novato, CA: New World Library, 2004).

49 **Studies show that men are more:** See Andrew J. Elliot, Tobias Greitemeyer, and Adam D. Pazda, "Women's Use of Red Clothing As a Sexual Signal in Intersexual Interaction," *Journal of Experimental Social Psychology* 49, no. 3 (2013): 599–602, for a review.

49 **Greater feelings of attractiveness:** Juan J. Tarín and Vanessa Gómez-Piquer, "Do Women Have a Hidden Heat Period?" *Human Reproduction* 17, no. 9 (2002): 2243–48.

49 **Oxytocin peaks:** M. D. Mitchell et al., "Plasma Oxytocin Concentrations During the Menstrual Cycle," *European Journal of Obstetrics & Gynecology and Reproductive Biology* 12, no. 3 (1981): 195–200.

49 **pupils even dilate:** Bruno Laeng and Liv Falkenberg, "Women's Pupillary Responses to Sexually Significant Others During the Hormonal Cycle," *Hormones and Behavior* 52, no. 4 (2007): 520–30.

49 **Women who are ovulating:** Christopher Ryan and Cacilda Jethá, *Sex at Dawn: The Prehistoric Origins of Modern Sexuality* (New York: HarperCollins, 2010).

49 **Women feel more attractive:** Tarín and Gómez-Piquer, "Do Women Have a Hidden Heat Period?" 2243–48.

49 **men are able to tell which women:** Martie G. Haselton et al., "Ovulatory Shifts in Human Female Ornamentation: Near Ovulation, Women Dress to Impress," *Hormones and Behavior* 51, no. 1 (2007): 40–45.

49 **In studies, men pay strippers:** Ryan and Jethá, *Sex at Dawn*.

50 **Women prefer men with a lower voice:** Jillian J. M. O'Connor et al., "Perceptions of Infidelity Risk Predict Women's Preferences for Low Male Voice Pitch in Short-Term over Long-Term Relationship Contexts," *Personality and Individual Differences* 56 (2014): 73–77.

50 **When women are ovulating:** Ian S. Penton-Voak et al. "Menstrual Cycle Alters Face Preference," *Nature* 399, no. 6738 (1999): 741–42.

50 **When not fertile, women still:** Randy Thornhill and Steven W. Gangestad, *The Evolutionary Biology of Human Female Sexuality* (Oxford University Press, 2008); Steven W. Gangestad and Randy Thornhill, "Human Oestrus," *Proceedings of the Royal Society B: Biological Sciences* 275, no. 1638 (2008): 991–1000.

50   **Women find classically masculine faces:** Tarín and Gómez-Piquer, "Do Women Have a Hidden
         Heat Period?" 2243–48.

50   **Fertile women are also more attracted:** Jan Havlíček et al., "Women's Preference for Dominant
         Male Odor: Effects of Menstrual Cycle and Relationship Status," *Biology Letters* 1, no. 3 (2005):
         256–59; Steven W. Gangestad et al., "Women's Preferences for Male Behavioral Displays Change
         Across the Menstrual Cycle," *Psychological Science* 15, no. 3 (2004): 203–7.

51   **Partnered women are more likely:** Havlíček et al., "Women's Preference for Dominant Male
         Odor," 256–59.

51   **There's no midcycle peak:** Andrea Salonia et al., "Menstrual Cycle-Related Changes in Plasma
         Oxytocin Are Relevant to Normal Sexual Function in Healthy Women," *Hormones and Behavior*
         47, no. 2 (2005): 164–69.

51   **As far as the brain is concerned:** Penton-Voak et al., "Menstrual Cycle Alters Face Preference,"
         741–42; Benedict C. Jones et al., "Effects of Menstrual Cycle Phase on Face Preferences," *Archives of
         Sexual Behavior* 37, no. 1 (2008): 78–84; Alexandra Alvergne and Virpi Lummaa, "Does the Con-
         traceptive Pill Alter Mate Choice in Humans?" *Trends in Ecology & Evolution* 25, no. 3 (2010):
         171–79.

51   **weaker or no preferences for facial:** A. C. Little et al., "Partnership Status and the Temporal Con-
         text of Relationships Influence Human Female Preferences for Sexual Dimorphism in Male Face
         Shape," *Proceedings of the Royal Society of London, Series B: Biological Sciences* 269, no. 1496
         (2002): 1095–1100.

51   **vocal masculinity:** Penton-Voak et al., "Menstrual Cycle Alters Face Preference," 741–42.

51   **Men are actually more likely to fall in love:** Arthur Aron et al., "Reward, Motivation, and Emo-
         tion Systems Associated with Early-Stage Intense Romantic Love," *Journal of Neurophysiology* 94,
         no. 1 (2005): 327–37.

52   **Women have a more:** Brizendine, *The Female Brain.*

52   **more brain space devoted:** M. Bensafi et al., "Sex-Steroid Derived Compounds Induce Sex-Spe-
         cific Effects on Autonomic Nervous System Function in Humans," *Behavioral Neuroscience* 117, no.
         6 (2003): 1125; Suma Jacob et al., "Context-Dependent Effects of Steroid Chemosignals on Human
         Physiology and Mood," *Physiology & Behavior* 74, no. 1 (2001): 15–27.

53   **Too-similar immune systems:** Christine E. Garver-Apgar et al., "Major Histocompatibility Com-
         plex Alleles, Sexual Responsivity, and Unfaithfulness in Romantic Couples," *Psychological Science*
         17, no. 10 (2006): 830–35.

53   **if a woman partners with a man:** Ibid.

54   **they like her scent more:** Jan Havlíček et al., "Non-Advertized Does Not Mean Concealed: Body
         Odor Changes Across the Human Menstrual Cycle," *Ethology* 112, no. 1 (2006): 81–90.

54   **If she's on the Pill:** Seppo Kuukasjärvi et al., "Attractiveness of Women's Body Odors over the Men-
         strual Cycle: The Role of Oral Contraceptives and Receiver Sex," *Behavioral Ecology* 15, no. 4
         (2004): 579–84.

54   **In a replay of the sweaty T-shirt experiment:** C. Wedekind et al., "MHC-Dependent Mate Prefer-
         ences in Humans," *Proceedings of the Royal Society of London* 260 (1995): 245–49; Randy Thorn-
         hill and Steven W. Gangestad, "Do Women Have Evolved Adaptation for Extra-Pair Copulation?" in
         Evolutionary Aesthetics, Springer Berlin Heidelber (2003): 341–68; Jan Havlíček and S. Craig Rob-
         erts, "MHC-Correlated Mate Choice in Humans: A Review," *Psychoneuroendocrinology* 34, no. 4
         (2009): 497–512.

54   **Women who were on oral contraceptives:** S. Craig Roberts et al., "Relationship Satisfaction and
         Outcome in Women Who Meet Their Partner While Using Oral Contraception," *Proceedings of the
         Royal Society B: Biological Sciences* 279, no. 1732 (2012): 1430–36.

Chapter Three: This Is Your Brain on Love

59   **falling in love is the neural mechanism:** Helen Fisher, *Why We Love: The Nature and Chemistry
         of Romantic Love* (New York: Macmillan), 2004.

60   **Experiments with prairie voles:** Brandon J. Aragona et al., "A Critical Role for Nucleus Accum-
         bens Dopamine in Partner-Preference Formation in Male Prairie Voles," *Journal of Neuroscience*
         23, no. 8 (2003): 3483–90.

60   **Helen Fisher's brain scans:** Helen Fisher et al., "Romantic Love: An fMRI Study of a Neural
         Mechanism for Mate Choice," *Journal of Comparative Neurology* 493, no. 1 (2005): 58–62.

60   **"motor of the mind":** J. R. Villablanca, "Why Do We Have a Caudate Nucleus?" *Acta Neurobiol Exp
         (Wars)* 70, no. 1 (2010): 95–105.

61   **The Rules:** Ellen Fein and Sherrie Schneider, *The Rules: Time-Tested Secrets for Capturing the
         Heart of Mr. Right* (New York: Warner Books, 1996).

61 **getting the reward too early:** Shunsuke Kobayashi and Wolfram Schultz, "Influence of Reward Delays on Responses of Dopamine Neurons," *Journal of Neuroscience* 28, no. 31 (2008): 7837–46.

61 **Increased levels of these two chemicals:** Anne M. Etgen et al., "Estradiol and Progesterone Modulation of Norepinephrine Neurotransmission: Implications for the Regulation of Female Reproductive Behavior," *Journal of Neuroendocrinology* 4, no. 3 (1992): 255–71.

62 **the "molecule of attraction":** Fisher, *Why We Love.*

62 **also found in a group of drugs:** Alexander Shulgin and Ann Shulgin, *Pihkal: A Chemical Love Story* (Berkeley: Transform Press, 1991).

62 **a short-term antidepressant:** Hector Sabelli et al., "Sustained Antidepressant Effect of PEA Replacement," *Journal of Neuropsychiatry and Clinical Neurosciences* 8, no. 2 (1995): 168–71.

62 **present in good chocolates:** John P. Chaytor et al., "The Identification and Significance of 2-Phenylethylamine in Foods," *Journal of the Science of Food and Agriculture* 26, no. 5 (1975): 593–98.

62 **may also spike during orgasm:** Hoyle Leigh, "Basic Foundations of Diagnosis, Psychiatric Diagnosis and Final Common Pathway Syndromes," in *Handbook of Consultation-Liaison Psychiatry* (New York: Springer, 2007), 53–73.

62 **The levels of the sex hormones:** Fisher, *Why We Love.*

62 **Estrogen and progesterone:** Schumacher, 1990.

62–63 **higher levels of circulating testosterone:** Rainer Knussmann et al., "Relations Between Sex Hormone Levels and Sexual Behavior in Men," *Archives of Sexual Behavior* 15, no. 5 (1986): 429–45; Jan L. Shifren et al., "Transdermal Testosterone Treatment in Women with Impaired Sexual Function After Oophorectomy," *New England Journal of Medicine* 343, no. 10 (2000): 682–88; Adriaan Tuiten et al., "Time Course of Effects of Testosterone Administration on Sexual Arousal in Women," *Archives of General Psychiatry* 57, no. 2 (2000): 149–53; Andrea M. Isidori et al., "Effects of Testosterone on Sexual Function in Men: Results of a Meta-Analysis," *Clinical Endocrinology* 63, no. 4 (2005): 381–94.

63 **inhaling male pheromones:** Erin D. Gleason et al., "Testosterone Release and Social Context: When It Occurs and Why," *Frontiers in Neuroendocrinology* 30, no. 4 (2009): 460–69.

63 **Just thinking about your new guy:** Katherine L. Goldey and Sari M. van Anders, "Sexy Thoughts: Effects of Sexual Cognitions on Testosterone, Cortisol, and Arousal in Women," *Hormones and Behavior* 59, no. 5 (2011): 754–64.

63 **men who are falling in love:** D. Marazziti et al., "Alteration of the Platelet Serotonin Transporter in Romantic Love," *Psychological Medicine* 29, no. 3 (1999): 741–45.

63 **same-sex couples can and do:** Michael W. Johnston and Alan P. Bell, "Romantic Emotional Attachment: Additional Factors in the Development of the Sexual Orientation of Men," *Journal of Counseling & Development* 73, no. 6 (1995): 621–25; Letitia Anne Peplau, "Rethinking Women's Sexual Orientation: An Interdisciplinary, Relationship-Focused Approach," *Personal Relationships* 8, no. 1 (2001): 1–19.

64 **Smiling babies and hugs:** Tracey A. Baskerville, "Dopamine and Oxytocin Interactions Underlying Behaviors: Potential Contributions to Behavioral Disorders," *CNS Neuroscience & Therapeutics* 16, no. 3 (2010): e92–e123.

64 **it can help to speed healing:** Kerstin Uvnas Moberg and Roberta Francis, *The Oxytocin Factor: Tapping the Hormone of Calm, Love, and Healing* (Cambridge, MA: Da Capo Press, 2003); Courtney E. Detillion et al., "Social Facilitation of Wound Healing," *Psychoneuroendocrinology* 29, no. 8 (2004): 1004–11.

64 **Women have more oxytocin receptors:** M. M. McCarthy, "Estrogen Modulation of Oxytocin and Its Relation to Behavior," *Advances in Experimental Medicine and Biology* 395 (1994): 235–45.

64 **In experiments, people given oxytocin:** Michael Kosfeld et al., "Oxytocin Increases Trust in Humans," *Nature* 435, no. 7042 (2005): 673–76; Paul J. Zak et al., "Oxytocin Increases Generosity in Humans," *PLoS One* 2, no. 11 (2007): e1128.

64 **people who are touched while spoken to:** Paul J. Zak, *The Moral Molecule: How Trust Works.* (New York: Penguin, 2012).

64 **When people fall in love, their fear circuitry:** Fisher, *Why We Love.*

64 **brain-derived neurotrophic factor:** E. Emanuele et al., "Raised Plasma Nerve Growth Factor Levels Associated with Early-Stage Romantic Love," *Psychoneuroendocrinology*, September 5, 2005.

65 **"obliterated and replaced":** Norman Doidge, *The Brain That Changes Itself* (New York: Penguin, 2007), 113.

65 **Blood serotonin levels in those newly in love:** Marazziti et al., "Alteration of the Platelet Serotonin Transporter in Romantic Love," *Psychological Medicine* 29, no. 3 (1999): 741–45.

66 **SSRIs interfere with mating:** Helen E. Fisher and J. Anderson Thomson Jr., "Lust, Romance,

Attachment: Do the Side Effects of Serotonin-Enhancing Antidepressants Jeopardize Romantic Love, Marriage, and Fertility?" *Evolutionary Cognitive Neuroscience* (2007): 245.

66   **Female rats treated chronically with SSRIs:** J. V. Matuszczyk et al., "Subchronic Administration of Fluoxetine Impairs Estrous Behavior in Intact Female Rats," *Neuropsychopharmacology* 19 (1998): 492–98.

66   **women on SSRIs rate men as less attractive:** Justin Garcia, e-mail message to author, September 8, 2014, September 9, 2014, September 10, 2014.

66   **"less likely to find those":** Justin Garcia, e-mail message to the author, September 8, 2014.

67   **"Scientists think the fickle female orgasm":** Helen Slater, "True Love," *National Geographic*, February 2006.

67   **But with lust, a biological drive:** Fisher, *Why We Love*.

67   **Even flirting seems to have some basis:** Sari M. van Anders and Katherine L. Goldey, "Testosterone and Partnering Are Linked Via Relationship Status for Women and 'Relationship Orientation' for Men," *Hormones and Behavior* 58, no. 5 (2010): 820–26.

67   **"almost any semi-appropriate partner":** Fisher, *Why We Love*, 78.

68   **surging testosterone levels in an adolescent girl:** C. T. Halpern and J. R. Udry, "Testosterone Predicts Initiation of Coitus in Adolescent Females," *Psychosomatic Medicine* 59, no. 2 (1997): 161–71.

68   **Rising testosterone levels:** M. I. Gonzalez et al., "Interactions Between 5-Hydroxytryptamine (5-HT) and Testosterone in the Control of Sexual and Nonsexual Behavior in Male and Female Rats," *Pharmacology Biochemistry and Behavior* 47, no. 3 (1994): 591–601.

69   **There is a strong desire in women:** Marc H. Hollender, "The Need or Wish to Be Held," *Archives of General Psychiatry* 22, no. 5 (1970): 445.

69   **Many of us will use sex as a means:** Marc H. Hollender et al., "Body Contact and Sexual Enticement," *Archives of General Psychiatry* 20, no. 2 (1969): 188.

69   **A common complaint among men:** Pat Love and J. T. Brown, "Creating Passion and Intimacy," in *The Intimate Couple*, ed. Jon Carlson and Len Sperry (Psychology Press, 1999): 55–65.

71   **mounting evidence that sexual pleasure:** James G. Pfaus, "Reviews: Pathways of Sexual Desire," *Journal of Sexual Medicine* 6, no. 6 (2009): 1506–33; Carolin Klein et al., "Circulating Endocannabinoid Concentrations and Sexual Arousal in Women," *Journal of Sexual Medicine* 9, no. 6 (2012): 1588–1601.

71   **The beginning of sexual pleasure:** Daniel Bergner, *What Do Women Want?: Adventures in the Science of Female Desire* (New York: Ecco, 2013).

71   **Peaking at orgasm, oxytocin:** D. L. Lefebvre et al., "Uterine Oxytocin Gene Expression. I. Induction During Pseudopregnancy and the Estrous Cycle," *Endocrinology* 134, no. 6 (1994): 2556–61.

72   **(They can, as long as their vagus nerve):** Barry R. Komisaruk et al., "Brain Activation During Vaginocervical Self-Stimulation and Orgasm in Women with Complete Spinal Cord Injury: fMRI Evidence of Mediation by the Vagus Nerves," *Brain Research* 1024, no. 1 (2004): 77–88.

72   **Leading up to orgasm, a series of brain blood flow changes:** B. R. Komisaruk et al., "An fMRI Time-Course Analysis of Brain Regions Activated During Self-Stimulation to Orgasm in Women," *Society for Neuroscience* (2010): 285.6.

73   **release of oxytocin:** The paraventricular nucleus.

73   **underlies reward seeking:** The nucleus accumbens.

Chapter Four: Marriage and Its Discontents

75   **study comparing the serotonin levels:** Donatella Marazziti, "The Neurobiology of Love," *Current Psychiatry Reviews* 1, no. 3 (2005): 331–35.

75   **Men's testosterone levels are lower:** Peter B. Gray et al., "Human Male Pair Bonding and Testosterone," *Human Nature* 15, no. 2 (2004): 119–31.

76   **Birds that are given an extra dose:** Kathleen E. Hunt et al., "Endocrine Influences on Parental Care During a Short Breeding Season: Testosterone and Male Parental Care in Lapland Longspurs (Calcarius Lapponicus)," *Behavioral Ecology and Sociobiology* 45, no. 5 (1999): 360–69.

76   **men with lower testosterone levels more responsive:** Anne E. Story et al., "Hormonal Correlates of Paternal Responsiveness in New and Expectant Fathers," *Evolution and Human Behavior* 21, no. 2 (2000): 79–95.

76   **"paternal effort":** Peter B. Gray et al., "Marriage and Fatherhood Are Associated with Lower Testosterone in Males," *Evolution and Human Behavior* 23, no. 3 (2002): 193–201; Christopher W.

Kuzawa et al., "Fatherhood, Pairbonding and Testosterone in the Philippines," *Hormones and Behavior* 56, no. 4 (2009): 429–35.

76 **Emotional connectedness:** Both men and women have each hormone, but because of estrogen and testosterone, oxytocin is more of an issue in women and vasopressin is more of an issue in men.

77 **In monogamous prairie voles:** Miranda M. Lim et al., "Ventral Striatopallidal Oxytocin and Vasopressin V1a Receptors in the Monogamous Prairie Vole (Microtus Ochrogaster)," *Journal of Comparative Neurology* 468, no. 4 (2004): 555–70.

77 **the "monogamy gene":** Brizendine, *The Female Brain.*

77 **the shorter gene is seen in autism:** A. Meyer-Lindenberg et al, "Genetic Variants in AVPR1A Linked to Austism Predict Amygdala Activation and Personality Traits in Healthy Humans," *Molecular Psychiatry* 14, no. 10 (2008): 968–75.

77 **In Helen Fisher's brain-imaging studies:** Arthur Aron et al., "Reward, Motivation, and Emotion Systems Associated with Early-Stage Intense Romantic Love," *Journal of Neurophysiology* 94, no. 1 (2005): 327–37.

77 **the "anchoring gaze":** Deborah Tannen, *Talking from 9 to 5!: How Women's and Men's Conversational Styles Affect Who Gets Heard, Who Gets Credit, and What Gets Done at Work* (New York: Simon & Schuster Audio, 1994).

77 **Looking away, turning away:** Ned H. Kalin et al., "The Role of the Central Nucleus of the Amygdala in Mediating Fear and Anxiety in the Primate," *Journal of Neuroscience* 24, no. 24 (2004): 5506–15.

77 **trigger stress hormones:** Cortisol and norepinephrine.

77 **We are wired to connect:** Matthew D. Lieberman, *Social: Why Our Brains Are Wired to Connect* (Oxford University Press, 2013).

77 **to need other people:** Myron A. Hofer, "The Psychobiology of Early Attachment," *Clinical Neuroscience Research* 4, no. 5 (2005): 291–300; Myron A. Hofer, "Psychobiological Roots of Early Attachment," *Current Directions in Psychological Science* 15, no. 2 (2006): 84–88.

77 **In more than ninety countries surveyed:** Helen E. Fisher, *Anatomy of Love: The Natural History of Monogamy, Adultery, and Divorce* (New York: Simon & Schuster, 1992).

78 **Since 2000 that number has risen:** Jackie Calmes, "To Hold Senate, Democrats Rely on Single Women," *New York Times,* July 2, 2014.

78 **First-time marriages end in divorce:** Natalie Angier, "The Changing American Family," *New York Times,* November 25, 2013.

78 **The Maslow hierarchy of human needs:** Abraham Harold Maslow, "A Theory of Human Motivation," *Psychological Review* 50, no. 4 (1943): 370.

78 **we're looking for our partnership:** Eli Finkel, "The All-or-Nothing Marriage," *New York Times,* February 14, 2014.

78 **The quality of a marriage:** Mark A. Whisman and Martha L. Bruce, "Marital Dissatisfaction and Incidence of Major Depressive Episode in a Community Sample," *Journal of Abnormal Psychology* 108, no. 4 (1999): 674; Mark A. Whisman, "The Association Between Depression and Marital Dissatisfaction," in *Marital and Family Processes in Depression: A Scientific Foundation for Clinical Practice,* Steven R. H. Beach (Washington, DC: American Psychological Association, 2001), 3–24.

78 **the positive effects of a strong union:** Linda Waite and Maggie Gallagher, *The Case for Marriage: Why Married People Are Happier, Healthier and Better Off Financially* (New York: Random House, 2002).

78 **strengthen over time:** Christine M. Proulx et al., "Marital Quality and Personal Well-Being: A Meta-Analysis," *Journal of Marriage and Family* 69, no. 3 (2007): 576–93.

80 **Any reminder of an early attachment failure:** Marion Solomon and Stan Tatkin, *Love and War in Intimate Relationships: Connection, Disconnection, and Mutual Regulation in Couple Therapy,* Norton Series on Interpersonal Neurobiology (New York: W. W. Norton & Company, 2011); Harville Hendrix, *Getting the Love You Want: A Guide for Couples* (New York: Macmillan, 2007).

80 **Higher cognitive functions are shut down:** Daniel J. Siegel, "An Interpersonal Neurobiology Approach to Psychotherapy," *Psychiatric Annals* 36, no. 4 (2006): 248.

81 **conscious couples enable positive, healthy aspects:** Harville Hendrix and Helen LaKelly Hunt, *Making Marriage Simple: 10 Truths for Changing the Relationship You Have into the One You Want* (New York: Random House, 2013).

81 **The number of women who are:** Pew Research Center, "Mothers as the Sole or Primary Provider," May 29, 2013.

81 **A recent business school survey:** Iraj Mahdavi, "Comparing Men's and Women's Definition of Success," *Journal of Behavioral Studies in Business* 3 (2010): 1–8.

82   **Sharing earnings and household chores:** Lynn Prince Cooke, "'Doing' Gender in Context: House-
      hold Bargaining and Risk of Divorce in Germany and the United States," *American Journal of So-
      ciology* 112, no. 2 (2006): 442–72.

82   **more likely to report marital troubles:** Marianne Bertrand et al., "Gender Identity and Relative
      Income Within Household," (working paper, National Bureau of Economic Research, number
      19023, 2013).

82   **if the wife earns around 40 percent:** Cooke, "'Doing' Gender in Context," 442–72.

82   **the egalitarian marriage:** Lori Gottlieb, "Does a More Equal Marriage Mean Less Sex?" *New York
      Times*, February 6, 2014.

82   **When our husbands are doing dishes:** Sabino Kornrich et al., "Egalitarianism, Housework, and
      Sexual Frequency in Marriage," *American Sociological Review* 78, no. 1 (2013): 26–50.

83   **the longer a couple stays together:** Gary L. Hansen, "Extradyadic Relations During Courtship,"
      Journal of Sex Research 23 (1987): 382–90.

83   **a spike in the numbers:** James D. Wiggins and Doris A. Lederer, "Differential Antecedents of
      Infidelity in Marriage," *American Mental Health Counselors Association Journal*, no. 6 (1984):
      152–61.

83   **Women are more likely to cheat:** Pamela Druckerman, *Lust in Translation: The Rules of Infidel-
      ity from Tokyo to Tennessee* (New York: Penguin Press, 2007).

84   **For men, the likelihood of an affair:** Chien Liu, "A Theory of Marital Sexual Life," *Journal of
      Marriage and Family* 62, no. 2 (2000): 363–74.

84   **High-risk times for men:** Mark A. Whisman et al., "Predicting Sexual Infidelity in a Population-
      Based Sample of Married Individuals," *Journal of Family Psychology* 21, no. 2 (2007): 320–24.

84   **Very few animals:** Ryan and Jethá, *Sex at Dawn*.

84   **Pair-bonding is rare:** I. Tsapelas, H. E. Fisher, and A. Aron, "Infidelity: When, Where, Why," in
      The Dark Side of Close Relationships II, W. R. Cupach and B. H. Spitzberg (New York: Routledge,
      2010), 175–96.

84   **Penguins are monogamous only:** J. F. Wittenberger and R. L. Tilson, "The Evolution of Monog-
      amy: Hypotheses and Evidence," *Annual Review of Ecology and Systematics* 11 (1980): 197–232; D.
      W. Mock and M. Fujioka, "Monogamy and Long-Term Bonding in Vertebrates," *Trends in Ecology
      and Evolution* 5, no. 2 (1990): 39–43.

84   **we didn't descend from apes:** Michael J. Benton, *Vertebrate Paleontology* (Wiley-Blackwell,
      2005).

85   **Chimps and bonobos:** Anne E. Pusey, "Of Genes and Apes: Chimpanzee Social Organization and
      Reproduction," *Tree of Origin: What Primate Behavior Can Tell Us About Human Social Evolution*
      (2001): 9–38.

85   **Humans and bonobos:** Ryan and Jethá, *Sex at Dawn*.

85   **In bonobo troops:** Barbara Fruth and Gottfried Hohmann, "Social Grease for Females? Same-Sex
      Genital Contacts in Wild Bonobos," in Volker Sommer and Paul L. Vasey, eds., *Homosexual Behav-
      iour in Animals: An Evolutionary Perspective* (New York: Cambridge University Press, 2006):
      294–315.

85   **the bonobo clitoris:** Katarina Nolte, *Mystery Revealed: Female Sexuality Redefined for the 21st
      Century, Volume One—Primates* (Katarina Nolte, 2009).

85   **one ape that is monogamous:** Ryan and Jethá, *Sex at Dawn*.

86   **Chimps, bonobos, and human males:** Ibid.

86   **The meadow voles:** Sherrie Gruder-Adams and Lowell L. Getz, "Comparison of the Mating System
      and Paternal Behavior in Microtus Ochrogaster and M. Pennsylvanicus," *Journal of Mammalogy*
      66, no. 1 (1985): 165–67.

86   **The vasopressin receptor:** Thomas R. Insel et al., "Patterns of Brain Vasopressin Receptor Distri-
      bution Associated with Social Organization in Microtine Rodents," *Journal of Neuroscience* 14, no.
      9 (1994): 5381–92.

86   **When genes from the monogamous male prairie voles:** Lim et al., "Ventral Striatopallidal Oxy-
      tocin and Vasopressin V1a Receptors," 555–70.

86   **Men who have a gene variant:** Hasse Walum et al., "Genetic Variation in the Vasopressin Recep-
      tor 1a Gene (AVPR1A) Associates with Pair-Bonding Behavior in Humans," 105, no. 37 (2008):
      14153–56.

86   **Married men and fathers:** Sari M. van Anders and Neil V. Watson, "Relationship Status and
      Testosterone in North American Heterosexual and Non-Heterosexual Men and Women: Cross-
      sectional and Longitudinal Data," *Psychoneuroendocrinology* 31, no. 6 (2006): 715–23.

86   **Right after his child is born:** Gray et al., "Marriage and Fatherhood," 193–201.

86   **Men who maintain multiple female partners:** Alexandra Alvergne et al., "Variation in Testosterone Levels and Male Reproductive Effort: Insight from a Polygynous Human Population," *Hormones and Behavior* 56, no. 5 (2009): 491–97.

87   **married men with higher testosterone:** Lee T. Gettler et al., "Do Testosterone Declines During the Transition to Marriage and Fatherhood Relate to Men's Sexual Behavior? Evidence from the Philippines," *Hormones and Behavior* 64, no. 5 (2013): 755–63.

87   **men who cheat:** Peter T. Ellison, "Social Relationships and Reproductive Ecology," in *Endocrinology of Social Relationships* (Cambridge, MA: Harvard University Press, 2009), 54–73.

87   **women rated men with lower voices:** Jillian J. M. O'Connor et al., "Perceptions of Infidelity Risk Predict Women's Preferences for Low Male Voice Pitch in Short-Term over Long-Term Relationship Contexts," *Personality and Individual Differences* 56 (2014): 73–77.

87   **"The search for the unfamiliar":** Meredith F. Small, *Female Choices: Sexual Behavior of Female Primates* (Ithaca, NY: Cornell University Press, 1993), 153.

87   **Nature has bred philandering:** Fisher, *Anatomy of Love.*

88   **Research suggests that people who cheat:** T. Orzeck and E. Lung, "Big-Five Personality Differences of Cheaters and Non-Cheaters," *Current Psychology* 24 (2005): 274–86.

88   **more easily bored:** S. Hendrick and C. Hendrick, "Multidimensionality of Sexual Attitudes," *The Journal of Sex Research* 23 (1987): 502–26.

88   **Couples who spend all their time:** Esther Perel, *Mating in Captivity: Unlocking Erotic Intelligence* (New York: Harper, 2007).

88   **one partner will be clingier:** Stan Tatkin, *Wired for Love: How Understanding Your Partner's Brain and Attachment Style Can Help You Defuse Conflict and Build a Secure Relationship* (Oakland, CA: New Harbinger Publications, 2012).

89   **Couples who spend weekly time:** W. Bradford Wilcox and Jeffrey Dew, "The Date Night Opportunity: What Does Couple Time Tell Us About the Potential Value of Date Nights?" National Marriage Project, 2012, www.virginia.edu/marriageproject.

89   **Spouses who share friends:** P. R. Amato and S. J. Rogers, "A Longitudinal Study of Marital Problems and Subsequent Divorce," *Journal of Marriage and the Family* 59 (1997): 612–24.

89   **For couples with kids:** Jeffrey Dew, "Has the Marital Time Cost of Parenting Changed Over Time?" *Social Forces* 88, no. 2 (2009): 519–41.

89   **Nearly a third of marriages:** Tammy Nelson, *The New Monogamy: Redefining Your Relationship After Infidelity* (Oakland: New Harbinger Publications, 2013).

89   **Sometimes the discovery:** Bruce Roscoe et al., "Dating Infidelity: Behaviors, Reasons and Consequences," *Adolescence* 89 (1988) 35–43; Druckerman, *Lust in Translation.*

89   **improve communication:** Michael M. Olson et al., "Emotional Processes Following Disclosure of an Extramarital Affair," *Journal of Marital and Family Therapy* 28, no. 4 (2002): 423–34.

89   **quality of the partnership:** Hansen, "Extradyadic Relations During Courtship," 382–90.

90   **One of you went outside:** Solomon and Tatkin, *Love and War in Intimate Relationships.*

90   **Sometimes people have sex:** D. Easton and C. Liszt, *The Ethical Slut: A Guide to Infinite Sexual Possibilities* (Eugene: Greenery Press, 1997).

90   **"couples who negotiate . . . long-term love":** Perel, *Mating in Captivity,* 179.

92   **Dopamine injected into the male rat's:** F. Ferrari and D. Giuliani, "Sexual Attraction and Copulation in Male Rats: Effects of the Dopamine Agonist SND 919," *Pharmacology Biochemistry and Behavior* 50, no. 1 (1995): 29–34.

92   **horny rats that copulate:** D. Wenkstern et al., "Dopamine Transmission Increases in the Nucleus Accumbens of Male Rats During Their First Exposure to Sexually Receptive Female Rats," *Brain Research* 618, no. 1 (1993): 41–46.

92   **excitation transfer:** J. Bancroft et al., "The Relation Between Mood and Sexuality in Heterosexual Men," *Archives of Sexual Behavior* 32 (2003): 217–30.

92   **Regular exposure to male pheromones:** Winnifred B. Cutler et al., "Sexual Behavior Frequency and Menstrual Cycle Length in Mature Premenopausal Women," *Psychoneuroendocrinology* 4, no. 4 (1979): 297–309.

93   **"almost all individuals":** Fisher, *Why We Love.*

93   **Negativity is invisible abuse:** Hendrix and Hunt, *Making Marriage Simple.*

94   **Mirror, validate:** Ibid.

94   **we may be physiologically built:** David G. Blanchflower, and Andrew J. Oswald, "Money, Sex and Happiness: An Empirical Study," *The Scandinavian Journal of Economics* 106, no. 3 (2004): 393–415.

94   **Cultivating and maintaining:** D. Kahnman, "Objective Happiness," in *Well-Being: The Founda-*

tions of Hedonic Psychology, ed. Daniel Kahneman, Ed Diener, and Norbert Schwarz (New York: Russell Sage Foundation, 2003), 3–26.

Chapter Five: Motherhead

95 **massive neuronal reorganization:** Doidge, *The Brain That Changes Itself.*

95 **neurons multiply at a rate:** Craig Howard Kinsley, "The Neuroplastic Maternal Brain," *Hormones and Behavior* 54, no. 1 (2008): 1–4; Cindy K. Barha and Liisa A. M. Galea, "Influence of Different Estrogens on Neuroplasticity and Cognition in the Hippocampus," *Biochimica et Biophysica Acta (BBA)—General Subjects* 1800, no. 10 (2010): 1056–67.

95 **"baby brain suck":** Carrie Cuttler et al., "Everyday Life Memory Deficits in Pregnant Women," *Canadian Journal of Experimental Psychology/Revue Canadienne de Psychologie Expérimentale* 65, no. 1 (2011): 27; Charles M. Poser et al., "Benign Encephalopathy of Pregnancy Preliminary Clinical Observations," *Acta Neurologica Scandinavica* 73, no. 1 (1986): 39–43; Peter M. Brindle et al., "Objective and Subjective Memory Impairment in Pregnancy," *Psychological Medicine* 21, no. 03 (1991): 647–53.

96 **Parental-induced neuroplasticity:** Craig Kinsley and Kelly Lambert, "Reproduction-Induced Neuroplasticity: Natural Behavioral and Neuronal Alterations Associated with the Production and Care of Offspring," *Journal of Neuroendocrinology* 20, no. 4 (2008a): 515–25.

96 **The hormone responsible:** Doidge, *The Brain That Changes Itself.*

96 **During conception, oxytocin:** G. Kunz et al., "Uterine Peristalsis During the Follicular Phase of the Menstrual Cycle: Effects of Estrogen, Antioestrogen and Oxytocin," *Human Reproduction Update* 4, no. 5 (1998): 647–54.

96 **During childbirth, oxytocin:** Anna-Riitta Fuchs et al., "Oxytocin Receptors and Human Parturition: A Dual Role for Oxytocin in the Initiation of Labor," *Science* 215, no. 4538 (1982): 1396–98.

96 **In some experiments:** Carsten De Dreu et al., "The Neuropeptide Oxytocin Regulates Parochial Altruism in Intergroup Conflict Among Humans," *Science* 328, no. 5984 (2010): 1408–11.

96 **Motherhood brings a whole new:** A. Ferreira et al., "Role of Maternal Behavior on Aggression, Fear and Anxiety," *Physiology & Behavior* 77, no. 2 (2002): 197–204.

96 **Sometimes existing attachments:** Walter J. Freeman, *Neurodynamics: An Exploration in Mesoscopic Brain Dynamics* (New York: Springer, 2000).

97 **Though we're starting later:** Natalie Angier, "The Changing American Family," *New York Times,* November 25, 2013.

97 **The quality of eggs:** Lewis Krey et al., "Fertility and Maternal Age," *Annals of the New York Academy of Sciences* 943, no. 1 (2001): 26–33.

98 **Fertility drugs:** Linda Hammer Burns, "Psychiatric Aspects of Infertility and Infertility Treatments," *Psychiatric Clinics of North America* 30, no. 4 (2007): 689–716; J. L. Blenner, "Clomiphene-Induced Mood Swings," *Journal of Obstetric, Gynecologic, & Neonatal Nursing* 20, no. 4 (1991): 321–27; So-Hyun Choi et al., "Psychological Side-Effects of Clomiphene Citrate and Human Menopausal Gonadotrophin," *Journal of Psychosomatic Obstetrics & Gynecology* 26, no. 2 (2005): 93–100.

98 **Rare cases of psychosis:** F. Siedentopf et al., "Clomiphene Citrate as a Possible Cause of a Psychotic Reaction During Infertility Treatment," *Human Reproduction* 12, no. 4 (1997): 706–7.

98 **mania:** Rainer N. Persaud and Raymond C. Lam, "Manic Reaction After Induction of Ovulation with Gonadotropins," *American Journal of Psychiatry* 155, no. 3 (1998): 447–48.

98 **Nesting:** J. Johnston, "The Nesting Instinct," *Midwifery Today with International Midwife* 71 (2003): 36–37.

98 **Gynecologists will sometimes:** V. Hendrick et al., "Antidepressant Medications, Mood and Male Fertility," *Psychoneuroendocrinology* 25, no. 1 (2000): 37–51.

98 **melatonin tablets:** M. Juszczak and M. Michalska. "The Effect of Melatonin on Prolactin, Luteinizing Hormone (LH), and Follicle-Stimulating Hormone (FSH) Synthesis and Secretion," *Postepy higieny i medycyny doswiadczalnej* (online) 60 (2005): 431–38.

98 **the high levels of stress:** Elysia Poggi Davis et al., "Prenatal Exposure to Maternal Depression and Cortisol Influences Infant Temperament," *Journal of the American Academy of Child & Adolescent Psychiatry* 46, no. 6 (2007): 737–46; R. L. Huot et al., "Negative Affect in Offspring of Depressed Mothers Is Predicted by Infant Cortisol Levels at 6 Months and Maternal Depression During Pregnancy, But Not Postpartum," *Annals of the New York Academy of Sciences* 1032, no. 1 (2004): 234–36.

98 **The risks are low but present:** K. A. Yonkers et al., "The Management of Depression During Pregnancy: A Report from the American Psychiatric Association and the American College of Obstetricians and Gynecologists," *Obstetrics and Gynecology* 114 (2009): 703–13; Rachel M. Hayes et al.,

"Maternal Antidepressant Use and Adverse Outcomes: A Cohort Study of 228,876 Pregnancies," *American Journal of Obstetrics and Gynecology* 207, no. 1 (2012): 49.e1-49.e9.

98-99 **link between SSRI exposure:** Rebecca A. Harrington et al., "Serotonin Hypothesis of Autism: Implications for Selective Serotonin Reuptake Inhibitor Use During Pregnancy," *Autism Research* 6, no. 3 (2013): 149-68.

99 **another said it was twice as likely:** Lisa A. Croen et al., "Antidepressant Use During Pregnancy and Childhood Autism Spectrum Disorders," *Archives of General Psychiatry* 68, no. 11 (2011): 1104-12.

99 **other studies don't bear this out:** Anders Hviid et al., "Use of Selective Serotonin Reuptake Inhibitors During Pregnancy and Risk of Autism," *New England Journal of Medicine* 369, no. 25 (2013): 2406-15; Merete Juul Sørensen et al., "Antidepressant Exposure in Pregnancy and Risk of Autism Spectrum Disorders," *Clinical Epidemiology* 5 (2013): 449.

99 **women with bipolar disorder:** Yonkers et al., "The Management of Depression During Pregnancy," 703-13.

99 **Rates of depression:** Lori L. Altshuler et al., "An Update on Mood and Anxiety Disorders During Pregnancy and the Postpartum Period," *Primary Care Companion to the Journal of Clinical Psychiatry* 2, no. 6 (2000): 217.

99 **in women who are younger:** Ibid.

100 **Many women report the worst sleep:** Kathryn A. Lee and Aaron B. Caughey, "Evaluating Insomnia During Pregnancy and Postpartum," in *Sleep Disorders in Women* (Totowa, NJ: Humana Press, 2006), 185-98.

100 **Insomnia comes:** Jodi A. Mindell and Barry J. Jacobson, "Sleep Disturbances During Pregnancy," *Journal of Obstetric, Gynecologic, & Neonatal Nursing* 29, no. 6 (2000): 590-97.

100 **we're given an epidural:** Ellice Lieberman and Carol O'Donoghue, "Unintended Effects of Epidural Analgesia During Labor: A Systematic Review," *American Journal of Obstetrics and Gynecology* 186, no. 5 (2002): S31-S68.

101 **(Endocannabinoids):** Osama M. H. Habayeb et al., "Plasma Levels of the Endocannabinoid Anandamide in Women—A Potential Role in Pregnancy Maintenance and Labor?" *Journal of Clinical Endocrinology & Metabolism* 89, no. 11 (2004): 5482-87.

101 **Endocannabinoids:** The endocannabinoid system is well represented in the reproductive tissues and is involved in ovulation and implantation as well.

101 **peak during labor induction:** V. Nallendran et al., "The Plasma Levels of the Endocannabinoid, Anandamide, Increase with the Induction of Labor," *BJOG: An International Journal of Obstetrics & Gynecology* 117, no. 7 (2010): 863-69.

101 **breast-fed babies:** Dale L. Johnson et al., "Breast Feeding and Children's Intelligence," *Psychological Reports* 79, no. 3f (1996): 1179-85.

101 **lower incidences of breast cancer:** Polly A. Newcomb et al., "Lactation and a Reduced Risk of Premenopausal Breast Cancer," *New England Journal of Medicine* 330, no. 2 (1994): 81-87.

101 **ovarian cancer:** Marta L. Gwinn et al., "Pregnancy, Breast Feeding, and Oral Contraceptives and the Risk of Epithelial Ovarian Cancer," *Journal of Clinical Epidemiology* 43, no. 6 (1990): 559-68.

101 **They also have lower:** Elizabeth Sibolboro Mezzacappa, "Breastfeeding and Maternal Stress Response and Health." *Nutrition Reviews* 62, no. 7 (2004): 261-68.

101 **Oxytocin turns down:** S. C. Gammie et al., "Role of Corticotropin Releasing Factor-Related Peptides in the Neural Regulation of Maternal Defense," *Neurobiology of the Parental Brain* (San Diego, CA: Elsevier, 2008).

101 **Breast milk has tryptophan:** W. E. Heine, "The Significance of Tryptophan in Infant Nutrition," *Adv Exp Med Biol* 467 (1999): 705-10.

102 **stimulates endorphin production:** T. Barrett et al., "Does Melatonin Modulate Beta-Endorphin, Corticosterone, and Pain Threshold?" *Life Sciences* 66, no. 6 (2000): 467-76.

102 **endorphins called galattorphins:** Ibid., Zanardo.

102 **have higher endorphin levels:** V. Zanardo et al., "Beta Endorphin Concentrations in Human Milk," *J Pediatr Gastroenterol Nutr* 33, no. 2 (2001): 160-64; R. Franceschini et al., "Plasma Beta-Endorphin Concentrations During Suckling in Lactating Women," *Br J Obstet Gynaecol* 96, no. 6 (1989): 711-13.

102 **also contains cannabinoids:** Timothy H. Marczylo et al., "A Solid-Phase Method for the Extraction and Measurement of Anandamide from Multiple Human Biomatrices," *Analytical Biochemistry* 384, no. 1 (2009): 106-13.

102 **Goat milk has:** R. Mechoulam et al., "Endocannabinoids, Feeding and Suckling—from Our Perspective," *International Journal of Obesity* 30 (2006): S24-S28.

102 **human breast milk:** V. Di Marzo et al., "Trick or Treat from Food Endocannabinoids?" *Nature* 396

(1998): 636–37; Florence Williams, *Breasts: A Natural and Unnatural History* (New York: W. W. Norton & Company, 2012).

102 **cannabinoid receptors:** Ester Fride, "The Endocannabinoid-CB1 Receptor System in Pre- and Postnatal Life," *European Journal of Pharmacology* 500, no. 1 (2004): 289–97.

102 **given to newborn mice:** Ester Fride et al., "Critical Role of the Endogenous Cannabinoid System in Mouse Pup Suckling and Growth," *European Journal of Pharmacology* 419, no. 2 (2001): 207–14.

102 **babies may get fatter:** Y. Le Strat and B. Le Foll, "Obesity and Cannabis Use: Results from 2 Representative National Surveys," *American Journal of Epidemiology* 174, no. 8 (2011): 929.

102 **Even though stoners:** N. Rodondi et al., "Marijuana Use, Diet, Body Mass Index, and Cardiovascular Risk Factors (from the CARDIA Study)," *American Journal of Cardiology* 98, no. 4 (2006): 478–84.

102 **Cannabinoids in breast milk:** Williams, *Breasts*.

102 **appreciable levels of pollutants:** Ibid.

102 **you burn about thirty calories:** Linda S. Adair and Ernesto Pollitt, "Energy Balance During Pregnancy and Lactation," *Lancet* 320, no. 8291 (1982): 219; F. Kramer et al., "Breast-Feeding Reduces Maternal Lower-Body Fat," *Journal of the American Dietetic Association* 93, no. 4 (1993): 429–33.

102 **breast milk into a bottle:** Avent Isis gets my vote for best breast pump.

103 **Cuddling and nurturing:** Thomas R. Insel, "Oxytocin—a Neuropeptide for Affiliation: Evidence from Behavioral, Receptor Autoradiographic, and Comparative Studies," *Psychoneuroendocrinology* 17, no. 1 (1992): 3–35.

103 **cohabiting parents share:** Ilanit Gordon et al., "Oxytocin and the Development of Parenting in Humans," *Biological Psychiatry* 68, no. 4 (2010): 377–82.

103 **his bond will be stronger:** Linda F. Palmer, "The Chemistry of Attachment," *Attachment Parenting International News* 5, no. 2 (2002).

103 **Vasopressin is the biggest factor:** Thomas R. Insel et al., "Oxytocin, Vasopressin, and the Neuroendocrine Basis of Pair Bond Formation," in *Vasopressin and Oxytocin* (U.S.: Springer, 1998), 215–24.

103 **Men have prolactin:** Alison S. Fleming et al., "Testosterone and Prolactin Are Associated with Emotional Responses to Infant Cries in New Fathers," *Hormones and Behavior* 42, no. 4 (2002): 399–413.

103 **Monkeys reared without physical contact:** John Bowlby, "Maternal Care and Mental Health," *Journal of Consulting Psychology* 16, no. 3 (1952): 232.

103 **their brain chemicals imbalanced:** Maté, *When the Body Says No.*

103 **In laboratory animals:** Myron A. Hofer, "Physiological and Behavioral Processes in Early Maternal Deprivation," *Physiology, Emotion and Psychosomatic Illness*, Elsevier (1972): 175–86.

103 **Maternal care in infancy:** Christian Caldji et al., "Maternal Care During Infancy Regulates the Development of Neural Systems Mediating the Expression of Fearfulness in the Rat," *PNAS* 95, no. 9 (1998): 5335–40; Christian Caldji et al., "Variations in Maternal Care in Infancy Regulate the Development of Stress Reactivity," *Biological Psychiatry* 48, no. 12 (2000): 1164–74.

103 **disruption of attachment in infancy:** Maté, *When the Body Says No.*

104 **When we give our children:** Daniel J. Siegel and Mary Hartzell, *Parenting from the Inside Out* (New York: Penguin, 2003).

104 **As many as 50 to 80 percent of women:** Michael W. O'Hara, "Post-partum Blues, Depression, and Psychosis: A Review," *Journal of Psychosomatic Obstetrics & Gynecology* 7, no. 3 (1987): 205–27.

105 **But roughly 10 to 15 percent:** Joanna L. Workman et al., "Endocrine Substrates of Cognitive and Affective Changes During Pregnancy and Postpartum," *Behavioral Neuroscience* 126, no. 1 (2012): 54.

105 **energy, appetite, sleep, and libido:** Zachary N. Stowe and Charles B. Nemeroff, "Women at Risk for Postpartum-Onset Major Depression," *American Journal of Obstetrics and Gynecology* 173, no. 2 (1995): 639–45.

105 **postpartum psychosis:** O'Hara, "Post-partum Blues, Depression," 205–27.

105 **Prolactin can make us:** Maureen W. Groer and Katherine Morgan, "Immune, Health and Endocrine Characteristics of Depressed Postpartum Mothers," *Psychoneuroendocrinology* 32, no. 2 (2007): 133–39.

105 **the postpartum blues:** Michael W. O'Hara et al., "Prospective Study of Postpartum Blues: Biologic and Psychosocial Factors," *Archives of General Psychiatry* 48, no. 9 (1991): 801.

105 **a quick drop-off of estrogen:** O'Hara, "Post-partum Blues, Depression," 205–27.

105 **The peak time for postpartum depression:** Victor J. M. Pop et al., "Prevalence of Post Partum Depression: or Is It Post-Puerperium Depression?" *Acta obstetricia et gynecologica Scandinavica* 72, no. 5 (1993): 354–58.

106   **Breast-feeding reliably reduces**: Cristina Borra, Maria Iacovou, and Almudena Sevilla, "New Evidence on Breastfeeding and Postpartum Depression: The Importance of Understanding Women's Intentions," *Maternal and Child Health Journal* (2014): 1–11.

106   **if your baby is colicky**: Jenny S. Radesky et al., "Inconsolable Infant Crying and Maternal Postpartum Depressive Symptoms," *Pediatrics* 131, no. 6 (2013): e1857–e1864.

106   **A history of a previous depression**: Miki Bloch et al., "Risk Factors Associated with the Development of Postpartum Mood Disorders," *Journal of Affective Disorders* 88, no. 1 (2005): 9–18.

106   **The rational frontal lobes**: Sandra Aamodt and Sam Wang, *Welcome to Your Child's Brain: How the Mind Grows, from Birth to University* (London: Oneworld Publications, 2012).

106   **for your teenage daughter**: Sil Reynolds and Eliza Reynolds, *Mothering and Daughtering: Keeping Your Bond Strong Through the Teenage Years* (Boulder, CO: Sounds True, 2013).

107   **Mothering is as much about**: Ibid.

107   **Since the 1970s**: Angier, "The Changing American Family," *New York Times*.

108   **Three-quarters of women today**: Ibid.; Pew Research Center analysis of 2011 American Community Survey.

108   **40 percent of us**: Ibid., Angier.

108   **They learn from their peers**: Gordon Neufeld and Gabor Maté, *Hold On to Your Kids: Why Parents Need to Matter More Than Peers* (Toronto: Vintage, 2013).

108   **"cooperative breeders"**: Sarah Blaffer Hrdy, "Mothers and Others," *Natural History* 110, no. 4 (2001): 50–62.

108   **In tribal societies**: Ryan and Jethá, *Sex at Dawn*.

108   **"inappropriate for our species"**: Ibid., 109

109   **In a survey of married women**: Brooke Showell, "The State of Married Sex," iVillage.com, May 8, 2010.

109   **women in early pregnancy**: Kay Mordecai Robson et al., "Maternal Sexuality During First Pregnancy and After Childbirth," *BJOG: An International Journal of Obstetrics & Gynecology* 88, no. 9 (1981): 882–89; A. Don Solberg et al., "Sexual Behavior in Pregnancy," in *Handbook of Sex Therapy* (U.S.: Springer, 1978), 361–71.

109–110   **marital satisfaction plummets**: Carolyn Pape Cowan and Philip A. Cowan, *When Partners Become Parents: The Big Life Change for Couples* (Hillsdale, NJ: Lawrence Erlbaum Associates, 2000).

110   **"the quality of the mother role"**: Margaret A. De Judicibus and Marita P. McCabe, "Psychological Factors and the Sexuality of Pregnant and Postpartum Women," *Journal of Sex Research* 39, no. 2 (2002): 94–103.

110   **The first three months postpartum**: Virginia L. Larsen, "Stresses of the Childbearing Year," *American Journal of Public Health and the Nations Health* 56, no. 1 (1966): 32–36.

110   **a few reasons for lackluster libido**: Berman, and Berman, *For Women Only*.

110   **Having little kids climbing all over you**: Ibid.

110   **married women have lower testosterone**: Emily S. Barrett et al., "Marriage and Motherhood Are Associated with Lower Testosterone Concentrations in Women," *Hormones and Behavior* 63, no. 1 (2013): 72–79.

111   **Your children end up being**: Perel, *Mating in Captivity*.

111   **"virtual annihilation of the self"**: Sheila Kitzinger, *Ourselves as Mothers: The Universal Experience of Motherhood* (Reading, MA: Addison-Wesley, 1995).

111   **Our frustration about**: John Mordechai Gottman and Nan Silver, *The Seven Principles for Making Marriage Work* (New York: Random House, 1999).

111   **And until nonsexual issues**: Winks and Semans, *Sexy Mamas*.

112   **more men than women complain**: Patricia Love and Jo Robinson, *Hot Monogamy: Essential Steps to More Passionate, Intimate Lovemaking* (Dutton, 1994).

112   **For men, sex can be the only way**: Perel, *Mating in Captivity*.

112   **A desire discrepancy**: Love and Robinson, *Hot Monogamy*.

112   **In an iVillage survey**: Showell, *The State of Married Sex*.

113   **The book *Sexy Mamas* recommends**: winks and semans, *Sexy Mamas*.

114   **Sometimes what's hot is**: Ibid.

115   **"authentic eroticism"**: Ibid., 191

Chapter Six: Perimenopause: The Storm Before the Calm

117   **The average age for menopause**: Berman and Berman, *For Women Only*.

118   **Nearly a quarter of women**: Jennifer Senior, *All Joy and No Fun: The Paradox of Modern Parenthood* (New York: HarperCollins, 2014).

118 **one Gallup poll from 1998:** Jim Duffy, "Lifting the Fog," *Hopkins Medicine*, October 1, 2013, 31–37.

119 **Complaints during this stretch:** Sara Gottfried, *The Hormone Cure: Reclaim Balance, Sleep, Sex Drive and Vitality Naturally with the Gottfried Protocol* (New York: Simon and Schuster, 2013); Berman and Berman, *For Women Only.*

119 **three-quarters of women:** Laura E. Corio, *The Change Before the Change* (New York: Bantam, 2000).

119 **Hot flashes affect 80 percent of women:** Ibid.

119 **last between one and five minutes:** Ellen W. Freeman et al., "Temporal Associations of Hot Flashes and Depression in the Transition to Menopause," *Menopause* 16, no. 4 (2009): 728.

119 **Sudden dips in estrogen levels:** D. R. Meldrum et al., "Pituitary Hormones During the Menopausal Hot Flash," *Obstetrics and Gynecology* 64, no. 6 (1984): 752–56.

120 **The closer you get toward menopause** Mary G. Metcalf, "Incidence of Ovulatory Cycles in Women Approaching the Menopause," *Journal of Biosocial Science* 11, no. 1 (1979): 39–48.

121 **A menopausal woman has 5 percent:** Steven F. Hotze, *Hormones, Health, and Happiness* (Houston, TX: Forrest Publishing, 2005).

121 **This means estrogen dominance:** Gottfried, *Hormone Cure.*

121 **Estrogen promotes fat storage:** Hotze, *Hormones, Health, and Happiness.*

121 **Add to this the xenoestrogens:** Ibid.

121 **Unopposed estrogen:** Corio, *The Change Before the Change.*

121 **Estrogen dominance is gone:** Christiane Northrup, *The Wisdom of Menopause*, rev. ed. (Hay House, Inc., 2012).

122 **belly and back fat:** The hippy gynoid shape is normal in 80 percent of premenopausal women, but as the years tick by, more of us turn from pear-shaped to apple-shaped (called android), chipping that number down to 50 percent of perimenopausal women, and then to 40 percent of postmenopausal women.

122 **hippy synoid shape:** Corio, *The Change Before the Change.*

122 **Your risk for diabetes rises:** Rebecca C. Thurston et al., "Vasomotor Symptoms and Insulin Resistance in the Study of Women's Health Across the Nation," *Journal of Clinical Endocrinology & Metabolism* 97, no. 10 (2012): 3487–94.

122 **So can stress:** Stress causes the release of cortisol from the adrenal glands, which sit atop the kidneys. Cortisol counteracts insulin, causing higher blood sugar levels. It also stimulates sugar production in the liver, called gluconeogenesis, and stops the production of a transporter (called GLUT4) that sugar needs to get into the cell. All this excess glucose that isn't burned as energy or stored for later use in the liver gets stored as belly fat.

122 **increase in abdominal fat:** André Tchernof et al., "Menopause, Central Body Fatness, and Insulin Resistance: Effects of Hormone-Replacement Therapy," *Coronary Artery Disease* 9, no. 8 (1998): 503–12.

122 **Progesterone can help with weight loss:** Hotze, *Hormones, Health, and Happiness.*

122 **If you don't ovulate:** Corio, *The Change Before the Change.*

122 **high estrogen levels signal the liver:** Hotze, *Hormones, Health, and Happiness.*

122 **free thyroid hormone:** Pregnancy, birth control pills, and estrogen supplementation can further increase the protein that gobbles up free thyroid hormone.

123 **An underactive thyroid:** Gottfried, *Hormone Cure.*

123 **Fifty-year-old women produce:** Hotze, *Hormones, Health, and Happiness.*

123 **Rats that have their ovaries removed:** Lori Asarian and Nori Geary, "Modulation of Appetite by Gonadal Steroid Hormones," *Philosophical Transactions of the Royal Society B: Biological Sciences* 361, no. 1471 (2006): 1251–63.

123 **one of the first symptoms:** Freeman et al., "Temporal Associations of Hot Flashes and Depression," 728.

124 **Your risk of depression:** E. W. Freeman et al., "Hormones and Menopausal Status as Predictors of Depression in Women in Transition to Menopause," *Archives of General Psychiatry* 61 (2004): 62–70.

124 **The prevalence of depression:** "QuickStats: Prevalence of Current Depression Among Persons Aged 12 Years, by Age Group and Sex—United States, National Health and Nutrition Examination Survey, 2007–2010," *Morbidity and Mortality Weekly Report (MMWR)* 60, no. 51 (2012): 1747.

124 **When you remove a female rat's ovaries:** Erika Estrada-Camarena et al., "Antidepressant-like Effect of Different Estrogenic Compounds in the Forced Swimming Test," *Neuropsychopharmacology: Official Publication of the American College of Neuropsychopharmacology* 28, no. 5 (2003): 830–38.

124 **Lower estrogen levels:** Zenab Amin et al., "Effect of Estrogen-Serotonin Interactions on Mood and Cognition," *Behavioral and Cognitive Neuroscience Reviews* 4, no. 1 (2005): 43–58.

124 **overall serotonin activity:** Estrogen increases the expression of the gene for the enzyme that makes serotonin, and it also directly increases serotonin activity. If you want a sense of how estrogen and progesterone work as opposites, consider this: while estrogen creates high levels of serotonin by blocking its breakdown by the enzyme MAO, high progesterone levels increase MAO activity, thus lowering serotonin levels. High progesterone also inhibits testosterone's mood-elevating effects, which is why in the second half of your cycle, when progesterone dominates, you can feel depressed, sedated, and lackadaisical.

124 **major depressions need to be treated:** M. F. Morrison et al., "Lack of Efficacy of Estradiol for Depression in Post-Menopausal Women: A Randomized, Controlled Trial," *Biological Psychiatry* 55 (2004): 406–12; Jennifer L. Payne et al., "A Reproductive Subtype of Depression: Conceptualizing Models and Moving Toward Etiology," *Harvard Review of Psychiatry* 17, no. 2 (2009): 72–86.

124 **High estrogen:** Zenab Amin et al., "The Interaction of Neuroactive Steroids and GABA in the Development of Neuropsychiatric Disorders in Women," *Pharmacology Biochemistry and Behavior* 84, no. 4 (2006): 635–43.

124 **When the brain's hormone control center:** Corio, *The Change Before the Change.*

125 **Women experience insomnia more than men:** Ibid.

125 **when cortisol levels drop:** Theresa M. Buckley and Alan F. Schatzberg, "On the Interactions of the Hypothalamic-Pituitary-Adrenal (HPA) Axis and Sleep: Normal HPA Axis Activity and Circadian Rhythm, Exemplary Sleep Disorders," *Journal of Clinical Endocrinology & Metabolism* 90, no. 5 (2005): 3106–14.

125 **restless leg syndrome:** Leg spasms occur in 40 percent of perimenopausal women, likely due to these low magnesium levels.

125 **Estrogen dominance exacerbates:** Hotze, *Hormones, Health, and Happiness.*

125 **Estrogen is involved in:** Bruce S. McEwen and Stephen B. Alves, "Estrogen Actions in the Central Nervous System 1." *Endocrine Reviews* 20, no. 3 (1999): 279–307.

126 **memory and concentration:** Nouns are the first to go; people's names or the title of the movie you saw last night will escape you when your estrogen levels dip. Verbal memory seems the specific domain of estrogen, though some menopausal women report less fine-motor coordination and longer reaction times.

126 **Giving women estrogen can:** Barbara B. Sherwin and Susana Phillips, "Estrogen and Cognitive Functioning in Surgically Menopausal Women," *Annals of the New York Academy of Sciences* 592, no. 1 (1990): 474–75; Barbara B. Sherwin, "Estrogen and Cognitive Functioning in Women," *Endocrine Reviews* 24, no. 2 (2003): 133–51.

126 **vigilance, reasoning:** E. S. LeBlanc et al., "Hormone Replacement Therapy and Cognition: Systematic Review and Metaanalysis," *JAMA* 285 (2001): 1489–99.

126 **Testosterone is essential for learning:** Elizabeth Barrett-Connor and Deborah Goodman-Gruen, "Cognitive Function and Endogenous Sex Hormones in Older Women," *Journal of the American Geriatrics Society* (1999); Jeri S. Janowsky, "Thinking with Your Gonads: Testosterone and Cognition," *Trends in Cognitive Sciences* 10, no. 2 (2006): 77–82.

126 **Testosterone can directly influence:** David R. Rubinow and Peter J. Schmidt, "Androgens, Brain, and Behavior," *American Journal of Psychiatry* 153, no. 8 (1996): 974–84.

126 **Postmenopausal women score better:** Barbara B. Sherwin, "Estrogen and/or Androgen Replacement Therapy and Cognitive Functioning in Surgically Menopausal Women," *Psychoneuroendocrinology* 13, no. 4 (1988): 345–57.

126 **Postmenopausal women who take estrogen:** Peter P. Zandi et al., "Hormone Replacement Therapy and Incidence of Alzheimer Disease in Older Women: The Cache County Study," *JAMA* 288, no. 17 (2002): 2123–29.

126 **Testosterone also reduces:** Gunnar K. Gouras et al., "Testosterone Reduces Neuronal Secretion of Alzheimer's B-Amyloid Peptides," *PNAS* 97, no. 3 (2000): 1202–5.

126 **plays a neuroprotective role:** Janowsky, "Thinking with Your Gonads," 77–82.

126 **estrogen increases BDNF levels:** V. Luine and M. Frankfurt, "Interactions Between Estradiol, BDNF and Dendritic Spines in Promoting Memory," *Neuroscience* 239 (2013): 34–45.

127 **that number drops to 38 percent:** Joey Sprague and David Quadagno, "Gender and Sexual Motivation: An Exploration of Two Assumptions," *Journal of Psychology & Human Sexuality* 2, no. 1 (1989): 57–76.

127 **minus the sexual attraction:** Lori Gottlieb, "Does a More Equal Marriage Mean Less Sex?" *New York Times*, February 6, 2014.

127 **sexy thoughts can trigger:** Katherine L. Goldey and Sari M. van Anders, "Sexy Thoughts: Effects of Sexual Cognitions on Testosterone, Cortisol, and Arousal in Women," *Hormones and Behavior* 59, no. 5 (2011): 754–64.

127 **Sexual function may rely more:** Lorraine Dennerstein et al., "The Relative Effects of Hormones

and Relationship Factors on Sexual Function of Women Through the Natural Menopausal Transition," *Fertility and Sterility* 84, no. 1 (2005): 174–80.

128 **Younger eggs are more likely:** D. T. Armstrong, "Effects of Maternal Age on Oocyte Developmental Competence," *Theriogenology* 55, no. 6 (2001): 1303–22.

128 **The risk of autism and schizophrenia rises:** Abraham Reichenberg et al., "Advancing Paternal Age and Autism," *Archives of General Psychiatry* 63, no. 9 (2006): 1026–32; Dolores Malaspina et al., "Advancing Paternal Age and the Risk of Schizophrenia," *Archives of General Psychiatry* 58, no. 4 (2001): 361–67.

128 **Men's testosterone begins to wane:** S. M. Harman et al., "Longitudinal Effects of Aging on Serum Total and Free Testosterone Levels in Healthy Men," Baltimore Longitudinal Study of Aging, *J Clin Endocrinol Metabol* 86 (2001): 724–31.

128 **older men end up having twice as much estrogen:** Joel S. Finkelstein et al., "Gonadal Steroids and Body Composition, Strength, and Sexual Function in Men," *New England Journal of Medicine* 369, no. 11 (2013): 1011–22.

128 **testosterone levels:** Two androgens, testosterone and androstenedione, are still made in the ovaries up to five years after menopause.

128 **testosterone dominance:** Uwe D. Rohr, "The Impact of Testosterone Imbalance on Depression and Women's Health," *Maturitas* 41 (2002): 25–46.

128 **A steep decline occurs:** Rohr, "The Impact of Testosterone Imbalance," 25–46.

128 **When estrogen levels are high:** Hotze, *Hormones, Health, and Happiness.*

129 **libido bump:** Tibolone, a medicine that raises free testosterone and estrogen level, but, more important, lowers SHBG levels, improves mood and libido in menopausal women.

129 **High testosterone levels in women correlate positively:** Sari M. van Anders, "Testosterone and Sexual Desire in Healthy Women and Men," *Archives of Sexual Behavior* 41, no. 6 (2012): 1471–84.

129 **whether the levels are too low:** Rebecca Goldstat et al., "Transdermal Testosterone Therapy Improves Well-Being, Mood, and Sexual Function in Premenopausal Women," *Menopause* 10, no. 5 (2003): 390–98.

129 **or too high:** Joyce T. Bromberger et al., "Longitudinal Change in Reproductive Hormones and Depressive Symptoms Across the Menopausal Transition: Results from the Study of Women's Health Across the Nation (SWAN)," *Archives of General Psychiatry* 67, no. 6 (2010): 598–607.

129 **15 to 20 percent of American couples:** Bob Berkowitz and Susan Yager-Berkowitz, *He's Just Not Up for It Anymore: Why Men Stop Having Sex, and What You Can Do About It* (New York: Harper-Collins, 2007).

130 **Lack of interest in sex:** Edward O. Laumann et al., "Sexual Dysfunction in the United States: Prevalence and Predictors," *JAMA* 281, no. 6 (1999): 537–44; Alan Riley and Elizabeth Riley, "Controlled Studies on Women Presenting with Sexual Drive Disorder: I. Endocrine Status," *Journal of Sex & Marital Therapy* 26, no. 3 (2000): 269–83.

130 **A badly functioning thyroid:** Berman and Berman, *For Women Only.*

130 **When magnesium levels are depleted:** Hotze, *Hormones, Health, and Happiness.*

130 **in the later stages of the transition:** Brian W. Somerville, "The Role of Estradiol Withdrawal in the Etiology of Menstrual Migraine," *Neurology* 22, no. 4 (1972): 355–55.

130 **migraines can result:** Low estrogen and low magnesium levels are also the cause of premenstrual migraines during PMS.

130 **synthetic progestins such as Provera:** Ann E. MacGregor, "Contraception and Headache," *Headache: The Journal of Head and Face Pain* 53, no. 2 (2013): 247–76.

130 **Natural, bioidentical progesterones:** Corio, *The Change Before the Change.*

130 **decreased blood flow to the vagina:** Berman and Berman, *For Women Only.*

131 **orgasms become weaker:** Corio, *The Change Before the Change.*

131 **Nipple sensation wanes:** Berman and Berman, *For Women Only.*

131 **may have more anovulatory cycles:** Britt-Marie Landgren et al., "Menopause Transition: Annual Changes in Serum Hormonal Patterns over the Menstrual Cycle in Women During a Nine-Year Period Prior to Menopause," *Journal of Clinical Endocrinology & Metabolism* 89, no. 6 (2004): 2763–69; Henry G. Burger et al., "Cycle and Hormone Changes During Perimenopause: The Key Role of Ovarian Function," *Menopause* 15, no. 4 (2008): 603–12.

131 **Testosterone levels begin to wane:** A. Guay et al., "Serum Androgen Levels in Healthy Premenopausal Women with and without Sexual Dysfunction: Part A. Serum Androgen Levels in Women Aged 20–49 Years with No Complaints of Sexual Dysfunction," *International Journal of Impotence Research* 16, no. 2 (2004): 112–20.

131 **Testosterone supplementation:** Corio, *The Change Before the Change.*

131 **A study of menopausal women:** R. D. Gambrell Jr. and R. B. Greenblatt, "Hormone Therapy for the Menopause," *Geriatrics* 36, no. 7 (1981): 53–61.

131 **"If women care about their bones":** Irwin Goldstein (director, Sexual Medicine, Alvarado Hospital, San Diego, CA), interview conducted by phone, June 4, 2014.

131 **Testosterone supplementation reduces osteoporosis:** Susan R. Davis et al., "Testosterone Enhances Estradiol's Effects on Postmenopausal Bone Density and Sexuality," *Maturitas* 21, no. 3 (1995): 227–36.

131 **estrogen's effects:** In women with higher SHBG taking oral estrogens, muscle mass is reduced.

131 **increases muscle mass:** S. Bhasin et al., "Proof of the Effect of Testosterone on Skeletal Muscle," *Journal of Endocrinology* 170, no. 1 (2001): 27–38.

132 **Ditch the oral contraceptives:** Peter R. Casson et al., "Effect of Postmenopausal Estrogen Replacement on Circulating Androgens," *Obstetrics & Gynecology* 90, no. 6 (1997): 995–98.

132 **synthetic progesterones drive down:** N. Van der Vange et al., "Effects of Seven Low-Dose Combined Oral Contraceptives on Sex Hormone Binding Globulin, Corticosteroid Binding Globulin, Total and Free Testosterone," *Contraception* 41, no. 4 (1990): 345–52.

132 **Drinking more leads to more conversion:** Judith S. Gavaler and David H. Thiel, "The Association Between Moderate Alcoholic Beverage Consumption and Serum Estradiol and Testosterone Levels in Normal Postmenopausal Women: Relationship to the Literature," *Alcoholism: Clinical and Experimental Research* 16, no. 1 (1992): 87–92.

132 **the xenoestrogens in plastics:** Hotze, *Hormones, Health, and Happiness.*

132 **Vaginal atrophy:** D. W. Sturdee and N. Panay, "Recommendations for the Management of Postmenopausal Vaginal Atrophy," *Climacteric* 13, no. 6 (2010): 509–22.

132 **"senile vagina":** Sandra Leiblum et al., "Vaginal Atrophy in the Postmenopausal Woman: The Importance of Sexual Activity and Hormones," *JAMA* 249, no. 16 (1983): 2195–98.

133 **vaginal itching, dryness, and burning:** Corio, *The Change Before the Change.*

133 **alterations in the vaginal pH:** Berman and Berman, *For Women Only.*

133 **Regular sex may help to maintain:** Winnifred B. Cutler et al., "Sexual Behavior Frequency and Menstrual Cycle Length in Mature Premenopausal Women," *Psychoneuroendocrinology* 4, no. 4 (1979): 297–309.

133 **If lubrication is a problem:** Berman and Berman, *For Women Only.*

133 **Vaginal estrogen is superior:** Corio, *The Change Before the Change.*

133 **Local hormone treatment:** Sturdee and Panay, "Recommendations for the Management of Postmenopausal Vaginal Atrophy," 509–22.

133 **sex becomes more goal oriented:** Berman and Berman, *For Women Only.*

134 **Viagra did help them:** Ibid.

134 **VENIS (very erotic, noninsertive sex):** Ibid.

135 **estrogen lowers the risk for diabetes:** Youhua Xu et al., "Combined Estrogen Replacement Therapy on Metabolic Control in Postmenopausal Women with Diabetes Mellitus," *The Kaohsiung Journal of Medical Sciences* 30, no. 7 (2014): 350–61.

135 **HRT attenuates:** A. O. Mueck, "Postmenopausal Hormone Replacement Therapy and Cardiovascular Disease: The Value of Transdermal Estradiol and Micronized Progesterone," *Climacteric* 15, no. S1 (2012): 11–17.

135 **normalize weight and appetite:** Gail A. Greendale et al., "Symptom Relief and Side Effects of Postmenopausal Hormones: Results from the Postmenopausal Estrogen/Progestin Interventions Trial," *Obstetrics & Gynecology* 92, no. 6 (1998): 982–88.

135 **biodentical hormones:** Bioidentical products are derived from plant hormones. Soybeans and Mexican wild yams contain diosgenin, which is converted into progesterone in a lab. It can be further converted into estrogen. One caveat: bioequivalent is not bioidentical. Equivalence has to do with potency only, and is a marketing strategy meant to confuse the consumer.

135 **Provera and other synthetic progestins:** Corio, *The Change Before the Change.*

135 **Synthetic hormones can also deplete:** Hotze, *Hormones, Health, and Happiness.*

135 **Pills get broken down by the liver:** Marinka S. Post et al., "Effect of Oral and Transdermal Estrogen Replacement Therapy on Hemostatic Variables Associated with Venous Thrombosis: A Randomized, Placebo-Controlled Study in Postmenopausal Women," *Arteriosclerosis, Thrombosis, and Vascular Biology* 23, no. 6 (2003): 1116–21.

135 **For testosterone supplementation:** Hotze, *Hormones, Health, and Happiness.*

136 **The Women's Health Initiative:** Ellen C. G. Grant, "Hormone Replacement Therapy and Risk of Breast Cancer," *JAMA* 287, no. 18 (2002): 2360–61.

136 **"million women study":** V. Beral et al., "Evidence from Randomized Trials on the Long-Term Effects of Hormone Replacement Therapy," *Lancet* 360 (2002): 942–44.

136 **women who started the hormones within months:** Rowan T. Chlebowski et al., "Estrogen Plus Progestin and Breast Cancer Incidence and Mortality in the Women's Health Initiative Observational Study," *Journal of the National Cancer Institute* 105, no. 8 (2013): 526–35.

136 **If a woman has her:** Ronald K. Ross, et al.,"Effect of Hormone Replacement Therapy on Breast Cancer Risk: Estrogen Versus Estrogen Plus Progestin," Journal of the National Cancer Institute 92, no. 4 (2000): 328–32; Catherine Schairer et al., "Menopausal Estrogen and Estrogen-Progestin Replacement Therapy and Breast Cancer Risk," *JAMA* 283, no. 4 (2000): 485–91.

136 **A study of infertile women:** Linda D. Cowan et al., "Breast Cancer Incidence in Women with a History of Progesterone Deficiency," *American Journal of Epidemiology* 114, no. 2 (1981): 209–17.

137 **women have opted:** Within a year of its publication, the number of prescriptions for Premarin and Prempro dropped to half of what they were. The good news is that large drops in breast cancer diagnoses followed suit over the next several years.

138 **Procter & Gamble invested millions:** Lila Nachtigall et al., "Safety and Tolerability of Testosterone Patch Therapy for Up to 4 Years in Surgically Menopausal Women Receiving Oral or Transdermal Estrogen," *Gynecological Endocrinology* 27, no. 1 (2011): 39–48.

138 **Obesity increases your risk:** A. J. Hartz et al., "The Association of Obesity with Infertility and Related Menstural Abnormalities in Women," *International Journal of Obesity* 3, no. 1 (1978): 57–73.

138 **and hot flashes:** Lisa Gallicchio et al., "Body Mass, Estrogen Levels, and Hot Flashes in Midlife Women," *American Journal of Obstetrics and Gynecology* 193, no. 4 (2005): 1353–60.

138 **Yoga and Pilates can help improve:** T. Ivarsson et al., "Physical Exercise and Vasomotor Symptoms in Postmenopausal Women," *Maturitas* 29 (1998): 139–46; Corio, *The Change Before the Change.*

138 **Exercise . . . helps to make you horny:** Tierney Ahrold Lorenz and Cindy May Meston, "Exercise Improves Sexual Function in Women Taking Antidepressants: Results from a Randomized Crossover Trial," *Depression and Anxiety* 99 (2013):1–8.

139 **a healthy activity that you do:** Berman and Berman, *For Women Only.*

139 **Having sex may help you:** Michael F. Roizen and Elizabeth Anne Stephenson, *Realage: Are You As Young As You Can Be?* (New York: Cliff Street Books, 1999).

139 **there is a correlation between orgasms:** George Davey Smith et al., "Sex and Death: Are They Related? Findings from the Caerphilly Cohort Study," *British Medical Journal* 315, no. 7123 (1997): 1641–44.

139 **Vitamin D is crucial:** Keiko Kinuta et al., "Vitamin D Is an Important Factor in Estrogen Biosynthesis of Both Female and Male Gonads." *Endocrinology* 141, no. 4 (2000): 1317–24.

139 **Soy milk has components:** David T. Zava et al., "Estrogen and Progestin Bioactivity of Foods, Herbs, and Spices," *Experimental Biology and Medicine* 217, no. 3 (1998): 369–78.

139 **If you're estrogen dominant:** Berman and Berman, *For Women Only.*

139 **The highest-binding herbs for progesterone-like:** Zava et al., "Estrogen and Progestin Bioactivity of Foods," 369–78.

139 **one study found that it worked even better:** G. Warnecke, "Influencing of Menopausal Complaints with a Phytodrug: Successful Therapy with Cimicifuga Monoextract," *Medizinische Welt* 36 (1985): 871–74.

139 **Pine bark extract:** S. Errichi et al., "Supplementation with Pycnogenol® Improves Signs and Symptoms of Menopausal Transition," *Panminerva Medica* 53, no. 3, suppl 1 (2011): 65–70; Han-Ming Yang et al., "A Randomised, Double-Blind, Placebo-Controlled Trial on the Effect of Pycnogenol® on Tte Climacteric Syndrome in Peri-Menopausal Women," *Acta Obstetricia Et Gynecologica Scandinavica* 86, no. 8 (2007): 978–85.

139 **Then there's maca:** H. O. Meissner et al., "Therapeutic Effects of Pre-Gelatinized Maca (Lepidium peruvianum Chacon) Used as a Non-Hormonal Alternative to HRT in Perimenopausal Women—Clinical Pilot Study," *IJBS* 2, no. 2 (2006): 143; Julius Goepp, "A New Way to Manage Menopause Regain Hormonal Balance with a Cutting-edge Adaptogen," *Reprod Biol Endocrinol* 3 (2005): 16; Nicole A. Brooks et al., "Beneficial Effects of Lepidium Meyenii (Maca) on Psychological Symptoms and Measures of Sexual Dysfunction in Postmenopausal Women Are Not Related to Estrogen or Androgen Content," *Menopause* 15, no. 6 (2008): 1157–62.

140 **well tolerated and may also be used:** Christina M. Dording et al., "A Double-Blind, Randomized, Pilot Dose-Finding Study of Maca Root (L. Meyenii) for the Management of SSRI-Induced Sexual Dysfunction," *CNS Neuroscience & Therapeutics* 14, no. 3 (2008): 182–91.

140 **maca works its wonders without changing:** Yali Wang et al., "Maca: An Andean Crop with Multi-Pharmacological Functions," *Food Research International* 40, no. 7 (2007): 783–92.

140 **protect against brain damage:** Alejandro Pino-Figueroa et al., "Mechanism of Action of Lepidium

Meyenii (Maca): An Explanation for Its Neuroprotective Activity," *American Journal of Neuroprotection and Neuroregeneration* 3, no. 1 (2011): 87–92.

140 **Chasteberry, also known as vitex:** Jianghua Liu et al., "Evaluation of Estrogenic Activity of Plant Extracts for the Potential Treatment of Menopausal Symptoms," *Journal of Agricultural and Food Chemistry* 49, no. 5 (2001): 2472–79; M. Blumenthal, *The Complete German Commission E Monographs: Therapeutic Guide to Herbal Medicines* (Austin, TX: American Botanical Council, 1998).

140 **good for PMS:** For more on using herbs for perimenopause, please see WomenToWomen.com.

140 **compounds in cannabis:** Kazuhito Watanabe et al., "Marijuana Extracts Possess the Effects Like the Endocrine Disrupting Chemicals," *Toxicology* 206, no. 3 (2005): 471–78.

140 **a variety of perimenopausal complaints:** H. Diana van Die, "Herbal Medicine and Menopause: An Historical Perspective," *Australian Journal of Medical Herbalism* 22, no. 4 (2010); Ethan Russo, "Cannabis Treatments in Obstetrics and Gynecology: A Historical Review," *Journal of Cannabis Therapeutics* 2, no. 3–4 (2002): 5–35.

140 **Cannabis increases luteinizing hormone levels:** J. H. Mendelson et al., "Acute Effects of Marijuana on Luteinizing Hormone in Menopausal Women," *Pharmaco. Biochem Behav* 23 (1985): 765.

140 **Hemp seeds added to the diet of rats:** A. Saberivand et al., "The Effects of Cannabis Sativa L. Seed (Hempseed) in the Ovariectomized Rat Model of Menopause," *Methods Find Exp Clin Pharmacol* 32, no. 7 (2010): 467–73.

140 **Cannabidiol (CBD), the component of cannabis:** M. A. Sauer et al., "Marijuana: Interaction with the Estrogen Receptor," *J Pharmacol Exp Ther* 224, no. 2 (1983): 404–7.

141 **there are cannabinoid receptors:** Aymen I. Idris et al., "Regulation of Bone Mass, Bone Loss and Osteoclast Activity by Cannabinoid Receptors," *Nature Medicine* 11, no. 7 (2005): 774–79; Orr Ofek et al., "Peripheral Cannabinoid Receptor, CB2, Regulates Bone Mass," *PNAS* 103, no. 3 (2006): 696–701.

141 **Animal studies show that a synthetic CB2 agonist:** Idris et al., "Regulation of Bone Mass,"; Antonia Sophocleous et al., "The Type 2 Cannabinoid Receptor Regulates Bone Mass and Ovariectomy-Induced Bone Loss by Affecting Osteoblast Differentiation and Bone Formation," *Endocrinology* 152, no. 6 (2011): 2141–49.

141 **people who have a genetic problem:** Itai Bab et al., "Cannabinoids and the Skeleton: From Marijuana to Reversal of Bone Loss," *Annals of Medicine* 41, no. 8 (2009): 560–67.

141 **a third of our lives being postmenopausal:** Duffy, "Lifting the Fog," 31–37.

142 **delineated downtime:** Perhaps the new or full moon can serve as a reminder of spiritual growth and rebirth, of honoring the divine feminine.

142 **our version of the midlife crisis:** Ibid.

143 **The majority of divorces in America:** Xenia P. Montenegro, *The Divorce Experience: A Study of Divorce at Midlife and Beyond Conducted for AARP The Magazine*, AARP, Knowledge Management, National Member Research, 2004.

143 **wrote about her experience in *Vital Aging*:** Sara Wolff, *Vital Aging: Seven Years of Building Community and Enhancing Health* (Amherst, MA: Levelers Press, 2010).

Chapter Seven: Inflammation, The Key to Everything

148 **Chronic stressors:** Borja García-Bueno et al., "Stress as a Neuroinflammatory Condition in Brain: Damaging and Protective Mechanisms," *Neuroscience & Biobehavioral Reviews* 32, no. 6 (2008): 1136–51.

149 **Chronic stress can precede:** Maté, *When the Body Says No;* K. S. Kendler and L. M. Karkowski, "Causal relationship Between Stressful Life Events and the Onset of Major Depression," *American Journal of Psychiatry* 156 (1999): 837–41.

149 **If you induce inflammatory reactions:** C. L. Raison et al., "A Randomized Controlled Trial of the Tumor Necrosis Factor Antagonist Infliximab for Treatment-Resistant Depression: The Role of Baseline Inflammatory Biomarkers," *JAMA Psychiatry* 70 (2013): 31–41; Neil A. Harrison et al., "Inflammation Causes Mood Changes Through Alterations in Subgenual Cingulate Activity and Mesolimbic Connectivity," *Biological Psychiatry* 66, no. 5 (2009): 407–14; Naomi I. Eisenberger et al., "Inflammation-Induced Anhedonia: Endotoxin Reduces Ventral Striatum Responses to Reward," *Biological Psychiatry* 68, no. 8 (2010): 748–54.

149 **Chronically stress a laboratory animal:** P. Willner, "Chronic Mild Stress (CMS) Revisited: Consistency and Behavioral-Neurobiological Concordance in the Effects of CMS," *Neuropsychobiology* 52 (2005): 90–110.

149 **anti-inflammatory agents:** Michael Maes, "The Cytokine Hypothesis of Depression: Inflammation, Oxidative & Nitrosative Stress (IO&NS) and Leaky Gut as New Targets for Adjunctive Treatments in Depression," *Neuro Endocrinol Lett* 29, no. 3 (2008a): 287–91.

149　**Depressed people:** Charles L. Raison et al., "Cytokines Sing the Blues: Inflammation and the Pathogenesis of Depression," *Trends in Immunology* 27, no. 1 (2006): 24–31.

149　**markers, called cytokines, are higher:** Y. Dowlati et al., "A Meta-analysis of Cytokines in Major Depression," *Biological Psychiatry* 67, no. 5 (2010): 446–57; Janice K. Kiecolt-Glaser et al., "Depressive Symptoms, Omega-6: Omega-3 Fatty Acids, and Inflammation in Older Adults," *Psychosomatic Medicine* 69, no. 3 (2007): 217–24; A. H. Miller et al., "Inflammation and Its Discontents: The Role of Cytokines in the Pathophysiology of Major Depression," *Biological Psychiatry* 65 (2009): 732–41.

149　**lower in those who've been successfully treated:** Miller, *Inflammation and It's Discontens*; Beatriz M. Currier and Charles B. Nemeroff, "Inflammation and Mood Disorders: Proinflammatory Cytokines and the Pathogenesis of Depression," *Anti-Inflammatory & Anti-Allergy Agents in Medicinal Chemistry* 9, no. 3 (2010): 212–20.

149　**intense suicidal ideation:** A. O'Donovan et al., "Suicidal Ideation Is Associated with Elevated Inflammation in Patients with Major Depressive Disorder," *Depress Anxiety* 30 (2013): 307–14.

149　**Stressed-out patients with anxiety:** Michael Maes et al., "The Effects of Psychological Stress on Humans: Increased Production of Pro-Inflammatory Cytokines and Th1-Like Response in Stress-Induced Anxiety," *Cytokine* 10, no. 4 (1998): 313–18.

149　**hepatitis drug interferon:** Hitoshi Miyaoka et al., "Depression from Interferon Therapy in Patients with Hepatitis C," *American Journal of Psychiatry* 156, no. 7 (1999): 1120.

149　**neural circuitry of depression:** K. J. Ressler and H. S. Mayberg, "Targeting Abnormal Neural Circuits in Mood and Anxiety Disorders: From the Laboratory to the Clinic," *Nature Neuroscience* 10 (2007): 1116–24.

149　**Giving proinflammatory cytokines:** Raison et al., "A Randomized Controlled Trial of the Tumor Necrosis Factor Antagonist Infliximab," 31-41.

149　**Stress causing inflammation:** Dantzer et al., "From Inflammation to Sickness and Depression," 46–56.

150　**looking at sick people:** Mark Schaller et al., "Mere Visual Perception of Other People's Disease Symptoms Facilitates a More Aggressive Immune Response," *Psychological Science* 21, no. 5 (2010): 649–52.

150　**inflammation leads to greater amygdala response:** Tristen K. Inagaki et al., "Inflammation Selectively Enhances Amygdala Activity to Socially Threatening Images," *Neuroimage* 59, no. 4 (2012): 3222–26.

150　**cytokines target and sabotage:** C. B. Zhu et al., "Interleukin-1 Receptor Activation by Systemic Lipopolysaccharide Induces Behavioral Despair Linked to MAPK Regulation of CNS Serotonin Transporters," *Neuropsychopharmacology* 35 (2010): 2510–20

150　**Cytokines also break down tryptophan:** A. J. Rush et al., "Acute and Longer-Term Outcomes in Depressed Outpatients Requiring One or Several Treatment Steps: A STAR*D Report," *American Journal of Psychiatry* 163 (2006): 1905–17; J. Couzin-Frankel, "Inflammation Bares a Dark Side," *Science* 330 (2010): 1621.

151　**make matters worse:** By disrupting dopamine levels.

151　**cytokines diminish motivation:** T. Kumal et al., "Effects of Interferon-Alpha on Tyrosine Hydroxylase and Catecholeamine Levels in the Brains of Rats," *Life Sciences* 67 (2000): 663–69; H. Shuto et al., "Repeated Interferon-Alpha Administration Inhibits Dopaminergic Neural Activity in the Mouse Brain," *Brain Research* 747 (1997): 348–51.

151　**also antagonize glutamate:** L. McNally et al., "Inflammation, Glutamate, and Glia in Depression: A Literature Review," *CNS Spectrums* 13 (2008): 501–10.

151　**Nearly a third of depressed people:** Brian E. Leonard, "The Immune System, Depression and the Action of Antidepressants," *Progress in Neuro-Psychopharmacology and Biological Psychiatry* 25, no. 4 (2001): 767–80.

151　**higher levels of proinflammatory markers:** S. Lanquillon et al., "Cytokine Production and Treatment Response in Major Depressive Disorder," *Neuropsychopharmacology* 22 (2000): 370–79; T. Eller et al., "Pro-Inflammatory Cytokines and Treatment Response to Escitalopram in Major Depressive Disorder," *Prog Neuropsychopharmacol Biol Psychiatry* 32 (2008): 445–50; Raison et al., "A Randomized Controlled Trial of the Tumor Necrosis Factor Antagonist Infliximab," 31–41.

151　**Some researchers have used anti-inflammatory medications:** Miller et al., "Inflammation and Its Discontents," 732–41; Raison et al., "A Randomized Controlled Trial of the Tumor Necrosis Factor Antagonist Infliximab," 31–41; E. Haroon et al., "Psychoneuroimmunology Meets Neuropsychopharmacology: Translational Implications of the Impact of Inflammation on Behavior," *Neuropsychopharmacology* 37 (2012): 137–62.

151　**Leaky barriers play a role:** M. Maes et al., "The Gut-Brain Barrier in Major Depression: Intestinal

Mucosal Dysfunction with an Increased Translocation of LPS from Gram Negative Enterobacteria (Leaky Gut) Plays a Role in the Inflammatory Pathophysiology of Depression," *Neuro Endocrinology Letters* 29 (2008): 117–24.

151 **and anxiety:** D. O'Malley et al., "Distinct Alterations in Colonic Morphology and Physiology in Two Rat Models of Enhanced Stress-Induced Anxiety and Depression-like Behavior," *Stress* 13 (2010): 114–22.

151 **Infections and autoimmune diseases make the blood-brain barrier leaky:** Dantzer et al., "From Inflammation to Sickness and Depression," 46–56.

152 **Increased inflammatory reactivity:** Christoph Laske, et al., "Autoantibody Reactivity in Serum of Patients with Major Depression, Schizophrenia and Healthy Controls," *Psychiatry Research* 158, no. 1 (2008): 83–86; Betty Diamond et al., "Losing Your Nerves? Maybe It's the Antibodies," *Nature Reviews Immunology* 9, no. 6 (2009): 449–56.

152 **Several autoimmune diseases:** Michael E. Benros et al., "Autoimmune Diseases and Severe Infections as Risk Factors for Mood Disorders: A Nationwide Study," *JAMA Psychiatry* (2013): 1–9.

152 **if you have infections or autoimmune disorders:** Ibid.

<u>152</u> **higher risk:** In looking at the timing of medical illnesses and mood disorders, one study showed that a prior infection occurred before the mood disorder in 32 percent of patients. A prior autoimmune illness, though far less common in the general population, occurred in 5 percent. Any history of hospitalization for infection increased the risk of a subsequent mood disorder by 62 percent. If you're unlucky enough to have been felled by both an infection and an autoimmune illness, especially within the past year, then the risk for depression quadruples.

152 **Chronic stress increases the risk:** Anette Pedersen et al., "Influence of Psychological Stress on Upper Respiratory Infection—A Meta-analysis of Prospective Studies," *Psychosomatic Medicine* 72, no. 8 (2010): 823–32.

152 **Natural killer cells:** Michael Irwin et al., "Depression and Reduced Natural Killer Cytotoxicity: A Longitudinal Study of Depressed Patients and Control Subjects," *Psycholocal Medicine* 22 (1992): 1045–1045; Steven J. Schleifer et al., "Depression and Immunity: Clinical Factors and Therapeutic Course," *Psychiatry Research* 85, no. 1 (1999): 63–69.

152 **antidepressants augment their invader-fighting abilities:** Matthew Gerald Frank et al., "Antidepressants Augment Natural Killer Cell Activity: In Vivo and in Vitro," *Neuropsychobiology* 39, no. 1 (1999): 18–24.

152 **Stress creates inflammation:** Hans Selye, *The Stress of Life* (New York: McGraw-Hill, 1956).

152 **People under extreme stress:** Gary M. Franklin et al., "Stress and Its Relationship to Acute Exacerbations in Multiple Sclerosis," *Neurorehabilitation and Neural Repair* 2, no. 1 (1988): 7–11.

152 **In asthmatic kids:** Glenn Affleck et al., "Mood States Associated with Transitory Changes in Asthma Symptoms and Peak Expiratory Flow," *Psychosomatic Medicine* 62, no. 1 (2000): 61–68.

152 **In premenopausal women who have heart attacks:** Viola Vaccarino et al., "Sex Differences in Mental Stress–Induced Myocardial Ischemia in Young Survivors of an Acute Myocardial Infarction," *Psychosomatic Medicine* (2014): 45–53.

152 **women have greater coronary artery reactivity:** B. Ostadal and P. Ostadal, "Sex-Based Differences in Cardiac Ischaemic Injury and Protection: Therapeutic Implications," *British Journal of Pharmacology* 171, no. 3 (2014): 541–54.

153 **The main factors that can trigger:** H. Ursin, E. Baade, and S. Levine, *The Psychobiology of Stress: A Study of Coping Men* (New York: Academic Press, 1978).

153 **Inescapable shocks:** Mark L. Laudenslager et al., "Coping and Immunosuppression: Inescapable but Not Escapable Shock Suppresses Lymphocyte Proliferation," *Science* 221, no. 4610 (1983): 568–70.

153 **If you block a rat's ability:** Ewa Chelmicka-Schorr and Barry G. Arnason, "Nervous System–Immune System Interactions and Their Role in Multiple Sclerosis," *Annals of Neurology* 36, no. S1 (1994): S29–S32.

153 **control over their health-care issues:** Carsten Wrosch et al., "Health Stresses and Depressive Symptomatology in the Elderly: The Importance of Health Engagement Control Strategies," *Health Psychology* 21, no. 4 (2002): 340.

153 **Subordinate female monkeys:** Carol A. Shively et al., "Behavior and Physiology of Social Stress and Depression in Female Cynomolgus Monkeys," *Biological Psychiatry* 41, no. 8 (1997): 871–82.

153 **The higher your social position:** Michael Marmot and Eric Brunner, "Epidemiological Applications of Long-Term Stress in Daily Life," *Everyday Biological Stress Mechanisms* 22 (2004): 80–90.

153 **social networking like Facebook:** Ethan Kross, et al., "Facebook Use Predicts Declines in Subjective Well-Being in Young Adults," *PloS One* 8, no. 8 (2013): e69841.

153 **Certain repressive behaviors in women:** Maté, *When the Body Says No.*

153 **"rationality and anti-emotionality":** Ronald Grossarth-Maticek et al., "Psychosocial Factors as Strong Predictors of Mortality from Cancer, Ischaemic Heart Disease and Stroke: The Yugoslav Prospective Study," *Journal of Psychosomatic Research* 29, no. 2 (1985): 167–76.

153 **emotional factors are potentially more important to survival:** S. M. Levy and B. D. Wise, "Psychosocial Risk Factors in Cancer Prognosis," *Stress and Breast Cancer* (Chichester, UK: John Wiley, 1988).

154 **Let your true feelings show:** Lissa Rankin, TED Talks, 2011, https://www.youtube.com/watch?v=7tu9nJmr4Xs.

154 **Resilience is a key component:** Daphne Simeon et al., "Factors Associated with Resilience in Healthy Adults," *Psychoneuroendocrinology* 32, no. 8 (2007): 1149–52.

154 **Exposure to mild or moderate stressors:** D. M. Lyons and K. J. Parker, "Stress Inoculation-Induced Indications of Resilience in Monkeys," *Journal of Traumatic Stress* 20 (2007): 423–33; Laura Anderko et al., "Peer Reviewed: Promoting Prevention Through the Affordable Care Act: Workplace Wellness," *Preventing Chronic Disease* 9 (2012). E175–E190.

154 **Students cocooned by protective helicopter parents:** Holly Rogers, "Mindfulness Meditation for Increasing Resilience in College Students," *Psychiatric Annals* 43, no. 12 (2013): 545–48.

154 **Rat pups separated from their mothers:** B. P. Rutten et al., "Resilience in Mental Health: Linking Psychological and Neurobiological Perspectives," *Acta Psychiatrica Scandinavica* 128, no. 1 (2013): 3–20.

154 stressful event: Rats actually secrete corticosterone, their version of cortisol.

154 **A secure early attachment:** Simeon et al., "Factors Associated with Resilience in Healthy Adults," 1149–52; Maté, *When the Body Says No.*

154 **sustained activation of the panic/stress circuitry:** Christine D. Heim et al., "The Link Between Childhood Trauma and Depression: Insights from HPA Axis Studies in Humans," *Psychoneuroendocrinology* 33, no. 6 (2008): 693–710.

154 **People who've been traumatized:** Lisa M. Shin et al., "Amygdala, Medial Prefrontal Cortex, and Hippocampal Function in PTSD," *Annals of the New York Academy of Sciences* 1071, no. 1 (2006): 67–79.

155 **baseline inflammation:** A. Danese et al., "Elevated Inflammation Levels in Depressed Adults with a History of Childhood Maltreatment," *Archives of General Psychiatry* 65 (2008): 409–415

155 **higher inflammatory responses:** Ibid., 2008; Miller et al., "Inflammation and Its Discontents," 732–41.

155 **The quality of early parenting:** Maté, *When the Body Says No.*

155 **How a mother cares for her infant:** Christian Caldji et al., "Variations in Maternal Care in Infancy Regulate the Development of Stress Reactivity," *Biological Psychiatry* 48, no. 12 (2000): 1164–74.

155 **Adult rats who had been licked:** Christian Caldji et al., "Maternal Care During Infancy Regulates the Development of Neural Systems Mediating the Expression of Fearfulness in the Rat," *PNAS* 95, no. 9 (1998): 5335–40.

155 **A recent study showed definitively that children:** Gregory E. Miller et al., "A Family-Oriented Psychosocial Intervention Reduces Inflammation in Low-SES African American Youth," *Proceedings of the National Academy of Sciences* 111, no. 31 (2014): 11287–92.

155 **early parenting environment can strongly influence:** Dong Liu et al., "Maternal Care, Hippocampal Glucocorticoid Receptors, and Hypothalamic-Pituitary-Adrenal Responses to Stress," *Science* 277, no. 5332 (1997): 1659–62; Michael J. Meaney, and Moshe Szyf, "Environmental Programming of Stress Responses Through DNA Methylation: Life at the Interface Between a Dynamic Environment and a Fixed Genome," *Dialogs in Clinical Neuroscience* 7, no. 2 (2005): 103.

155 **In studies of rhesus monkeys:** Michael Marmot and Richard Wilkinson, eds., *Social Determinants of Health* (New York: Oxford University Press, 2005).

156 **Anxious mothers are likely:** Gabor Maté, *In the Realm of Hungry Ghosts: Close Encounters with Addiction* (New York: Random House, 2008).

156 **Mothers with severe PTSD:** Rachel Yehuda et al., "Cortisol Levels in Adult Offspring of Holocaust Survivors: Relation to PTSD Symptom Severity in the Parent and Child," *Psychoneuroendocrinology* 27, no. 1 (2002): 171–80.

156 **Children, and even grandchildren:** Lea Baider et al., "Transmission of Response to Trauma? Second-Generation Holocaust Survivors' Reaction to Cancer," *American Journal of Psychiatry* 157, no. 6 (2000): 904–10; Rachel Yehuda, and Linda M. Bierer, "Transgenerational Transmission of Cortisol and PTSD Risk." *Progress in Brain Research* 167 (2007): 121–35.

156 **You see this in laboratory animals:** Micah Leshem and Jay Schulkin, "Transgenerational Effects of Infantile Adversity and Enrichment in Male and Female Rats," *Developmental Psychobiology* 54, no. 2 (2012): 169–86; Alice Shachar-Dadon et al., "Adversity Before Conception Will Affect Adult Progeny in Rats," *Developmental Psychology* 45, no. 1 (2009): 9.

156 **If you mate a stressed-out rat:** Hiba Zaidan et al., "Prereproductive Stress to Female Rats Alters Corticotropin Releasing Factor Type 1 Expression in Ova and Behavior and Brain Corticotropin Releasing Factor Type 1 Expression in Offspring," *Biological Psychiatry* 74, no. 9 (2013): 680–87.

156 **serotonin production:** The enzyme that makes serotonin, tryptophan dehydroxylase.

156 **your risk for depression, suicidality, or aggression:** David A. Nielsen et al., "Suicidality and 5-Hydroxyindoleacetic Acid Concentration Associated with a Tryptophan Hydroxylase Polymorphism," *Archives of General Psychiatry* 51, no. 1 (1994): 34; Stephen B. Manuck et al., "Aggression and Anger-Related Traits Associated with a Polymorphism of the Tryptophan Hydroxylase Gene," *Biological Psychiatry* 45, no. 5 (1999): 603–14.

156 **after you've been stressed-out:** Derick E. Vergne and Charles B. Nemeroff, "The Interaction of Serotonin Transporter Gene Polymorphisms and Early Adverse Life Events on Vulnerability for Major Depression," *Current Psychiatry Reports* 8, no. 6 (2006): 452–57; Avshalom Caspi et al., "Influence of Life Stress on Depression: Moderation by a Polymorphism in the 5-HTT Gene," *Science Signaling* 301, no. 5631 (2003): 386.

156 **genes that control the SSRI docking space:** Elaine Fox et al., "Looking on the Bright Side: Biased Attention and the Human Serotonin Transporter Gene," *Proceedings of the Royal Society B: Biological Sciences* 276, no. 1663 (2009): 1747–51; Jan-Emmanuel De Neve, "Functional Polymorphism (5-HTTLPR) in the Serotonin Transporter Gene Is Associated with Subjective Well-Being: Evidence from a U.S. Nationally Representative Sample," *Journal of Human Genetics* 56, no. 6 (2011): 456–59; Stefanie Wagner et al., "The 5-HTTLPR Polymorphism Modulates the Association of Serious Life Events (SLE) and Impulsivity in Patients with Borderline Personality Disorder," *Journal of Psychiatric Research* 43, no. 13 (2009): 1067–72.

156 **patients who are more vulnerable to depression:** Carolyn A. Fredericks et al., "Healthy Young Women with Serotonin Transporter SS Polymorphism Show a Pro-inflammatory Bias Under Resting and Stress Conditions," *Brain, Behavior, and Immunity* 24, no. 3 (2010): 350–57.

156 **getting depressed when they're medically:** K. Karg et al., "The Serotonin Transporter Promoter Variant (5-HTTLPR), Stress, and Depression Meta-analysis Revisited: Evidence of Genetic Moderation," *Archives of General Psychiatry* 68 (2011): 444–54.

157 **Change your mind about stress:** Jeremy P. Jamieson et al., "Mind Over Matter: Reappraising Arousal Improves Cardiovascular and Cognitive Responses to Stress," *Journal of Experimental Psychology: General* 141, no. 3 (2012): 417.

157 **One study showed a whopping 43 percent risk:** Abiola Keller et al., "Does the Perception That Stress Affects Health Matter? The Association with Health and Mortality," *Health Psychology* 31, no. 5 (2012): 677.

157 **Positive emotions prevent or undo:** Barbara L. Fredrickson et al., "The Undoing Effect of Positive Emotions," *Motivation and Emotion* 24, no. 4 (2000): 237–58; Barbara L. Fredrickson, "The Role of Positive Emotions in Positive Psychology: The Broaden-and-Build Theory of Positive Emotions," *American Psychologist* 56, no. 3 (2001): 218.

157 **Develop your ability to experience positive emotions:** Inez Myin-Germeys et al., "Evidence That Moment-to-Moment Variation in Positive Emotions Buffer Genetic Risk for Depression: A Momentary Assessment Twin Study," *Acta Psychiatrica Scandinavica* 115, no. 6 (2007): 451–57; Nicole Geschwind et al., "Meeting Risk with Resilience: High Daily Life Reward Experience Preserves Mental Health," *Acta Psychiatrica Scandinavica* 122, no. 2 (2010): 129–38.

157 **Women with more day-to-day positive emotions:** Anthony D. Ong et al., "Psychological Resilience, Positive Emotions, and Successful Adaptation to Stress in Later Life," *Journal of Personality and Social Psychology* 91, no. 4 (2006): 730.

157 **More resilient folks are more likely:** Michele M. Tugade and Barbara L. Fredrickson, "Resilient Individuals Use Positive Emotions to Bounce Back from Negative Emotional Experiences," *Journal of Personality and Social Psychology* 86, no. 2 (2004): 320.

157 **For patients with depression:** Suzanne Meeks et al., "The Pleasant Events Schedule–Nursing Home Version: A Useful Tool for Behavioral Interventions in Long-Term Care," *Aging and Mental Health* 13, no. 3 (2009): 445–55.

158 **Chronic stress chips away:** Rita B. Effros, "Telomere/telomerase Dynamics Within the Human Immune System: Effect of Chronic Infection and Stress," *Experimental Gerontology* 46, no. 2 (2011): 135–40.

158 **In a study of women taking care:** Elissa S. Epel et al., "Accelerated Telomere Shortening in Response to Life Stress," *PNAS* 101, no. 49 (2004): 17312–15.

158 **telomere length:** Also the lower her level of the enzyme telomerase, which is responsible for adding length to the telomere.

158 **Chronic inflammation can shorten:** Elissa Epel, personal communication via telephone, March 25, 2014.

158 **As immune cells age:** R. B. Effros et al., "The Role Of CD8 T Cell Replicative Senescence in Human Aging," *Immunological Reviews* 205 (2005): 147–57.

158 **predict the onset of diseases such as cancer:** P. Willeit et al., "Fifteen-Year Follow-up of Association Between Telomere Length and Incident Cancer and Cancer Mortality," *JAMA* 306 (2011): 42–44.

158 **dementia:** L. S. Honig et al., "Association of Shorter Leukocyte Telomere Repeat Length with Dementia and Mortality," *Archives of Neurology* (2012): 1–8.

158 **Abdominal obesity shortens:** R. Farzaneh-Far et al., "Association of Marine Omega-3 Fatty Acid Levels with Telomeric Aging in Patients with Coronary Heart Disease," *JAMA* 303 (2010): 250–57.

158 **exercise will help to keep them long:** C. Werner et al., "Physical Exercise Prevents Cellular Senescence in Circulating Leukocytes and in the Vessel Wall," *Circulation* 120 (2009): 2438–47; Eli Puterman and Elissa Epel, "An Intricate Dance: Life Experience, Multisystem Resiliency, and Rate of Telomere Decline Throughout the Lifespan," *Social and Personality Psychology Compass* 6, no. 11 (2012): 807–25.

158 **Less stress and better sleep:** J. Lin et al., "Telomeres and Lifestyle Factors: Roles in Cellular Aging," *Mutation Research* 730 (2012): 85–89; Puterman and Epel, "An Intricate Dance."

159 **mindfulness-based practices:** Tonya L. Jacobs et al., "Intensive Meditation Training, Immune Cell Telomerase Activity, and Psychological Mediators," *Psychoneuroendocrinology* 36, no. 5 (2011): 664–81; J. Daubenmier et al., "Changes in Stress, Eating, and Metabolic Factors Are Related to Changes In Telomerase Activity in a Randomized Mindfulness Intervention Pilot Study," *Psychoneuroendocrinology* 37 (2012): 917–28; H. Lavretsky et al., "A Pilot Study of Yogic Meditation for Family Dementia Caregivers with Depressive Symptoms: Effects on Mental Health, Cognition, and Telomerase Activity," *International Journal of Geriatric Psychiatry* 28, no. 1 (2013): 57–65.

159 **Expert meditators:** Perla Kaliman et al., "Rapid Changes in Histone Deacetylases and Inflammatory Gene Expression in Expert Meditators," *Psychoneuroendocrinology* 40 (2014): 96–107.

159 **Social connectedness improves resilience:** M. DeRosier et al., "The Potential Role of Resilience Education for Preventing Mental Health Problems for College Students," *Psychiatric Annals* 43, no. 12 (2013): 538–44.

159 **Positive social interactions:** Markus Heinrichs et al., "Social Support and Oxytocin Interact to Suppress Cortisol and Subjective Responses to Psychosocial Stress," *Biological Psychiatry* 54, no. 12 (2003): 1389–98.

160 **Social support can lower cortisol levels:** C. Kirschbaum et al., "The 'Trier Social Stress Test'—A Tool for Investigating Psychobiological Stress Responses in a Laboratory Setting," *Neuropsychobiology* 28 (1993): 76 –81; K. Sayal et al., "Effects of Social Support During Weekend Leave on Cortisol and Depression Ratings: A Pilot Study," *Journal of Affective Disorders* 71(2002): 153–57.

160 **lower cardiovascular reactivity:** S. J. Lepore et al., "Social Support Lowers Cardiovascular Reactivity to an Acute Stressor," *Psychosomatic Medicine* 55 (1993): 518–24.

160 **ameliorate symptoms of depression:** J. C. Hays et al., "Does Social Support Buffer Functional Decline in Elderly Patients with Unipolar Depression? *American Journal of Psychiatry* 158 (2001): 1850–55; Sayal et al., "Effects of Social Support During Weekend Leave," 153–57.

160 **Oxytocin has anti-inflammatory:** Martin Clodi et al., "Oxytocin Alleviates the Neuroendocrine and Cytokine Response to Bacterial Endotoxin in Healthy Men," *American Journal of Physiology-Endocrinology and Metabolism* 295, no. 3 (2008): E686–E691.

160 **relaxes blood vessels:** Sybil Lloyd and Mary Pickford, "The Effect of Oestrogens and Sympathetic Denervation on the Response to Oxytocin of the Blood Vessels in the Hind Limb of the Dog," *Journal of Physiology* 163, no. 2 (1962): 362–71.

160 **Frequent hugs:** Kathleen C. Light et al., "More Frequent Partner Hugs and Higher Oxytocin Levels Are Linked to Lower Blood Pressure and Heart Rate in Premenopausal Women," *Biological Psychology* 69, no. 1 (2005): 5–21.

160 **oxytocin receptors on the heart:** Marek Jankowski et al., "Anti-inflammatory Effect of Oxytocin in Rat Myocardial Infarction," *Basic Research in Cardiology* 105, no. 2 (2010): 205–18.

160 **Socially isolated adults:** Lisa F. Berkman and S. Leonard Syme, "Social Networks, Host Resistance, and Mortality: A Nine-Year Follow-up Study of Alameda County Residents," *American Journal of Epidemiology* 109, no. 2 (1979): 186–204; James S. House et al., "Social Relationships and Health," *Science* 241, no. 4865 (1988): 540–45.

160 **Lonely people have worse sleep:** John T. Cacioppo et al., "Loneliness and Health: Potential Mechanisms," *Psychosomatic Medicine* 64, no. 3 (2002): 407–17.

160 **more depressive symptoms:** John T. Cacioppo and William Patrick, *Loneliness: Human Nature and the Need For Social Connection* (New York: WW Norton & Company, 2008).

160 **Isolation also impairs immune functioning:** George M. Slavich et al., "Neural Sensitivity to Social Rejection Is Associated with Inflammatory Responses to Social Stress," *PNAS* 107, no. 33 (2010): 14817–22; W. B. Malarkey et al., "Behavior: The Endocrine-Immune Interface and Health Outcomes," *Advances in Psychosomatic Medicine* 22 (2001): 104–15; M. Irwin et al., "Neuropeptide Y and Natural Killer Cell Activity: Findings in Depression and Alzheimer Caregiver Stress," *The FASEB Journal* 5, no. 15 (1991): 3100–3107.

160 **Studies of stress, isolation, and neuroplasticity:** C. Pugh et al., "Role of Interleukin-1 Beta in Impairment of Contextual Fear Conditioning Caused by Social Isolation," *Behavioral Brain Research* 106, no. 1 (1999): 109–18; R. M. Barrientos et al., "Brain-Derived Neurotrophic Factor Mrna Downregulation Produced by Social Isolation Is Blocked by Intrahippocampal Interleukin-1 Receptor Antagonist," *Neuroscience* 121, no. 4 (2003): 847–53.

160 **memory formation:** If you stress lab rats, they release a proinflammatory cytokine called IL1-beta. If you take them away from their group housing, shock them in a separate space, and return them to their group, they're understandably stressed when you take them back to the shocking room; they remember where they got the pain. But if you take them away from their pals, shock them, but then put them in solitary confinement, they don't remember the shocking place. Being alone not only activates IL1-beta but also tanks the BDNF necessary to grow neuronal connections and learn something. Stress activates inflammation, which turns off the neurotrophic signals. If you block the IL1-beta, you block those changes, and you don't see the hippocampal shrinkage and stupidity.

160 **Isolation also leads to impaired top-down:** A. B. Silva-Gómez et al., "Decreased Dendritic Spine Density on Prefrontal Cortical and Hippocampal Pyramidal Neurons in Post-weaning Social Isolation Rats," *Brain Reearch* 983 (2003): 128–36 (2003).

161 **Not only are cannabinoids anti-inflammatory:** John M. McPartland and Ethan B. Russo, "Cannabis and Cannabis Extracts: Greater Than the Sum of Their Parts?" *Journal of Cannabis Therapeutics* 1, no. 3–4 (2001): 103–32; S. H. Burstein and R. B. Zurier, "Cannabinoids, Endocannabinoids, and Related Analogs in Inflammation," *AAPS Journal* 11 (2009): 109–19; Julie Holland, ed., *The Pot Book: A Complete Guide to Cannabis* (Rochester, VT: Inner Traditions/Bear & Co, 2010).

161 **Cannabinoids alter immune reactions:** Radu Tanasescu and Cris S. Constantinescu, "Cannabinoids and the Immune System: An Overview," *Immunobiology* 215, no. 8 (2010): 588–97.

161 **Anandamide, our main internal cannabis molecule:** M. N. Hill and J. G. Tasker, "Endocannabinoid Signaling, Glucocorticoid-Mediated Negative Feedback, and Regulation of the Hypothalamic-Pituitary-Adrenal Axis," *Neuroscience* 204 (2012): 5–16.

161 **Higher anandamide levels:** R. J. Bluett et al., "Central Anandamide Deficiency Predicts Stress-Induced Anxiety: Behavioral Reversal Through Endocannabinoid Augmentation," *Translational Psychiatry* 4, no. 7 (2014): e408.

161 **anandamide levels rise:** Matthew N. Hill et al., "Rapid Elevations in Limbic Endocannabinoid Content by Glucocorticoid Hormones in Vivo," *Psychoneuroendocrinology* 35, no. 9 (2010): 1333–38.

161 **pot affects memory:** Nadia Solowij and Robert Battisti, "The Chronic Effects of Cannabis on Memory in Humans: A Review," *Current Drug Abuse Reviews* 1, no. 1 (2008): 81–98.

161 **Boosting anandamide can promote this forgetting:** Ozge Gunduz-Cinar et al., "Amygdala FAAH and Anandamide: Mediating Protection and Recovery from Stress," *Trends in Pharmacological Sciences* 34, no. 11 (2013): 637–44.

161 **Veterans with PTSD may smoke cannabis:** Murdoch Leeies et al., "The Use of Alcohol and Drugs to Self-Medicate Symptoms of Posttraumatic Stress Disorder," *Depression and Anxiety* 27, no. 8 (2010): 731–36; George R. Greer et al., "PTSD Symptom Reports of Patients Evaluated for the New Mexico Medical Cannabis Program," *Journal of Psychoactive Drugs* 46, no. 1 (2014): 73–77.

161 **attempting to rebalance:** Matthew N. Hill et al., "Reductions in Circulating Endocannabinoid Levels in Individuals with Post-traumatic Stress Disorder Following Exposure to the World Trade Center Attacks," *Psychoneuroendocrinology* 38, no. 12 (2013): 2952–61.

161 **Many psychiatric disorders:** Ethan B. Russo, "Clinical Endocannabinoid Deficiency (Cecd): Can This Concept Explain Therapeutic Benefits of Cannabis In Migraine, Fibromyalgia, Irritable Bowel Syndrome and Other Treatment-Resistant Conditions?" *Neuroendocrinology Letters* 25, no. 1–2 (2003): 31–39.

161–162 **Endocannabinoid levels:** Matthew N. Hill et al., "Circulating Endocannabinoids and N-Acyl Ethanolamines Are Differentially Regulated in Major Depression and Following Exposure to Social Stress," *Psychoneuroendocrinology* 34, no. 8 (2009): 1257–62.

162 **Mice raised to have no cannabis receptors:** Matthew N. Hill et al., "Alterations in Corticolimbic Dendritic Morphology and Emotional Behavior in Cannabinoid CB1 Receptor–Deficient Mice Parallel the Effects of Chronic Stress," *Cerebral Cortex* 21, no. 9 (2011): 2056–64.

162 **may represent a good animal model:** O. Valverde and M. Torrens, "CB1 Receptor–Deficient Mice as a Model for Depression," *Neuroscience* 204 (2012): 193–206.

162 **Animal studies show that enhancing endocannabinoid:** Matthew N. Hill and Boris B. Gorzalka, "Pharmacological Enhancement of Cannabinoid CB1 Receptor Activity Elicits an Antidepressant-like Response in the Rat Forced Swim Test," *European Neuropsychopharmacology* 15, no. 6 (2005): 593–99.

162 **One potential site of action:** Jasmeer P. Chhatwal et al., "Enhancing Cannabinoid Neurotransmission Augments the Extinction of Conditioned Fear," *Neuropsychopharmacology* 30, no. 3 (2005): 516–24. O. Gunduz-Cinar et al., "Convergent Translational Evidence of a Role for Anandamide in Amygdala-Mediated Fear Extinction, Threat Processing and Stress-Reactivity," *Molecular Psychiatry* 18, no. 7 (2013a): 813–23.

162 **Inhibiting FAAH, which raises anandamide levels:** Gunduz-Cinar et al., "Amygdala FAAH and Anandamide," 637–44.

162 **Variations in the human FAAH gene:** Gunduz-Cinar et al., "Convergent Translational Evidence of a Role for Anandamide," 813–23.

162 **Women and cannabis:** Michelle Sexton, "The Female: Cannabis Relationship," Ladybud.com, February 25, 2014.

162 **Anandamide levels fluctuate:** N. H. Lazzarin et al., "Fluctuations of Fatty Acid Amide Hydrolase and Anandamide Levels During the Human Ovulatory Cycle," *Gynecological Endocrinology* 18, no. 4 (2004): 212–18.

162 **Estrogen inhibits FAAH activity:** Matthew N. Hill et al., "Estrogen Recruits the Endocannabinoid System to Modulate Emotionality," *Psychoneuroendocrinology* 32, no. 4 (2007): 350–57.

162–163 **This same estrogen-FAAH interaction:** Mauro Maccarrone et al., "Progesterone Up-Regulates Anandamide Hydrolase in Human Lymphocytes: Role of Cytokines and Implications for Fertility," *The Journal of Immunology* 166, no. 12 (2001): 7183–89.

163 **full of cannabinoid receptors:** Michael C. Dennedy et al., "Cannabinoids and the Human Uterus During Pregnancy," *American Journal of Obstetrics and Gynecology* 190, no. 1 (2004): 2–9.

163 **oldest known recommended use for cannabis:** Paul Ghalioungui, *The Ebers Papyrus: A New English Translation, Commentaries and Glossaries* (Cairo: Academy of Scientific Research and Technology, 1987).

163 **Queen Victoria was prescribed cannabis:** British Medical Association, *Therapeutic Uses of Cannabis* (UK: CRC Press, 1997).

163 **long-standing use of cannabinoids:** Wei-Ni Lin Curry, "Hyperemesis Gravidarum and Clinical Cannabis: To Eat or Not to Eat?" *Journal of Cannabis Therapeutics* 2, no. 3–4 (2002): 63–83; Rachel E. Westfall et al., "Survey of Medicinal Cannabis Use Among Childbearing Women: Patterns of Its Use in Pregnancy and Retroactive Self-Assessment of Its Efficacy Against 'Morning Sickness.'" *Complementary Therapies in Clinical Practice* 12, no. 1 (2006): 27–33.

Chapter Eight: Food: A Drug We Can't Resist

165 **Being loved, cared for, and fed:** Doidge, *The Brain That Changes Itself.*

166 **food issues:** When obese women are shown pictures of high-calorie foods, their brains show greater activity in regions associated with anticipating reward than do the brains of women with more normal weight.

166–167 **in a study pitting Oreos against cocaine:** Joseph Schroeder, "Oreos Trigger More Robust Dopamine Response and Place-Preference Than Cocaine in Rats," presented at Society for Neuroscience conference in San Diego, California, 2013.

167 **junk foods:** Rats fed junk-food diets need increasing amounts to trigger the release of dopamine and get the same brain boost. They become obese and lose control of their ability to stop eating, much like alcoholics who can't stop at one drink. Even when electric shocks are applied to their feet, which would stop control groups from eating rat chow, if the food is cheesecake, frosting, or bacon, the rats keep on eating. When the junk food is removed and replaced with healthy food, the rats stage a hunger strike, basically starving themselves for two weeks because they're so upset.

167 **Sugar creates a "bliss point":** Moss, *Salt, Sugar, Fat.*

167 **Fat content is difficult to discern:** Mirre Viskaal-van Dongen et al., "Hidden Fat Facilitates Passive Overconsumption," *Journal of Nutrition* 139, no. 2 (2009): 394–99; Drewnowski and Schwartz, "Invisible Fats," 203–17.

167 **Even artificial sweeteners can get us hooked:** M. D. Puhl et al., "Environmental Enrichment Protects Against the Acquisition of Cocaine Self-Administration in Adult Male Rats, But Does Not Eliminate Avoidance of a Drug-Associated Saccharin Cue," *Behavioural Pharmacology* 23 (2012): 43–53; D. J. Stairs, et al., "Effects of Environmental Enrichment on Extinction and Reinstatement

of Amphetamine Self-Administration and Sucrose-Maintained Responding," *Behavioural Pharmacology* 17 (2006): 597–604.

167 **interfere with self-admistration:** Rats show they prefer saccharine-sweetened water over cocaine.

167 **Rats fed a high-sugar diet:** Carlo Colantuoni et al., "Evidence That Intermittent, Excessive Sugar Intake Causes Endogenous Opioid Dependence," *Obesity Research* 10, no. 6 (2002): 478–88.

167 **Giving women who are binge eaters:** A. Drewnowski and M. Schwartz, "Invisible Fats: Sensory Assessment of Sugar/Fat Mixtures," *Appetite* 14, no. 3 (1990): 203–17.

167 **the endorphin system:** Walter Kaye, "Neurobiology of Anorexia and Bulimia Nervosa," *Physiology & Behavior* 94, no. 1 (2008): 121–35.

167 **Stress and emotions affect your gastrointestinal system:** Maté, *When the Body Says No.*

168 **having a gut feeling:** Emeran A. Mayer, "Gut Feelings: The Emerging Biology of Gut–Brain Communication," *Nature Reviews Neuroscience* 12, no. 8 (2011): 453–66.

168 **less inhibitory control in response to these reward cues:** Ashley Gearhardt and Kelly D. Brownell, "Neural Correlates of Food Addiction," *Archives of Geneneral Psychiatry* 68, no. 8 (2011): 808–16.

168 **The brain's ability to register dopamine surges:** Gene-Jack Wang et al, "Brain Dopamine and Obesity," *The Lancet* 357, no. 9253 (February 3, 2001): 354–57.

168 **Drugs and food compete in the brain:** Doug Brunk, "Neural Correlates of Addictive-Like Eating Behavior Studied," *Clinical Psychiatry News*, April 4, 2011.

169 **solid evidence that twelve-step programs:** Diane H. Wasson and Mary Jackson, "An Analysis of the Role of Overeaters Anonymous in Women's Recovery from Bulimia Nervosa," *Eating Disorders* 12, no. 4 (2004): 337–56; Nattie Ronel, Natti and Galit Libman, "Eating Disorders and Recovery: Lessons from Overeaters Anonymous," *Clinical Social Work Journal* 31, no. 2 (2003): 155–71.

169 **the dopamine reward pathway:** Brian Knutson et al., "Dissociation of Reward Anticipation and Outcome with Event-Related fMRI," *Neuroreport* 12, no. 17 (2001): 3683–87; John P. O'Doherty et al., "Neural Responses During Anticipation of a Primary Taste Reward," *Neuron* 33, no. 5 (2002): 815–26.

169 **don't stop eating:** The way to prevent the munchies is to simply keep food out of your mouth. The endocannabinoid system is designed to make you *keep* eating, so just don't start.

170 **The hormone leptin:** Ioannis Kyrou et al., "Stress, Visceral Obesity, and Metabolic Complications," *Annals of the New York Academy of Sciences* 1083, no. 1 (2006): 77–110.

170 **how fat you really are:** Leptin also lets your reproductive system know whether "all systems are go" and you have enough energy reserves to conceive.

170 **appetite suppressant:** In animals it was found to reduce all food intake, in particular "palatable" food intake, and obesity.

171 **Or drink them:** Michael G. Tordoff and Annette M. Alleva, "Effect of Drinking Soda Sweetened with Aspartame or High-Fructose Corn Syrup on Food Intake and Body Weight," *The American Journal of Clinical Nutrition* 51, no. 6 (1990): 963–69; Michael G. Tordoff and Annette M. Alleva, "Oral Stimulation with Aspartame Increases Hunger," *Physiology & Behavior* 47, no. 3 (1990): 555–59; J. H. Lavin et al., "The Effect of Sucrose- and Aspartame-Sweetened Drinks on Energy Intake, Hunger and Food Choice of Female, Moderately Restrained Eaters," *Int J Obes Relat Metab Disord* 21, no. 1 (1997): 37–42.

171 **Artificial sweeteners do not satiate:** Peter J. Rogers and John E. Blundell, "Separating the Actions of Sweetness and Calories: Effects of Saccharin and Carbohydrates on Hunger and Food Intake in Human Subjects," *Physiology & Behavior* 45, no. 6 (1989): 1093–99; Qing Yang, "Gain Weight by 'Going Diet?' Artificial Sweeteners and the Neurobiology of Sugar Cravings: Neuroscience 2010," *The Yale Journal of Biology and Medicine* 83, no. 2 (2010): 101.

171 **can make you fat:** G. A. Colditz et al., "Patterns of Weight Change and Their Relation to Diet in a Cohort of Healthy Women," *American Journal of Clinical Nutrition* 51, no. 6 (1990): 1100–1105; S. P. Fowler et al., "Fueling the Obesity Epidemic? Artificially Sweetened Beverage Use and Long-Term Weight Gain," *Obesity* 16, no. 8 (2008): 1894–1900.

172 **A high-protein, low-carb diet:** M. Hession et al., "Systematic Review of Randomized Controlled Trials of Low-Carbohydrate Vs. Low-Fat/Low- Calorie Diets in the Management of Obesity and Its Comorbiditie, "*Obesity Reviews* 10, no. 1 (2009): 36–50.

172 **lower your risk for heart disease:** L. A. Bazzano et al., "Effects of Low-Carbohydrate and Low-Fat Diets: A Randomized Trial," *Annals of Internal Medicine* 161 (2014): 309–18; T. Hu and L. A. Bazzano, "The Low-Carbohydrate Diet and Cardiovascular Risk Factors: Evidence from Epidemiologic Studies," *Nutrition, Metabolism and Cardiovascular Diseases* 24, no. 4 (2014): 337–43.

172 **Numerous studies suggest that the omega-3:** Da Young Oh et al., "GPR120 Is an Omega-3 Fatty Acid Receptor Mediating Potent Anti-inflammatory and Insulin-Sensitizing Effects," *Cell* 142, no. 5 (2010): 687–98.

172-173 **What else reverses insulin resistance? Cannabis:** T. C. Kirkham, "Endocannabinoids in the Regulation of Appetite and Body Weight," *Behavioral Pharmacology* 16, no. 5-6 (2005): 297-313.

173 **Chronic pot smokers:** Yann Le Strat and Bernard Le Foll, "Obesity and Cannabis Use: Results from 2 Representative National Surveys," *American Journal of Epidemiology* 174, no. 8 (2011): 929.

173 **better cholesterol and fatty acid levels:** Elizabeth A. Penner et al., "The Impact of Marijuana Use on Glucose, Insulin, and Insulin Resistance Among U.S. Adults," *American Journal of Medicine* 126, no. 7 (2013): 583-89.

173 **The third hormone, ghrelin:** S. Taheri et al., "Short Sleep Duration Is Associated with Reduced Leptin, Elevated Ghrelin, and Increased Body Mass Index," *PLoS Medicine* 1, no. 3 (2004): e62.

173 **In obese people:** P. J. English et al., "Food Fails to Suppress Ghrelin Levels in Obese Humans," *Journal of Clinical Endocrinology and Metabolism* 87, no. 6 (2002): 2984.

173 **Twins, whether they grow up together:** Albert J. Stunkard et al., "A Twin Study of Human Obesity," *JAMA* 256, no. 1 (1986): 51-54.

173 **or are separated at birth:** Albert J. Stunkard et al., "The Body-Mass Index of Twins Who Have Been Reared Apart," *New England Journal of Medicine* 322, no. 21 (1990): 1483-87.

173 **children adopted out have the BMIs:** Albert J. Stunkard et al., "An Adoption Study of Human Obesity," *New England Journal of Medicine* 314, no. 4 (1986a): 193-98.

173 **Australian researchers:** P. Sumithran et al., "Long-Term Persistence of Hormonal Adaptations to Weight Loss," *New England Journal of Medicine* 365, no. 17 (2011):1597-1604.

174 **whipped cream:** On the other hand, you don't want to make yourself crazy trying to eat local, pesticide free, organic, vegan, etc. There's a new eating disorder called orthorexia for people who are getting way too obsessive about what they eat.

174 **American-born children don't live as long:** Gopal K. Singh and Barry A. Miller, "Health, Life Expectancy, and Mortality Patterns Among Immigrant Populations in the United States," *Canadian Journal of Public Health* 95, no. 3 (2003): 114-21.

174 **One study that divided people into two diets:** Tasnime N. Akbaraly et al., "Dietary Pattern and Depressive Symptoms in Middle Age," *British Journal of Psychiatry* 195, no. 5 (2009): 408-13.

175 **diets high in fats and low in carbs:** Westman et al,. "Low-Carbohydrate Nutrition and Metabolism," 276-84; F. L. Santos et al., "Systematic Review and Meta-analysis of Clinical Trials of the Effects of Low Carbohydrate Diets on Cardiovascular Risk Factors," *Obesity Reviews* 13, no. 11 (2012): 1048-66.

175 **in particular belly fat loss:** Ronald M. Krauss et al., "Separate Effects of Reduced Carbohydrate Intake and Weight Loss on Atherogenic Dyslipidemia," *American Journal of Clinical Nutrition* 83, no. 5 (2006): 1025-31.

175 **lower blood sugar and insulin levels:** Westman et al., "Low-Carbohydrate Nutrition and Metabolism," 276-84; Hession et al., "Systematic Review of Randomized Controlled Trials," 36-50.

175 **Saturated fat and cholesterol don't increase:** Patty W. Siri-Tarino et al., "Meta-analysis of Prospective Cohort Studies Evaluating the Association of Saturated Fat with Cardiovascular Disease," *American Journal of Clinical Nutrition* 91, no. 3 (2010): 535-46.

175 **The countries eating the most saturated fat:** Robert Hoenselaar, "Saturated Fat and Cardiovascular Disease: The Discrepancy Between the Scientific Literature and Dietary Advice," *Nutrition* 28, no. 2 (2012): 118-23.

175 **Low-carb diets:** Bonnie J. Brehm et al., "A Randomized Trial Comparing a Very Low Carbohydrate Diet and a Calorie-Restricted Low Fat Diet on Body Weight and Cardiovascular Risk Factors in Healthy Women," *Journal of Clinical Endocrinology & Metabolism* 88, no. 4 (2003): 1617-23.

175 **cholestrol numbers:** High-density lipoprotein (HDL) is the "good" type of cholesterol. The low-density lipoproteins (LDL) have the reputation of being the "bad" cholesterol, but it's not that simple. There are smaller, dense LDLs that are bad for you, and larger, fluffy ones that are good for you, just like my mother's matzo balls. There is an unholy trinity, called pattern B, where you see dense LDLs, low levels of desirable HDLS, and high triglycerides, a setup for narrowing the arteries with plaques, causing heart attacks or strokes. The bad matzo balls—the dense LDLs—are linked to inflammation and many medical illnesses but are not even produced by eating fat. They're produced by excess sugars and carbs. That is a big shift from the old thinking on diet and cholesterol levels.

175 **okay again:** They increase LDLs, but the good, fluffy kind, and they also increase beneficial HDLs.

175 **Trans fats are still bad:** Esther Lopez-Garcia et al., "Consumption of Trans Fatty Acids Is Related to Plasma Biomarkers of Inflammation and Endothelial Dysfunction," *Journal of Nutrition* 135, no. 3 (2005): 562-66; Rajiv Chowdhur et al., "Association of Dietary, Circulating, and Supplement Fatty Acids with Coronary Risk: A Systematic Review and Meta-analysis," *Annals of Internal Medicine* 160, no. 6 (2014): 398-406.

175   **Monounsaturated fats, found in nuts:** Penny M. Kris-Etherton et al., "Nuts and Their Bioactive Constituents: Effects on Serum Lipids and Other Factors That Affect Disease Risk," *American Journal of Clinical Nutrition* 70, no. 3 (1999): 504s–511s.

176   **Now, it turns out:** Unique to coconut oil are its antiviral and antifungal properties. Around half the fat of coconut oil is lauric acid, a fatty acid rarely found in nature, though it is in human breast milk. Infants convert it to monolaurin, which kills some bacteria, giardia, measles, the flu, herpes, and HIV. Coconut oil is also great for your hair, cuticles, and dry skin. It can even clean your teeth. It is also a good lubricant for sex.

176   **coconut oil is the hot new thing:** Trent Gordon, *Coconut Oil—The Numerous Advantages: Hygiene, Diet and Weight Loss* (Newark, Del.: Speedy Publishing LLC, 2013).

176   **a way to add a bit of sweetener:** Monica L. Assunção et al., "Effects of Dietary Coconut Oil on the Biochemical and Anthropometric Profiles of Women Presenting Abdominal Obesity," *Lipids* 44, no. 7 (2009): 593–601.

176   **Raw vegetables are important:** Oyinlola Oyebode et al., "Fruit and Vegetable Consumption and All-Cause, Cancer and CVD Mortality: Analysis of Health Survey for England Data," *Journal of Epidemiology and Community Health* (2014): jech-2013.

176   **alkanize your body:** Animal products, grains, and processed foods can be acidic, while most vegetables, beans, and seeds are alkaline. Deep breathing, drinking spring water, and moderate exercise are also ways to alkalinize.

176   **maintaining bone health:** Tim Arnett, "Regulation of Bone Cell Function by Acid-Base Balance," *Proceedings of the Nutrition Society* 62, no. 2 (2003): 511–20.

176   **lowering your risk for obesity:** Mark Hyman, "Systems Biology, Toxins, Obesity, and Functional Medicine," *Altern Ther Health Med* 13, no. 2 (2007): S134–S139.

176   **diabetes, and heart disease:** R. Jaffe, "The Alkaline Way in Digestive Health," in *Bioactive Food as Dietary Interventions for Liver and Gastrointestinal Disease: Bioactive Foods in Chronic Disease States* (London: Academic Press, 2012): 1–21.

176   **strong evidence that ACV lowers insulin:** Y. Ostman et al., "Vinegar Supplementation Lowers Glucose and Insulin Responses and Increases Satiety After a Bread Meal in Healthy Subjects," *European Journal of Clinical Nutrition* 59 (2005): 983–88.

176   **keep diabetes in check:** Carol S. Johnston et al., "Preliminary Evidence That Regular Vinegar Ingestion Favorably Influences Hemoglobin A1c Values in Individuals with Type 2 Diabetes Mellitus," *Diabetes Research and Clinical Practice* 84, no. 2 (2009): e15–e17.

176   **drive weight loss:** Tomoo Kondo et al., "Acetic Acid Upregulates the Expression of Genes for Fatty Acid Oxidation Enzymes in Liver to Suppress Body Fat Accumulation," *Journal of Agricultural and Food Chemistry* 57, no. 13 (2009): 5982–86.

176   **improve cholesterol levels:** Nilgun H. Budak et al., "Effects of Apple Cider Vinegars Produced with Different Techniques on Blood Lipids in High-Cholesterol-Fed Rats," *Journal of Agricultural and Food Chemistry* 59, no. 12 (2011): 6638–44.

176   **reduce inflammation:** Christine M. Ross and John J. Poluhowich, "The Effect of Apple Cider Vinegar on Adjuvant Arthritic Rats," *Nutrition Research* 4, no. 4 (1984): 737–41.

176   **acetic acid in vinegar inhibits the digestion of starches:** Johnston et al., "Preliminary Evidence That Regular Vinegar Ingestion Favorably Influences Hemoglobin," e15–e17.

176   **won't be so bloated:** Apple cider vinegar is made from the alcohol obtained by the fermentation of apples by yeast and bacteria. If you can get raw ACV, it's even better, because pasteurization will kill off some of the good stuff, like enzymes. A tablespoon of ACV diluted in plenty of water before a meal is a common recommendation for people trying to lose weight. Dilution is crucial, because all vinegar is caustic to tooth enamel and stomach lining if not watered down.

177   **uses only the sugar glucose:** O. E. Owen et al., "Brain Metabolism During Fasting," *Journal of Clinical Investigation* 46, no. 10 (1967): 1589; A. Rao et al., "A Randomized, Double-Blind, Placebo-Controlled Pilot Study of a Probiotic in Emotional Symptoms of Chronic Fatigue Syndrome," *Gut Pathogens* 1, no. 1 (2009): 1–6.

177   **Chronic consumption of fructose:** Karen L. Teff et al., "Dietary Fructose Reduces Circulating Insulin and Leptin, Attenuates Postprandial Suppression of Ghrelin, and Increases Triglycerides in Women," *Journal of Clinical Endocrinology & Metabolism* 89, no. 6 (2004): 2963–72.

177   **It can also increase blood triglycerides:** Kimber L. Stanhope et al., "Consumption of Fructose and High Fructose Corn Syrup Increase Postprandial Triglycerides, LDL-Cholesterol, and Apolipoprotein-B in Young Men and Women," *Journal of Clinical Endocrinology & Metabolism* 96, no. 10 (2011): E1596–E1605.

177   **Estrogen may blunt some of these effects:** Caroline Couchepin et al., "Markedly Blunted Metabolic Effects of Fructose in Healthy Young Female Subjects Compared with Male Subjects." *Diabetes Care* 31, no. 6 (2008): 1254–56.

177   **male lab rats are more affected:** T. J. Horton et al., "Female Rats Do Not Develop Sucrose-Induced Insulin Resistance," *American Journal of Physiology* 272, no. 5 (1997): R1571–R1576.

177   **high triglyceride levels from high-fructose diets:** Hara Estoff Marano, "The Trouble with Fructose," *Psychology Today*, September/October 2012, 48.

178   **medicine that could cause memory loss:** Leslie R. Wagstaff et al., "Statin-Associated Memory Loss: Analysis of 60 Case Reports and Review of the Literature," *Pharmacotherapy: The Journal of Human Pharmacology and Drug Therapy* 23, no. 7 (2003): 871–880.

178   **increased blood-sugar levels, muscle damage:** Giuseppe Caso et al., "Effect of Coenzyme Q10 on Myopathic Symptoms in Patients Treated with Statins," *American Journal of Cardiology* 99, no. 10 (2007): 1409–12; Beatrice A. Golomb and Marcella A. Evans, "Statin Adverse Effects," *American Journal of Cardiovascular Drugs* 8, no. 6 (2008): 373–418.

178   **tingling and numbness in your extremities:** Y. L. Lo et al., "Statin Therapy and Small Fiber Neuropathy: A Serial Electrophysiological Study," *Journal of the Neurological Sciences* 208, no. 1 (2003): 105–8.

178   **deplete key nutrients:** Caso et al., "Effect of Coenzyme q10 on Myopathic Symptoms," 1409–12.

178   **eat more unhealthy foods:** Rita F. Redberg and Mitchell H. Katz, "Healthy Men Should Not Take Statins," *JAMA* 307, no. 14 (2012): 1491–92; Takehiro Sugiyama et al., "Different Time Trends of Caloric and Fat Intake Between Statin Users and Nonusers Among U.S. Adults: Gluttony in the Time of Statins?" *JAMA Internal Medicine*, April 24, 2014, pp. e1–e8.

178   **eggs are a great source of protein:** Maria Luz Fernandez, "Dietary Cholesterol Provided by Eggs and Plasma Lipoproteins in Healthy Populations," *Current Opinion in Clinical Nutrition & Metabolic Care* 9, no. 1 (2006): 8–12; Christopher N. Blesso et al., "Whole Egg Consumption Improves Lipoprotein Profiles and Insulin Sensitivity to a Greater Extent Than Yolk-Free Egg Substitute in Individuals with Metabolic Syndrome," *Metabolism* 62, no. 3 (2013): 400–410; Ying Rong et al., "Egg Consumption and Risk of Coronary Heart Disease and Stroke: Dose-Response Meta-analysis of Prospective Cohort Studies," *British Medical Journal* 346 (2013): e8539.

178   **eggs are high in choline:** Kristin L. Herron and Maria Luz Fernandez, "Are the Current Dietary Guidelines Regarding Egg Consumption Appropriate?" *Journal of Nutrition* 134, no. 1 (2004): 187–90.

178   **Many women aren't getting enough choline:** National Health and Nutrition Examination Survey (NHANES), 2005–2006 (ICPSR 25504), United States Department of Health and Human Services, Centers for Disease Control and Prevention, National Center for Health Statistics.

178   **low choline levels are associated with anxiety and depression:** I. Bjelland et al., "Choline in Anxiety and Depression: The Hordaland Health Study" *American Journal of Clinical Nutrition* 90, no. 4 (2009): 1056–60.

178   **Eat eggs:** Choline may be particularly crucial during pregnancy; mothers given choline supplements during their second trimester have babies with better brain function and less risk of schizophrenia.

179   **giving diet drinks to research subjects:** S. Fowler et al., "Diet Soft Drink Consumption Is Associated with Increased Incidence of Overweight and Obesity in the San Antonio Heart Study," *Diabetes* 54 (2005): A258; R. Dhingra et al., "Soft Drink Consumption and Risk of Developing Cardiometabolic Risk Factors and the Metabolic Syndrome in Middle-Aged Adults in the Community," *Circulation* 116 (2007): 480–88.

180   **Rats given aspartame:** Sharon P. Fowler et al., "Fueling the Obesity Epidemic? Artificially Sweetened Beverage Use and Long-term Weight Gain," *Obesity* 16, no. 8 (2008): 1894–1900.

180   **rats given saccharrine water:** Anthony Sclafani and Steven Xenakis, "Sucrose and Polysaccharide Induced Obesity in the Rat," *Physiology & Behavior* 32, no. 2 (1984): 169–74.

180   **Indigenous cultures with no processed food:** S. Lindeberg and B. Lundh, "Apparent Absence of Stroke and Ischaemic Heart Disease in a Traditional Melanesian Island: A Clinical Study in Kitava," *Journal of Internal Medicine* 233, no. 3 (1993): 269–75; Ami K. Patel, Jack T. Rogers, and Xudong Huang, "Flavanols, Mild Cognitive Impairment, and Alzheimer's Dementia," *International Journal of Clinical and Experimental Medicine* 1, no. 2 (2008): 181.

181   **Refined white flour and sugar:** David Perlmutter, *Grain Brain: The Surprising Truth About Wheat, Carbs, and Sugar—Your Brain's Silent Killers* (New York: Little, Brown and Company, 2013).

181   **fatty red meats:** Dorothy J. Pattison et al., "Dietary Risk Factors for the Development of Inflammatory Polyarthritis: Evidence for a Role of High Level of Red Meat Consumption," *Arthritis & Rheumatism* 50, no. 12 (2004): 3804–12.

181   **sweetened drinks:** Lawrence De Koning et al., "Sweetened Beverage Consumption, Incident Coronary Heart Disease, and Biomarkers of Risk in Men," *Circulation* 125, no. 14 (2012): 1735–41.

181   **diet sodas:** David S. Ludwig, "Artificially Sweetened Beverages: Cause for Concern," *JAMA* 302, no. 22 (2009): 2477–78.

181 **Ginger:** Reinhard Grzanna et al., "Ginger—An Herbal Medicinal Product with Broad Anti-inflammatory Actions," *Journal of Medicinal Food* 8, no. 2 (2005): 125–32.

181 **and turmeric:** Bharat B. Aggarwal and Kuzhuvelil B. Harikumar, "Potential Therapeutic Effects of Curcumin, the Anti-inflammatory Agent, Against Neurodegenerative, Cardiovascular, Pulmonary, Metabolic, Autoimmune and Neoplastic Diseases," *The International Journal of Biochemistry & Cell Biology* 41, no. 1 (2009): 40–59.

181 **catechins:** George L. Tipoe et al., "Green Tea Polyphenols as an Anti-oxidant and Anti-inflammatory Agent for Cardiovascular Protection," *Cardiovascular & Hematological Disorders—Drug Targets (Formerly Current Drug Targets—Cardiovascular & Hematological Disorders)* 7, no. 2 (2007): 135–44.

181 **theaflavin:** Rajesh Aneja et al., "Theaflavin, a Black Tea Extract, Is a Novel Anti-inflammatory Compound," *Critical Care Medicine* 32, no. 10 (2004): 2097–2103.

181 **Omega-3 fatty acids are antioxidants:** Maria Skouroliakou et al., "A Double-Blind, Randomized Clinical Trial of the Effect of Omega-3 Fatty Acids on the Oxidative Stress of Preterm Neonates Fed Through Parenteral Nutrition," *European Journal of Clinical Nutrition* 64, no. 9 (2010): 940–47.

181 **lower inflammation:** Philip C. Calder, "Omega-3 Polyunsaturated Fatty Acids, Inflammation, and Inflammatory Diseases," *American Journal of Clinical Nutrition* 83, no. 6 (2006): S1505–S1519.

182 **supplementation improves symptoms:** Anxious patients are more deficient in eicosapentaenoic acid (EPA, an omega-3) than depressed patients, who have lower-than-normal levels, and those with more severe social anxiety disorders have lower omega-3 fatty acid levels than those with less severe symptoms. Omega-3 supplementation decreases anxiety-like behaviors in rodents, nonhuman primates, and medical students. One important caveat for taking omega-3 supplements: they need to be high in EPA, at least 60 percent, and lower in docosahexaenoic acid (DHA) to have beneficial effects on psychiatric complaints.

182 **fish oils can be used to decrease impulsivity:** B. Hallahan and M. R. Garland, "Essential Fatty Acids and Their Role in the Treatment of Impulsivity Disorders," *Prostaglandins Leukot Essen. Fatty Acids* 71, no. 4 (2004): 211–16; Alexandra J. Richardson, "Omega-3 Fatty Acids in ADHD and Related Neurodevelopmental Disorders," *International Review of Psychiatry* 18, no. 2 (2006): 155–72; Jerome Sarris, et al., "Omega-3 for Bipolar Disorder: Meta-analyses of Use in Mania and Bipolar Depression," *Journal of Clinical Psychiatry* 73, no. 1 (2012): 81–86.

182 **some schizophrenia symptoms:** K. Akter et al., "A Review of the Possible Role of the Essential Fatty Acids and Fish Oils in the Etiology, Prevention or Pharmacotherapy of Schizophrenia," *Journal of Clinical Pharmacy and Therapeutics* 37, no. 2 (2012): 132–39.

182 **slow down telomere shortening:** R. Farzaneh-Far et al., "Association of Marine Omega-3 Fatty Acid Levels with Telomeric Aging in Patients with Coronary Heart Disease," *JAMA* 303 (2010): 250–57.

182 **can form endocannabinoids:** Iain Brown et al., "Cannabinoids and Omega-3/6 Endocannabinoids as Cell Death and Anticancer Modulators," *Progress in Lipid Research* 52, no. 1 (2013): 80–109.

182 **Hemp seeds:** J. C. Callaway, "Hempseed as a Nutritional Resource: An Overview," *Euphytica* 140, no. 1–2 (2004): 65–72.

182 **my morning muesli:** My mix: raw oats, chia seeds, flax seeds, hemp seeds, and sliced almonds, served with unsweetened almond milk and a splash of pure maple syrup from our woods, courtesy of Jeremy.

182 **Trillions of bacteria in our GI systems:** Hiroyuki Osawa et al., "Changes in Plasma Ghrelin Levels, Gastric Ghrelin Production, and Body Weight After Helicobacter Pylori Cure," *Journal of Gastroenterology* 41, no. 10 (2006): 954–61.

182 **How do you get a fat mouse thinner:** Peter J. Turnbaugh et al., "Diet-Induced Obesity Is Linked to Marked but Reversible Alterations in the Mouse Distal Gut Microbiome," *Cell Host & Microbe* 3, no. 4 (2008): 213–23.

182 **Gut bacteria have a lot to do with obesity:** John K. DiBaise et al., "Gut Microbiota and Its Possible Relationship with Obesity," in *Mayo Clinic Proceedings* 83, no. 4 (2008): 460–69.

182 **different levels of certain bacteria:** R. Mathur et al., "Methane and Hydrogen Positivity on Breath Test Is Associated with Greater Body Mass Index and Body Fat," *Journal of Clinical Endocrinology & Metabolism* 98, no. 4 (2013): E698–E702.

182 **In humans given a lean donor's microbes:** Anne Vrieze et al., "Transfer of Intestinal Microbiota from Lean Donors Increases Insulin Sensitivity in Individuals with Metabolic Syndrome," *Gastroenterology* 143, no. 4 (2012): 913–16.

182 **Probiotics help stop the weight gain... (Zyprexa):** K. J. Davey et al., "Antipsychotics and the Gut Microbiome: Olanzapine-Induced Metabolic Dysfunction Is Attenuated by Antibiotic Administration in the Rat," *Translational Psychiatry* 3, no. 10 (2013): e309.

183 **Smaller stomachs fill up more quickly:** David E. Cummings et al., "Plasma Ghrelin Levels After Diet-Induced Weight Loss or Gastric Bypass Surgery," *New England Journal of Medicine* 346, no. 21 (2002): 1623–30.

183 **nonsurgical recipients also lost weight:** Alice P. Liou et al., "Conserved Shifts in the Gut Microbiota Due to Gastric Bypass Reduce Host Weight and Adiposity," *Science of Translational Medicine* 5, no. 178 (2013): 178.

183 **Artificial sweeteners such as Splenda:** Mohamed B. Abou-Donia et al., "Splenda Alters Gut Microflora and Increases Intestinal P-Glycoprotein and Cytochrome P-450 in Male Rats," *Journal of Toxicology and Environmental Health, Part A* 71, no. 21 (2008): 1415–29.

183 **deranging glucose:** Jotham Suez et al. "Artificial Sweeteners Induce Glucose Intolerance by Altering the Gut Microbiota," *Nature*, published online, September 17, 2014, doi:10.1038/Nature13793.

183 **Probiotic supplements:** Michael Pollan, "Some of My Best Friends Are Germs," *New York Times Magazine*, May 15, 2013.

183 **encourage weight loss:** Nathalie M. Delzenne et al., "Targeting Gut Microbiota in Obesity: Effects of Prebiotics and Probiotics," *Nature Reviews Endocrinology* 7, no. 11 (2011): 639–46.

183 **Onions, artichokes, asparagus, and sunchokes:** Roya Kelishadi et al., "A Randomized Triple-Masked Controlled Trial on the Effects of Synbiotics on Inflammation Markers in Overweight Children," *Jornal de Pediatria* 90, no. 2 (2014): 161–67.

<u>183</u> **keep down inflammation:** Typically, prebiotics come from plant fiber, but unlike any other living tissue, breasts make prebiotics. Breast milk is the best source of prebiotics for a baby, and actually the only source, unless you're game to give a baby pureed Jerusalem artichokes and asparagus.

184 **when gut microbes from easygoing, adventurous mice:** Stephen M. Collins et al., "The Adoptive Transfer of Behavioral Phenotype Via the Intestinal Microbiota: Experimental Evidence and Clinical Implications," *Current Opinion in Microbiology* 16, no. 3 (2013): 240–45.

184 **In animal studies, LPS administration:** M. Maes et al., "The Gut-Brain Barrier in Major Depression: Intestinal Mucosal Dysfunction with an Increased Translocation of LPS from Gram Negative Enterobacteria (Leaky Gut) Plays a Role in the Inflammatory Pathophysiology of Depression," *Neuro Endocrinology Letters* 29, no. 1 (2008): 117–24.

184 **A person's immune response to LPS:** Robert Dantzer et al., "From Inflammation to Sickness and Depression: When the Immune System Subjugates the Brain," *Nature Reviews Neuroscience* 9, no. 1 (2008): 46–56.

184 **cytokines associated with depression:** Tumor necrosis factor alpha (TNF-alpha), IL-6, and IL-1beta.

184 **Ingesting probiotics may improve depression:** A. C. Logan and M. Katzman, "Major Depressive Disorder: Probiotics May Be an Adjuvant Therapy," *Medical Hypotheses* 64, no. 3 (2005): 533–38.

184 **By manipulating the bacteria found in the stomach:** N. Sudo et al., "Postnatal Microbial Colonization Programs the Hypothalamic-Pituitary-Adrenal System for Stress Response in Mice," *Journal of Physiology* 558 (2004): 263–75.

<u>184</u> **behavior can be altered:** Chronic treatment with the bacteria *Mycobacterium vaccae* improves quality-of-life scores by reducing levels of cytokines, thus lowering inflammation. Treatment with *bifidobacteria* increases brain levels of tryptophan, required for serotonin synthesis.

184 **Treatment with probiotics lowers scores:** M. Messaoudi et al., "Beneficial Psychological Effects of a Probiotic Formulation (Lactobacillus Helveticus R0052 and Bifidobacterium Longum R0175) in Healthy Human Volunteers," *Gut Microbes* 2, no. 4 (July/August 2011): 256–61.

184 **Women who eat probiotic yogurt:** Kirsten Tillisch et al., "Consumption of Fermented Milk Product with Probiotic Modulates Brain Activity," *Gastroenterology* 144, no. 7 (2013): 1394–140.

184 **They affect GABA:** Radhika Dhakal et al., "Production of Gaba (Γ-Aminobutyric Acid) by Microorganisms: A Review," *Brazilian Journal of Microbiology* 43, no. 4 (2012): 1230–41.

184–185 **calm the nervous system:** *Lactobacillus* creates more GABA receptors in the brain and produces the neurotransmitter itself in the gut.

<u>185</u> **junctions between the cells:** Called desmosomes.

185 **corkscrew shape:** Families *Spirochaetaceae* and *Spirillaceae*.

186 **Stress, obesity, poor diet, and a leaky gut:** E. Haroon et al., "Psychoneuroimmunology Meets Neuropsychopharmacology: Translational Implications of the Impact of Inflammation on Behavior," *Neuropsychopharmacology* 37, no. 1 (2012): 137–62.

<u>186</u> **proteins in gluten:** Gliadins and glutenins.

187 **gluteomorphin, which hits the endorphin receptors:** William Davis, *Wheat Belly: Lose the Wheat, Lose the Weight, and Find Your Path Back to Health* (New York: Rodale, 2011).

188 **Geneen Roth's books:** *Breaking Free from Emotional Eating, Feeding the Hungry Heart, When Food Is Love, Appetites.*

189 **Slow, deep breathing through your nose:** Ravinder Jerath et al., "Physiology of Long Pranayamic

Breathing: Neural Respiratory Elements May Provide a Mechanism That Explains How Slow Deep Breathing Shifts the Autonomic Nervous System," *Medical Hypotheses* 67, no. 3 (2006): 566–71.

189   **Stress, whether physical or emotional:** Donna L. Tempel and Sarah F. Leibowitz, "PVN Steroid Implants: Effect on Feeding Patterns and Macronutrient Selection," *Brain Research Bulletin* 23, no. 6 (1989): 553–60; Rouach et al., "The Acute Ghrelin Response to a Psychological Stress Challenge," 693–702; Cizza et al., "Low 24-hour Adiponectin and High Nocturnal Leptin Concentrations," 1079–87.

190   **a protein called peptide Y:** G. Cizza et al., "Low 24-Hour Adiponectin and High Nocturnal Leptin Concentrations in a Case-Control Study of Community-Dwelling Premenopausal Women with Major Depressive Disorder: The Premenopausal, Osteopenia/Osteoporosis, Women, Alendronate, Depression (POWER) Study," *Journal of Clinical Psychiatry* 71, no. 8 (2010): 1079–87.

190   **Subordinate, bossed-around monkeys:** V. Rouach et al., "The Acute Ghrelin Response to a Psychological Stress Challenge Does Not Predict the Post-stress Urge to Eat," *Psychoneuroendocrinology* 32 (2007): 693–702.

190   **Monkeys lower in the dominance hierarchy:** M. E. Wilson et al., "Quantifying Food Intake in Socially Housed Monkeys: Social Status Effects on Caloric Consumption," *Physiology & Behavior* 94, no. 4 (2008): 586–94.

190   **Lower-ranked British civil servants:** M. G. Marmot et al., "Health Inequalities Among British Civil The Whitehall II Study," *Lancet* 337, no. 8754 (1991): 1387–93.

190   **People who are more stressed out:** Janet A. Tomiyama et al., "Comfort Food Is Comforting to Those Most Stressed: Evidence of the Chronic Stress Response Network in High Stress Women," *Psychoneuroendocrinology* 36, no. 10 (2011): 1513–19.

190   **reducing stress through meditation or yoga can help you lose weight:** Jennifer Daubenmier et al., "Mindfulness Intervention for Stress Eating to Reduce Cortisol and Abdominal Fat Among Overweight and Obese Women: An Exploratory Randomized Controlled Study," *Journal of Obesity*, article ID 651936 (2011).

190   **high cortisol levels associated with stress cause higher blood sugar levels:** Paul E. Marik and Rinaldo Bellomo, "Stress Hyperglycemia: An Essential Survival Response," *Critical Care* 17, no. 2 (2013): 305.

192   **food tastes best for the first few bites:** Mary Abbott, "Taste: The Neglected Nutritional Factor," *Journal of the American Dietetic Association* 97, no. 10 (1997): S205–S207.

193   **intense feelings can affect our taste buds:** Petra Platte et al., "Oral Perceptions of Fat and Taste Stimuli Are Modulated by Affect and Mood Induction," *PloS One* 8, no. 6 (2013): e65006.

193   **stressed-out monkeys lower in the dominance hierarchy:** Wilson et al., "Quantifying Food Intake in Socially Housed Monkeys," 586–94.

Chapter Nine: So Tired We're Wired

195   **Women are more sensitive:** Michael Breus, *The Sleep Doctor's Diet Plan: Lose Weight Through Better Sleep* (New York: Rodale, 2011).

195   **Women are more prone to insomnia:** Andrew D. Krystal, "Insomnia in Women," *Clinical Cornerstone* 5, no. 3 (2003): 41–50.

195   **three out of four insomnia patients:** Medco Health Solutions, "America's State of Mind Report," November 2011.

195   **Nearly 30 percent of American women:** Fiona C. Baker et al., "Association of Sociodemographic, Lifestyle, and Health Factors with Sleep Quality and Daytime Sleepiness in Women: Findings from the 2007 National Sleep Foundation 'Sleep in America Poll,'" *Journal of Women's Health* 18, no. 6 (2009): 841–49.

196   **When sleep is off-kilter:** Edward C. Suarez, "Self-Reported Symptoms of Sleep Disturbance and Inflammation, Coagulation, Insulin Resistance and Psychosocial Distress: Evidence for Gender Disparity," *Brain, Behavior, and Immunity* 22, no. 6 (2008): 960–68; Mary Amanda Dew et al., "Healthy Older Adults' Sleep Predicts All-Cause Mortality at 4 to 19 Years of Follow-up," *Psychosomatic Medicine* 65, no. 1 (2003): 63–73; Swapnil N. Rajpathak, "Lifestyle Factors of People with Exceptional Longevity," *Journal of the American Geriatrics Society* 59, no. 8 (August 2011): 1509–12.

196   **Sleep deprivation:** Endocannabinoids, the anti-inflammatory chemicals that mimic the pharmacological actions of cannabis, are likely essential factors in sleep promotion. Other sleep-inducing molecules include orexin, pieces of proteins called peptides, various hormones, and pro- and anti-inflammatory cytokines.

196   **Higher resting heart rates:** Kylie J. Barnett, "The Effects of a Poor Night Sleep on Mood, Cognitive, Autonomic and Electrophysiological Measures," *Journal of Integrative Neuroscience* 7, no. 03 (2008): 405–20.

196 **Americans are sleep deprived:** T. S. Wiley with Bent Formby, *Lights Out: Sleep, Sugar, and Survival* (New York: Simon and Schuster, 2000), 4.

196 **lucky if we get seven:** In the 1970s, we worked thirty-five hours a week and enjoyed twenty-seven hours of leisure time. Now it's forty-eight and fifteen.

196 **One-quarter of American adults report:** Yinong Chong et al., "Prescription Sleep Aid Use Among Adults: United States, 2005–2010," *NCHS Data Brief* 127 (2013): 1–8.

197 **Chronic sleep deprivation does three things:** Kristen L. Knutson et al., "The Metabolic Consequences of Sleep Deprivation," *Sleep Medicine Reviews* 11, no. 3 (June 2007): 163–78.

197 **Animal studies and human studies:** A. V. Nedeltcheva et al., "Sleep Curtailment Is Accompanied by Increased Intake of Calories from Snacks," *American Journal of Clinical Nutrition* 89 (2009): 126–33.

197 **Obese research subjects show:** J. E. Gangwisch et al., "Inadequate Sleep as a Risk Factor for Obesity: Analyses of the NHANES I," *Sleep* 28, no. 10 (2005) 1289–96.

197 **Chronic sleep deprivation:** Mariana G. Figueiro et al., "Light Modulates Leptin and Ghrelin in Sleep-Restricted Adults," *International Journal of Endocrinology* 2012, article ID 530; S. Taheri et al., "Short Sleep Duration Is Associated with Reduced Leptin, Elevated Ghrelin, and Increased Body Mass Index," *PLoS Medicine* 1 (2004): e62; P. Schüssler et al., "Nocturnal Ghrelin, ACTH, GH and Cortisol Secretion After Sleep Deprivation in Humans," *Psychoneuroendocrinology* 31 (2006): 915–23.

197 **Even a single night of sleep deprivation:** S. M. Schmid et al., "A Single Night of Sleep Deprivation Increases Ghrelin Levels and Feelings of Hunger in Normal-Weight Healthy Men," *Journal of Sleep Research* 17 (2008): 331–34.

197 **Sleep deprivation has been linked:** Karine Spiegel et al., "Sleep Loss: A Novel Risk Factor for Insulin Resistance and Type 2 Diabetes," *Journal of Applied Physiology* 99, no. 5 (2005): 2008–19; H. K. Yaggi et al., "Sleep Duration as a Risk Factor for the Development of Type 2 Diabetes," *Diabetes Care* 29 (2006): 657–61.

197 **Less than one week of sleep restriction:** N. T. Ayas et al., "A Prospective Study of Self-Reported Sleep Duration and Incident Diabetes in Women," *Diabetes Care* 26 (2003): 380–84.

197 **Sleep deprivation creates horrendous performance:** Fulda and Schulz, "Cognitive Dysfunction in Sleep Disorders," *Sleep Medicine Reviews* 15, no. 6 (2001): 423–45.

197 **just over 4 percent of American drivers:** Centers for Disease Control and Prevention, *MMWR* 61, no. 51 (January 4, 2013): 1033–37.

198 **slow-wave sleep:** Delta waves predominate here.

198 **dreaming occurs:** Except in children who have night terrors in slow-wave sleep.

199 **the immune system uses sleep time:** Lulu Xie et al., "Sleep Drives Metabolite Clearance from the Adult Brain," *Science* 342, no. 6156 (2013): 373–77.

199 **clean out debris:** The space between brain cells in lab rats is 60 percent greater during sleep, enhancing spinal fluid flow by a factor of ten.

199 **proinflammatory state:** Michael R. Irwin et al., "Sleep Loss Activates Cellular Inflammatory Signaling," *Biological Psychiatry* 64, no. 6 (2008): 538–40.

199 **alters microglia function:** Mark R. Zielinski and James M. Krueger, "Sleep and Innate Immunity," *Frontiers in Bioscience (Scholar edition)* 3 (2011): 632.

199 **Sleep prevents seizures:** Harinder Jaseja, "Purpose of REM Sleep: Endogenous Anti-epileptogenesis in Man—a Hypothesis," *Medical Hypotheses* 62, no. 4 (2004): 546–48.

199 **three-quarters of our sleep:** In newborns, it's 80 percent REM and 20 percent non-REM.

200 **sleep deprivation:** In depressive disorders, insomnia is often one of the first symptoms to appear, sometimes occurring before the onset of mood symptoms, while in anxiety disorders, insomnia comes after other symptoms.

200 **Circadian manipulation and sleep deprivation:** Thomas A. Wehr, "Improvement of Depression and Triggering of Mania by Sleep Deprivation," *JAMA* 267, no. 4 (1992): 548–51; Blynn G. Bunney and William E. Bunney, "Mechanisms of Rapid Antidepressant Effects of Sleep Deprivation Therapy: Clock Genes and Circadian Rhythms," *Biological Psychiatry* 73, no. 12 (2013): 1164–71.

200 **Using bright light in the morning:** Michael Terman and Jiuan Su Terman, "Bright Light Therapy: Side Effects and Benefits Across the Symptom Spectrum," *Journal of Clinical Psychiatry* 60, no. 11 (1999): 799–808.

201 **Both slow-wave sleep and REM-phase sleep:** Jutta Backhaus et al., "Midlife Decline in Declarative Memory Consolidation Is Correlated with a Decline in Slow Wave Sleep," *Learning & Memory* 14, no. 5 (2007): 336–41; Susanne Diekelmann and Jan Born, "The Memory Function of Sleep," *Nature Reviews Neuroscience* 11, no. 2 (2010): 114–26.

201 **As much as a ninety-minute nap:** Matthew P. Walker and Robert Stickgold, "Overnight Alchemy: Sleep-Dependent Memory Evolution," *Nature Reviews Neuroscience* 11, no. 3 (2010): 218–218.

201 **Losing sleep repeatedly:** S. Fulda and H. Schulz, "Cognitive Dysfunction in Sleep Disorders," *Sleep Medicine Reviews* 5, no. 6 (2001): 423–45.

201 **One study showed that 100 percent of children with an ADHD:** N. Golan et al., "Sleep Disorders and Daytime Sleepiness in Children with Attention-Deficit/Hyperactivity Disorder," *Sleep* 27, no. 2 (2004): 261–66.

202 **Half the children undergoing tonsillectomies:** R. D. Chervin et al., "Sleep-Disordered Breathing, Behavior, and Cognition in Children Before and After Adenotonsillectomy," *Pediatrics* 117 (2006): 769–78.

202 **Our body cycles over the course:** D. J. Brambilla et al., "The Effect of Diurnal Variation on Clinical Measurement of Serum Testosterone and Other Sex Hormone Levels in Men." *Journal of Clinical Endocrinology and Metabolism* 94 (2009): 907–13.

202 **nighttime breast milk has more compounds:** Williams, *Breasts*.

203 **Melatonin:** Melatonin has a reputation as being an antiaging supplement. Consuming melatonin may neutralize oxidative damage and delay the neurodegenerative process of aging. D. Acuña-Castroviejo et al., "Melatonin, Mitochondria, and Cellular Bioenergetics," *Journal of Pineal Research* 30, no. 2 (March 2001): 65–74; M. Pohanka, "Alzheimer's Disease and Related Neurodegenerative Disorders: Implication and Counteracting of Melatonin," *Journal of Applied Biomedicine* 9 (2011): 185–96.

203 **Healthy serotonin levels:** Gregory M. Cahill and Joseph C. Besharse, "Circadian Regulation of Melatonin in the Retina of Xenopus Laevis: Limitation by Serotonin Availability," *Journal of Neurochemistry* 54, no. 2 (1990): 716–19; Venkataramanujan Srinivasan et al., "Melatonin in Mood Disorders," *World Journal of Biological Psychiatry* 7, no. 3 (2006): 138–51.

203 **jet lag:** Here's how to treat jet lag: Take 3 milligrams of melatonin between ten P.M. and eleven P.M. for three nights when you first arrive at your destination. When you return home, again, take 3 milligrams for three nights between ten P.M. and eleven P.M. Easy. And it makes a huge difference. Please note that 3 milligrams is not what is typically used for sleep. Melatonin for sleep should still be taken bewteen ten P.M. and eleven P.M., but it's wiser to use half a milligram or 1 milligram in this case.

203 **Breast cancer has been linked:** R. G. Stevens, "Light-at-Night, Circadian Disruption and Breast Cancer: Assessment of Existing Evidence," *International Journal of Epidemiology* 38 (2009): 963–70.

203 **women who are blind:** E. E. Flynn-Evans et al., "Total Visual Blindness Is Protective Against Breast Cancer," *Cancer Causes and Control* 20 (2009): 1753–56.

203 **Sleeping in a dark room:** D. E. Blask, "Melatonin, Sleep Disturbance and Cancer Risk," *Sleep Medicine Reviews* 13 (2008): 257–64.

204 **In seasonal-breeding mammals:** Dorota A. Zieba et al., "In Vitro Evidence That Leptin Suppresses Melatonin Secretion During Long Days and Stimulates Its Secretion During Short Days in Seasonal Breeding Ewes," *Domestic Animal Endocrinology* 33, no. 3 (2007): 358–65.

204 **Rising ghrelin levels:** B. O. Yildiz et al., "Alterations in the Dynamics of Circulating Ghrelin, Adiponectin, and Leptin in Human Obesity," *PNAS* 101 (2004): 10434–39.

204 **Melatonin may enhance:** M. I. Alonso-Vale et al., "Melatonin Enhances Leptin Expression by Rat Adipocytes in the Presence of Insulin," *Am J Physiol Endocrinol Metab* 288, no. 4 (April 2005): E805–E812.

204–205 **In lab rats fed high-calorie diets:** María J. Ríos-Lugo et al., "Melatonin Effect on Plasma Adiponectin, Leptin, Insulin, Glucose, Triglycerides and Cholesterol in Normal and High Fat-Fed Rats," *Journal of Pineal Research* 49, no. 4 (2010): 342–48.

205 **Sleep deprivation is associated:** G. Copinschi, "Metabolic and Endocrine Effects of Sleep Deprivation," *Essential Psychopharmacology* 6, no. 6 (2005): 341–47.

205 **Women with lower levels of melatonin:** C. J. McMullan et al., "Melatonin Secretion and the Incidence of Type 2 Diabetes," *JAMA* 309, no. 13 (April 2013): 1388–96.

205 **Bright-light exposure:** Mariana G. Figueiro et al., "Light Modulates Leptin and Ghrelin in Sleep-Restricted Adults," *International Journal of Endocrinology* 2012, article ID 530726.

205 **A full night's sleep:** A. N. Vgontzas et al., "Adverse Effects of Modest Sleep Restriction on Sleepiness, Performance, and Inflammatory Cytokines," *J Clin Endocrinol Metab* 89 (2004): 2119–26.

205 **If you sleep less than seven hours:** Sheldon Cohen et al., "Sleep Habits and Susceptibility to the Common Cold," *Archives of Internal Medicine* 169, no. 1 (2009): 62.

207 **Estrogen, in particular, is involved:** Yuki Tsuchiya et al., "Cytochrome P450-Mediated Metabolism of Estrogens and Its Regulation in Humans," *Cancer Letters* 227 (2005) 115–24.

207 **Caffeine triggers adrenaline:** Stuart R. Snider and Bertil Waldeck, "Increased Synthesis of Adrenomedullary Catecholamines Induced by Caffeine and Theophylline," *Naunyn-Schmiedeberg's Archives of Pharmacology* 281, no. 2 (1974): 257–60; William R. Lovallo et al., "Caffeine Stimulation

of Cortisol Secretion Across the Waking Hours in Relation to Caffeine Intake Levels," *Psychosomatic Medicine* 67, no. 5 (2005): 734–39.

207 **It also reduces REM sleep:** Hans-Peter Landolt et al., "Caffeine Intake (200 Mg) in the Morning Affects Human Sleep and EEG Power Spectra at Night," *Brain Research* 675, no. 1 (1995): 67–74.

207 **Caffeine constricts blood vessels:** Stacey C. Sigmon et al., "Caffeine Withdrawal, Acute Effects, Tolerance, and Absence of Net Beneficial Effects of Chronic Administration: Cerebral Blood Flow Velocity, Quantitative EEG, and Subjective Effects," *Psychopharmacology* 204, no. 4 (2009): 573–85.

207–208 **Just two hours of iPad use:** Mariana G. Figueiro et al., "The Impact of Light from Computer Monitors on Melatonin Levels in College Students," *Neuro Endocrinology Letters* 32, no. 2 (2011): 158.

208 **two hours of computer use:** Christian Cajochen et al., "Evening Exposure to a Light-Emitting Diodes (LED)-Backlit Computer Screen Affects Circadian Physiology and Cognitive Performance," *Journal of Applied Physiology* 110, no. 5 (2011): 1432–38.

208 **no glowing screens at least one hour:** Andrew B. Dollins et al., "Effects of Illumination on Human Nocturnal Serum Melatonin Levels and Performance," *Physiology & Behavior* 53, no. 1 (1993): 153–60; Mariana G. Figueiro et al., "The Impact of Light from Computer Monitors on Melatonin Levels in College Students," *Neuro Endocrinology Letters* 32, no. 2 (2011): 158.

208 **Even electronic readers can shift your circadian rhythm signals:** A. Chang et al., "Impact of Evening Use of Light-Emitting Electronic Readers on Circadian Timing and Sleep Latency," *SLEEP* 35, abstract supplement (2012): A205.

208 **program called flux:** Free download here: http://stereopsis.com/flux/research.html.

208 **circadian receptors:** http://www.blueblocker.com.

208 **Blue blockers can significantly improve sleep:** K. Burkhart and J. R. Phelps, "Amber Lenses to Block Blue Light and Improve Sleep: A Randomized Trial," *Chronobiology International* 26, no. 8 (2009):1602–12.

208 **Listen to music:** Marconi Union's eight-minute, trance-inducing tune "Weightless," at sixty beats per minute, is a good place to start.

208 **Write in your journal:** Ting Zhang et al., "A 'Present' for the Future: The Unexpected Value of Rediscovery," *Psychological Science* (2014): 0956797614542274.

208 **Gratitude is good for your mood:** Andrew Weil, *Spontaneous Happiness* (Little, Brown and Company, 2011).

209 **Well-timed sleep deprivation:** Burkhard Pflug, "The Effect of Sleep Deprivation on Depressed Patients," *Acta Psychiatrica Scandinavica* 53, no. 2 (1976): 148–58; D. A. Sack et al., "The Timing and Duration of Sleep in Partial Sleep Deprivation Therapy of Depression," *Acta Psychiatrica Scandinavica* 77, no. 2 (1988): 219–24.

210 **Women need lower doses:** David J. Greenblatt et al., "Gender Differences in Pharmacokinetics and Pharmacodynamics of Zolpidem Following Sublingual Administration," *Journal of Clinical Pharmacology* 54, no. 3 (2014): 282–90.

211 **dementia:** John Elwood Gallacher et al., "Benzodiazepine Use and Risk of Dementia: Evidence from the Caerphilly Prospective Study (CaPS)," *J Epidemiology and Community Health* 66 (2012): 869–73.

211 **five-fold increase in early death:** Daniel F. Kripke et al., "Hypnotics' Association with Mortality or Cancer: A Matched Cohort Study," *British Medical Journal Open* 2, no. 1 (2012).

212 **Alcohol might help you pass out:** Timothy Roehrs and Thomas Roth, "Sleep, Sleepiness, and Alcohol Use," *Alcohol Research and Health* 25, no. 2 (2001): 101–9.

212 **Even low doses of alcohol:** Pierce Geoghegan et al., "Investigation of the Effects of Alcohol on Sleep Using Actigraphy," *Alcohol and Alcoholism* 47, no. 5 (2012): 538–44.

212 **can also worsen sleep apnea:** Lawrence Scrima et al., "Increased Severity of Obstructive Sleep Apnea After Bedtime Alcohol Ingestion: Diagnostic Potential and Proposed Mechanism of Action," *Sleep: Journal of Sleep Research & Sleep Medicine* 5, no. 4 (1982): 318–28.

212 **Alcohol also delays and suppresses:** Irshaad O. Ebrahim et al., "Alcohol and Sleep I: Effects on Normal Sleep," *Alcoholism: Clinical and Experimental Research* 37, no. 4 (2013): 539–49.

213 **homeopathic remedies:** Deep Sleep by Herbs, Etc., Somnipure by Peak Life, and Quietude by Boiron are three I like.

Chapter Ten: A Sex Guide That Actually Works

215 **Good sex . . . helps you destress:** Stuart Brody, "Blood Pressure Reactivity to Stress Is Better for People Who Recently Had Penile–Vaginal Intercourse Than for People Who Had Other or No Sexual Activity," *Biological Psychology* 71, no. 2 (2006): 214–22.

215 **risk of heart disease:** Susan A. Hall et al., "Sexual Activity, Erectile Dysfunction, and Incident Cardiovascular Events," *American Journal of Cardiology* 105, no. 2 (2010): 192–97.

215 **stimulates your immune system:** Carl J. Charnetski and Francis X. Brennan, "Sexual Frequency and Salivary Immunoglobulin A (IgA)," *Psychological Reports* 94, no. 3 (2004): 839–44.

216 **43 percent of women have complaints:** Edward O. Laumann et al., "Sexual Dysfunction in the United States," *JAMA* 281, no. 6 (1999): 537–44.

216 **sexual dysfunction:** Medically, there are four categories of female sexual dysfunction: hypoactive sexual desire disorder (not thinking horny thoughts or wanting sex); sexual arousal disorder (not responding fully to sexual stimulation); sexual pain disorders, like dyspareunia (pain during intercourse) and vaginismus (muscle spasms during stimulation); and orgasmic disorder (not climaxing).

216 **higher cortisol levels that inhibit:** Lisa Dawn Hamilton et al., "Cortisol, Sexual Arousal, and Affect in Response to Sexual Stimuli," *Journal of Sexual Medicine* 5, no. 9 (2008): 2111–18.

216 **restrict circulation:** Diabetes, high cholesterol, cigarette smoking, crushed arteries from chronic bicycle riding, pelvic surgery, or sexual trauma.

216 **a medication like Viagra:** L. A. Berman et al., "Efficacy and Tolerability of Viagra (Sildenafil Citrate) in Women with Sexual Arousal Disorder: A Double-Blind, Placebo-Controlled Study," *Int J Impot Res* 14, no. 3 (2002): S27–S28.

218 **this stress and anxiety jams:** Berman and Berman, *For Women Only.*

218–219 **antidepressants that enhance serotonin levels:** Parks W. Walker et al., "Improvement in Fluoxetine-Associated Sexual Dysfunction in Patients Switched to Bupropion," *Journal of Clinical Psychiatry* (1993); Charles C. Coleman et al., "Sexual Dysfunction Associated with the Treatment of Depression: A Placebo-Controlled Comparison of Bupropion Sustained Release and Sertraline Treatment," *Annals of Clinical Psychiatry* 11, no. 4 (1999): 205–15.

219 **Some SSRIs:** Zoloft and Paxil have reputations as significant disrupters of sexual pleasure. Lexapro, in my experience, has less impact on sexual functioning than some of the other antidepressants, and there is a new medication, dubbed Viibryd, that seems to have even fewer sexual side effects than the others. (I know. The double *i* is pretty silly, but the potential side effects aren't: nausea, insomnia, and diarrhea. Sometimes depression doesn't seem so bad in comparison.) I have switched quite a few of my patients over from another SSRI to Lexapro or from Lexapro to Viibryd, and they do report that it's easier for them to achieve orgasm.

220 **diminish libido:** Lactation (nursing) and antipsychotics can also raise prolactin levels, killing sexual desire.

220 **Prolactin is likely part of the negative feedback mechanism:** Tillmann H. C. Krüger et al., "Orgasm-Induced Prolactin Secretion: Feedback Control of Sexual Drive?" *Neuroscience & Biobehavioral Reviews* 26, no. 1 (2002): 31–44.

220 **sex act:** SSRIs are often used to treat paraphilias or sexual fetishes, eliminating behaviors that are bothersome to patients or their communities.

220 **In laboratory animals, the SSRI fluoxetine:** N. Maswood et al., "Modest Effects of Repeated Fluoxetine on Estrous Cyclicity and Sexual Behavior in Sprague-Dawley Female Rats," *Brain Research* 1245 (2008): 52–60.

220 **Sex researcher Jim Pfaus explains:** James G. Pfaus, "Reviews: Pathways of Sexual Desire," *Journal of Sexual Medicine* 6, no. 6 (2009): 1506–33.

220 **sex holiday:** For my patients, I often recommend that they take their antidepressants five days out of the week, Sunday through Thursday. This will allow sexual side effects to diminish by Saturday night and Sunday morning, prime sex time for those who work weekdays. Studies find no increased depressive symptoms with this schedule. Brian E. Moore and Anthony J. Rothschild, "Treatment of Antidepressant-Induced Sexual Dysfunction," *Hospital Practice* 34, no. 1 (1999): 89–91; Matthew J. Taylor et al., "Strategies for Managing Antidepressant-Induced Sexual Dysfunction: Systematic Review of Randomized Controlled Trials," *Journal of Affective Disorders* 88, no. 3 (2005): 241–54.

221 **sexual side effects:** It is likely the most common combination in all of psychiatry for this reason. They also happen to work very nicely together, sort of like peanut butter and jelly. Between the two of them, they create one kick-ass antidepressant, because they cover most of the neurotransmitters that are implicated in depression. In the seventies and eighties, tricyclic antidepressants were used to combat anxiety and depression. They enhanced transmission of serotonin, norepinephrine, and dopamine, and they worked well, but the side effects were unbearable for many. Combining an SSRI with Wellbutrin mimics these old tricyclics, hitting the same trifecta of neurotransmitters, but without the dry mouth, constipation, and sedation of the old days. So why not just take Wellbutrin alone? I find that it's great for a low-energy, low-motivation depression, but it's not that good for anxiety symptoms or if you have a "short fuse."

221 **for a select few:** There are a lot of women out there with the variant of the serotonin transporter

gene (called SERT, where the SSRIs dock) that can make them more susceptible to the double whammy. If you are on SSRIs and have the genotype of two long genes (double-L), you're nearly eight times more likely to have trouble with sexual dysfunction when oral contraceptives are added. Double-SERT people are more likely to be seasonal in their symptoms and tend to be better responders to SSRIs than double-S people, who tend to be more depressed than double-L people. So if you're really having trouble with sexual side effects, please consider slowly tapering off your antidepressant altogether, with the help of your psychiatrist. You may be able to treat your depression in other ways, especially with phototherapy in the fall and winter if you're a seasonally responsive double L. Or try a nonhormonal type of birth control if you can't successfully taper.

222 **In rats given an opioid receptor blocker:** Tracy K. McIntosh et al., "Effects of Morphine, B-Endorphin and Naloxone on Catecholamine Levels and Sexual Behavior in the Male Rat," *Pharmacology Biochemistry and Behavior* 13, no. 3 (1980): 435–41.

222 **blunting sensations:** In experiments, THC led to delayed time in both erection and ejaculation in men. In the female rat, levels of brain endocannabinoids are lowest during estrus (their peak of sexual responsiveness and fertility) and higher during other parts of their cycle. Female rats receiving an endocannabinoid antagonist, blocking the cannabinoid receptors, had increased signs of sexual motivation, suggesting that these may be potential medications for boosting low desire in women.

223 **Cannabis can help you:** Barbara Lewis, *The Sexual Power of Marijuana* (New York: P. H. Wyden., 1970); Frank H. Gawin, "Pharmacologic Enhancement of the Erotic: Implications of an Expanded Definition of Aphrodisiacs," *Journal of Sex Research* 14, no. 2 (1978): 107–17.

223 **In a study of five hundred women:** Robert C. Kolodny et al., *Textbook of Sexual Medicine* (Boston: Little, Brown, 1979).

223 **Women are more consistent:** Boris B. Gorzalka et al., "Male–Female Differences in the Effects of Cannabinoids on Sexual Behavior and Gonadal Hormone Function," *Hormones and Behavior* 58, no. 1 (2010): 91–99.

224 **Grooves get laid down:** Researchers have known for decades that if you stimulate pleasure centers chemically or electrically, the learned behavior is reinforced. The dopamine and endorphin release that accompanies arousal and orgasm will further reinforce this computer-linked behavior.

224 **Most concerning is that oxytocin:** William Struthers, *Wired for Intimacy: How Pornography Hijacks the Male Brain* (Westmont, IL: Intervarsity Press, 2009).

225 **no longer do it for them:** Sociology researcher Philip Zimbardo, in his article "The Demise of Guys," describes a syndrome of arousal addiction that looks a bit like many of the conditions I treat in my office, incorporating aspects of ADHD, social anxiety disorder, depression, performance anxiety, and OCD. Philip Zimbardo and Nikita Duncan, "'The Demise of Guys': How Video Games and Porn Are Ruining a Generation," *CNN News*, 2012.

225 **"their appetite for porn":** Doidge, *The Brain That Changes Itself,* 131.

227 **external portion of the clitoris:** We all start out as girls in the womb before the testosterone surge makes the male parts. Penises are like oversized clitorises made large by testosterone. When women are given testosterone, enlarged clitorises, called clitoromegaly, can result.

227 **The glans of the clitoris:** Helen E. O'Connell et al., "Anatomical Relationship Between Urethra and Clitoris," *Journal of Urology* 159, no. 6 (1998): 1892–97; Helen E. O'Connell et al., "Anatomy of the Clitoris," *Journal of Urology* 174, no. 4 (2005): 1189–95.

227 **clitoral body:** See http://www.ericsbinaryworld.com/tag/clitoris/.

227 **Spread clitoracy:** Unfortunately, this is an uphill battle. Detailed accurate representations of female genitals are hard to come by. Even some recent textbooks of anatomy do not include the clitoris in diagrams of the female pelvis. R. S. Snell, *Clinical Anatomy for Medical Students,* 3rd ed. (London: Little, Brown and Co., 1986); P. L. Williams, *Grays Anatomy: The Anatomical Basis of Medicine and Surgery,* 38th ed. (Edinburgh: Churchill Livingstone, 1996).

227 **unique genitals:** See http://www.webburgr.com/400-vaginas-wall/.

228 **orgasmic meditation:** Nicole Daedone, *Slow Sex: The Art and Craft of the Female Orgasm* (New York: Hachette, 2011).

228 **Some women see themselves as attracted to:** Lisa M. Diamond, *Sexual Fluidity: Understanding Women's Love and Desire* (Cambridge, MA: Harvard University Press, 2009).

228 **Of self-identified straight women:** Qazi Rahman and Glenn D. Wilson, "Born Gay? The Psychobiology of Human Sexual Orientation," *Personality and Individual Differences* 34, no. 8 (2003): 1337–82.

228 **evolution has favored women:** Barry X. Kuhle and Sarah Radtke, "Born Both Ways: The Alloparenting Hypothesis for Sexual Fluidity in Women," *Evolutionary Psychology* 11, no. 2 (2013).

229 **Women gaze just as long at porn:** Heather A. Rupp and Kim Wallen, "Sex Differences in Viewing Sexual Stimuli: An Eye-Tracking Study in Men and Women," *Hormones and Behavior* 51, no. 4 (2007): 524–33.

229 **In studies measuring vaginal blood flow:** Meredith L. Chivers et al., "A Sex Difference in the Specificity of Sexual Arousal," *Psychological Science* 15, no. 11 (2004): 736–44.

229 **"sparked or sustained by":** Bergner, *What Do Women Want,* 7.

229 **In studies measuring women's lubrication:** Meredith L. Chivers et al., "Agreement of Self-Reported and Genital Measures of Sexual Arousal in Men and Women: A Meta-Analysis," *Archives of Sexual Behavior* 39, no. 1 (2010): 5–56.

229 **Women who are hooked up:** Michele G. Alexander and Terri D. Fisher, "Truth and Consequences: Using the Bogus Pipeline to Examine Sex Differences in Self-Reported Sexuality," *Journal of Sex Research* 40, no. 1 (2003): 27–35.

230 **The number of women who admit:** Joseph W. Critelli and Jenny M. Bivona, "Women's Erotic Rape Fantasies: An Evaluation of Theory and Research," *Journal of Sex Research* 45, no. 1 (2008): 57–70.

231 **shape of a man's penis:** The flared glans creates suction, pulling previous sperm away from the cervix. Humans have a larger testes-to-body ratio than most primates, and the longest, thickest penises of any primate. The largest genitals are found in species where many males copulate with one female. The human testicular volume and libido are far beyond what's needed for monogamous pairing, and having an external scrotum is associated with promiscuous mating. In a man's semen, the later ejaculate contains enzymes that kill whatever sperm come after his. To insure against "poachers," men create more sperm when they haven't seen their partner for a few days, even if they have ejaculated in her absence.

231 **From an evolutionary standpoint:** Ibid.

232 **bring about climax:** Sympathetic nervous system.

232 **sharing your fantasies:** Talk with your partner specifically about what role-playing might consist of and what the dos and don'ts are. Sometimes a good place to start is by reversing traditional gender roles (you be the man and he the woman), or playing doctor, or trying the old cowboy/schoolmarm scenario. Another option is to experiment with blindfolds and loose knots.

232 **first experience:** Even babies in the womb touch themselves, and, though rare, orgasms have been observed in children, and even in infants as young as six months old.

233 **female-friendly:** Try these female-friendly Web sites: http://www.femalefriendlyporn.com, http://www.goodvibrationsvod.com/main.jhtml, http://www.hotmoviesforher.com.

233 **"my success rate . . . has been zero":** Betty Dodson, *Orgasms for Two: The Joy of Partner Sex* (New York: Random House, 2002), 117.

234 **according to Alfred Kinsey:** Alfred Charles Kinsey et al., *Sexual Behavior in the Human Male* (Philadelphia: WB Saunders, 1948).

234 **Masters and Johnson:** William H. Masters and Virginia E. Johnson, Reproductive Biology Research Foundation, *Human Sexual Response* (New York: Little, Brown, 1966).

235 **Women shown porn after exercise:** Cindy M. Meston and Manuel Worcel, "The Effects of Yohimbine Plus L-Arginine Glutamate on Sexual Arousal in Postmenopausal Women with Sexual Arousal Disorder," *Archives of Sexual Behavior* 31, no. 4 (2002): 323–32.

235 **Frequent exercise is one strategy:** Tierney A. Lorenz and Cindy M. Meston, "Acute Exercise Improves Physical Sexual Arousal in Women Taking Antidepressants," *Annals of Behavioral Medicine* 43, no. 3 (2012): 352–61.

235 **exercise-induced orgasm:** Sexual pleasure from exercise that doesn't lead to orgasm is more often seen in biking or spinning classes as well as abdominal work and weight lifting.

235 **Women reported more frequent and earlier-timed orgasms:** David A. Puts et al., "Men's Masculinity and Attractiveness Predict Their Female Partners' Reported Orgasm Frequency and Timing," *Evolution and Human Behavior* 33, no. 1 (2012): 1–9.

235 **pelvic floor:** See medicalartlibrary.com/pelvic-floor-muscles.html.

236 **Kegelcizer:** Dodsonandross.com.

236 **"hysterical paroxysms" in women:** Maines, *The Technology of Orgasm.*

237 **heavily influenced by hormonal factors:** J. E. Robinson and R. V. Short, "Changes in Breast Sensitivity at Puberty, During the Menstrual Cycle, and at Parturition," *British Medical Journal* 1, no. 6070 (1977): 1188.

237 **Nursing women are often much less sexually aroused:** Melissa D. Avery et al., "The Experience of Sexuality During Breastfeeding Among Primiparous Women," *Journal of Midwifery & Women's Health* 45, no. 3 (2000): 227–37.

238 ***coital alignment technique*:** E. W. Eichel et al., "The Technique of Coital Alignment and Its Relation to Female Orgasmic Response and Simultaneous Orgasm," *Journal of Sex & Marital Therapy* 14, no. 2 (Summer 1988): 129–41.

238 **contact with your clitoris:** There are YouTube videos of fully clothed people or cartoons to show you the details.

240 **peters out:** There has been fascinating research on just how the uterus contracts, how the cervix dips down to suck the semen into the opening, and then how the semen is directed toward the fallopian tube where the most mature egg is located. This activity is all mediated by oxytocin, the hormone that is released after orgasm and causes uterine contractions in childbirth, as well as prosocial, trusting behaviors.

240 **Freud was a thirty-year-old virgin:** Ryan and Jethá, *Sex at Dawn.*

240 **Masters and Johnson determined:** Masters and Johnson, *Human Sexual Response.*

240 **different types of orgasm:** Other researchers feel that since the G-spot is the back side of the clitoris, called the root, this is still a clitoral orgasm.

240 **a "pelvic floor" orgasm:** Berman and Berman, *For Women Only.*

240 **toe sucking:** See Barry Kamisurak and Beverly Whipple, "Non-genital Orgasms," *Sexual and Relationship Theory* 26, no. 4 (2011): 356–72.

240 **orgasm even after their spinal cord has been severed:** Barry R. Komisaruk et al., "Brain Activation During Vaginocervical Self-Stimulation and Orgasm in Women with Complete Spinal Cord Injury: fMRI Evidence of Mediation by the Vagus Nerves," *Brain Research* 1024, no. 1 (2004): 77–88.

240 **can climax from nipple stimulation:** Barry R. Komisaruk and Beverly Whipple, "Non-Genital Orgasms," *Sexual and Relationship Therapy* 26, no. 4 (2011): 356–72.

240 **can orgasm simply from thinking about their breasts:** Beverly Whipple et al., "Physiological Correlates of Imagery-Induced Orgasm in Women," *Archives of Sexual Behavior* 21, no. 2 (1992): 121–33.

240 **the Kinsey study put the rate:** A. Kinsey et al., *Sexual Behavior in the Human Female* (Philadelphia: Saunders, 1953).

240 **spontaneous orgasms:** Smaller surveys have placed the number higher, at 64 percent. Gina Ogden, "I'll Have What She's Thinking," *New York Times,* September 29, 2013.

241 **Two researchers put the number:** Kinsey et al., *Sexual Behavior in the Human Female;* Barbara L. Wells, "Predictors of Female Nocturnal Orgasms: A Multivariate Analysis," *Journal of Sex Research* 22, no. 4 (1986): 421–37; G. Winokur et al., "Nocturnal Orgasm in Women: Its Relation to Psychiatric Illness, Dreams, and Developmental and Sexual Factors," *Archives of General Psychiatry* 1, no. 2 (1959): 180; Comradge L. Henton, "Nocturnal Orgasm in College Women: Its Relation to Dreams and Anxiety Associated with Sexual Factors," *Journal of Genetic Psychology* 129, no. 2 (1976): 245–51.

241 **The G-spot is more like:** A. Kilchevsky et al., "Is the Female G-Spot Truly a Distinct Anatomic Entity?" *Journal of Sexual Medicine* 2011, no. 3 (January 2012): 719–26.

241 **Zone:** YouTube has a video called "G-Spot Stimulation" that is helpful: https://www.youtube.com/watch?v=hwJElbadlK0.

242 **The MRI data comparing clitoral versus G-spot:** B. R. Komisaruk et al., "An fMRI Time-Course Analysis of Brain Regions Activated During Self-Stimulation to Orgasm in Women," *Society for Neuroscience,* 285 no. 6. (2010).

242 **rear entry:** Seeing enough spots yet? There's more: the U-spot is south of the clitoris and north of the urethra. There is plenty of erectile tissue surrounding the urethra, but it is above the urethral opening and on either side of it. The urethra itself, and the area between the urethra and the vagina, doesn't have the same pleasurable feel when stroked, so make sure you're in the right neighborhood when searching for this spot. The U-spot is best stimulated gently and wetly. Pressure typically is less pleasurable.

242 **cervical tapping:** Winnifred B. Cutler, *Love Cycles: The Science of Intimacy* (Philadelphia: Athena Institute, 1996).

243 **Lubricated condoms:** Please note that most latex condoms will break down with petroleum-based lubricants like Vaseline. Water-based lubes are safest with condoms.

243 **Weekly sex can help women:** Winnifred B. Cutler et al., "Sexual Behavior Frequency and Menstrual Cycle Length in Mature Premenopausal Women," *Psychoneuroendocrinology* 4, no. 4 (1979): 297–309.

244 **It contains endorphins:** Burt Sharp and A. Eugene Pekary, "β-Endorphin61–91 and Other β-Endorphin-Immunoreactive Peptides in Human Semen," *Journal of Clinical Endocrinology & Metabolism* 52, no. 3 (1981): 586–88.

244 college women's condom use: G. Gordon Jr. et al., "Does Semen Have Antidepressant Properties?" *Archives of Sexual Behavior* 31, no. 3 (2002): 289–93.

Chapter Eleven: Your Body: Love It or Leave It

245 increasingly sedentary lifestyles: Harold W. Kohl et al., "The Pandemic of Physical Inactivity: Global Action for Public Health," *Lancet* (2012). 380, no. 9838 (2012): 294–305.

245 Inactivity taxes the body: I-Min Lee et al., "Effect of Physical Inactivity on Major Non-Communicable Diseases Worldwide: An Analysis of Burden of Disease and Life Expectancy," *Lancet* 380, no. 9838 (2012): 219-29.

246 childhood fitness declined: J. Gahche et al., "Cardiorespiratory Fitness Levels Among U.S. Youth Aged 12–15 Years: United States, 1999–2004 and 2012." *NCHS Data Brief* 153 (2014): 1–8.

246 Centers for Disease Control recommends: Centers for Disease Control and Prevention, "Adult Participation in Aerobic and Muscle-Strengthening Physical Activities—United States, 2011," *MMWR* 62, no. 17 (2013): 326.

246 Exercise helps to prevent: Harmon Eyre et al., "Preventing Cancer, Cardiovascular Disease, and Diabetes: A Common Agenda for the American Cancer Society, the American Diabetes Association, and the American Heart Association," *CA: A Cancer Journal for Clinicians* 54, no. 4 (2004): 190–207; Ming Kai et al., "Exercise Interventions: Defusing the World's Osteoporosis Time Bomb," *Bulletin of the World Health Organization* 81, no. 11 (2003): 827–30.

246 Cardiorespiratory fitness: Steven N. Blair and Suzanne Brodney, "Effects of Physical Inactivity and Obesity on Morbidity and Mortality: Current Evidence and Research Issues," *Medicine and Science in Sports and Exercise* 31 (1999): S646–S662.

246 cardio can release endorphins: P. Hoffman, "The Endorphin Hypothesis," in *Physical Activity and Mental Health*, ed. W. P. Morgan (Washington, DC: Taylor & Francis, 1997), 161–77.

246 improves levels of serotonin: F. Chaouloff, "The Serotonin Hypothesis," in Morgan, *Physical Activity and Mental Health*.

246 dopamine: A. A. Bove et al., "Increased Conjugated Dopamine in Plasma After Exercise Training," *Journal of Laboratory and Clinical Medicine* 104, no. 1 (1984): 77–85.

246 norepinephrine: R. K. Dishman, "The Norepinephrine Hypothesis," in Morgan, *Physical Activity and Mental Health*, 1997.

246 Moderate aerobic: P. Salmon, "Effects of Physical Exercise on Anxiety, Depression, and Sensitivity to Stress: A Unifying Theory," *Clinical Psychology Review* 21 (2001): 33–61; Chad D. Rethorst et al., "The Antidepressive Effects of Exercise," *Sports Medicine* 39, no. 6 (2009): 491–511.

247 cognition, focuses attention: P. D. Tomporowski, "Effects of Acute Bouts of Exercise on Cognition," *Acta Psychologica* 112, 297–324.

247 enhances wellbeing: D. Scully et al., "Physical Exercise and Psychological Well Being: A Critical Review," *British Journal of Sports Medicine* 32 (1998): 111–20.

247 reverse or forestall aging effects: Zsolt Radak et al., "Exercise and Hormesis: Oxidative Stress-Related Adaptation for Successful Aging," *Biogerontology* 6, no. 1 (2005): 71–75; John J. Ratey with Eric Hagerman, *Spark: The Revolutionary New Science of Exercise and the Brain* (Little, Brown and Company, 2008).

247 effects of hormonal fluctuations: Jennifer Lange-Collett and Lorna Schumann, "Promoting Health Among Perimenopausal Women Through Diet and Exercise," *Journal of the American Academy of Nurse Practitioners* 14, no. 4 (2002): 172–79; J. E. Jurkowski et al., "Ovarian Hormonal Responses to Exercise," *Journal of Applied Physiology* 44, no. 1 (1978): 109–14.

247 Exercising immediately before sex: Tierney Ahrold Lorenz and Cindy May Meston, "Exercise Improves Sexual Function in Women Taking Antidepressants: Results from a Randomized Crossover Trial," *Depression and Anxiety* 99 (2013): 1–8.

247 Scheduling regular exercise before sex: Ibid.

247 exercise fosters this plasticity: Ratey with Hagerman, *Spark*.

248 beneficial effects on memory: Kirk I. Erickson et al., "Exercise Training Increases Size of Hippocampus and Improves Memory," *PNAS* 108, no. 7 (2011): 3017–22.

248 waiting for neuroplasticity: Chittaranjan Andrade and N. Sanjay Kumar Rao, "How Antidepressant Drugs Act: A Primer on Neuroplasticity as the Eventual Mediator of Antidepressant Efficacy," *Indian Journal of Psychiatry* 52, no. 4 (2010): 378.

248 elevated levels of the growth factor BDNF: Biao Chen et al., "Increased Hippocampal BDNF Immunoreactivity in Subjects Treated with Antidepressant Medication," *Biological Psychiatry* 50, no. 4 (2001): 260–65.

248 new neuronal connections: Carrol D'Sa and Ronald S. Duman, "Antidepressants and Neuroplasticity," *Bipolar Disorders* 4, no. 3 (2002): 183–94.

248 BDNF itself may well act: Heath D. Schmidt and Ronald S. Duman, "Peripheral BDNF Produces Antidepressant-Like Effects in Cellular and Behavioral Models," *Neuropsychopharmacology* 35, no. 12 (2010): 2378–2391.

248 combine exercise with antidepressants: Amelia Russo-Neustadt et al., "Physical Activity–Antidepressant Treatment Combination: Impact on Brain-Derived Neurotrophic Factor and Behavior in an Animal Model," *Behavioral Brain Research* 120, no. 1 (2001): 87–95.

248 chronic stress not only tanks your mood: Christopher Pittenger and Ronald S. Duman, "Stress, Depression, and Neuroplasticity: A Convergence of Mechanisms," *Neuropsychopharmacology* 33, no. 1 (2007): 88–109.

248 endocannabinoid system is a major influencer: Gregory L. Gerdeman and David M. Lovinger, "Emerging Roles for Endocannabinoids in Long-Term Synaptic Plasticity," *British Journal of Pharmacology* 140, no. 5 (2003): 781–89.

248 synapses connect: If the breakdown of the endocannabinoid 2-AG (2-arachidonoylglycerol) is blocked, you see more hippocampal neuroplasticity as well as antidepressant and antianxiety effects.

248 Fat cells release cytokines: R. C. Shelton and A. H. Miller, "Eating Ourselves to Death (and Despair): The Contribution of Adiposity and Inflammation to Depression," *Progress in Neurobiology* 91 (2010): 275–99.

248 fatter patients have a lamer response: N. Oskooilar et al., "Body Mass Index and Response to Antidepressants in Depressed Research Subjects," *Journal of Clinical Psychiatry* 70 (2009): 1609–10.

248 Obese individuals have the bad combo: Gregory F. Oxenkrug, "Metabolic Syndrome, Age-Associated Neuroendocrine Disorders, and Dysregulation of Tryptophan—Kynureninee Metabolism," *Annals of the New York Academy of Sciences* 1199, no. 1 (2010): 1–14.

248 When the weight is taken off: L. Breum et al., "Twenty-Four-Hour Plasma Tryptophan Concentrations and Ratios Are Below Normal in Obese Subjects and Are Not Normalized by Substantial Weight Reduction," *American Journal of Clinical Nutrition* 77 (2003): 1112–18; G. Brandacher et al., "Bariatric Surgery Cannot Prevent Tryptophan Depletion Due to Chronic Immune Activation in Morbidly Obese Patients," *Obesity Surgery* 16 (2006): 541–48.

248 Being obese (abdominal fat in particular): F. S. Luppino et al., "Overweight, Obesity, and Depression: A Systematic Review and Meta-analysis of Longitudinal Studies," *Archives of General Psychiatry* 67 (2010): 220–29; Kristy Sanderson et al., "Overweight and Obesity in Childhood and Risk of Mental Disorder: A 20-Year Cohort Study," *Australian and New Zealand Journal of Psychiatry* 45, no. 5 (2011): 384–92.

248 anxiety disorders: G. Gariepy et al., "The Association Between Obesity and Anxiety Disorders in the Population: A Systematic Review and Meta-analysis," *International Journal of Obesity* 34, no. 3 (2010): 407–19.

248–349 panic attacks, generalized anxiety: Nancy M. Petry et al., "Overweight and Obesity Are Associated with Psychiatric Disorders: Results from the National Epidemiologic Survey on Alcohol and Related Conditions," *Psychosomatic Medicine* 70, no. 3 (2008): 288–97.

249 People with severe depression: Arianne K. B. van Reedt Dortland et al., "Longitudinal Relationship of Depressive and Anxiety Symptoms with Dyslipidemia and Abdominal Obesity," *Psychosomatic Medicine* 75, no. 1 (2013): 83–89.

249 Obese laboratory animals: Gordon Winocur et al., "Memory Impairment in Obese Zucker Rats: An Investigation of Cognitive Function in an Animal Model of Insulin Resistance and Obesity," *Behavioral Neuroscience* 119, no. 5 (2005): 1389; Susan A. Farr et al., "Obesity and Hypertriglyceridemia Produce Cognitive Impairment," *Endocrinology* 149, no. 5 (2008): 2628–36.

249 Fat cells create a proinflammatory cytokine: Joanna R. Erion et al., "Obesity Elicits Interleukin 1-Mediated Deficits in Hippocampal Synaptic Plasticity," *Journal of Neuroscience* 34, no. 7 (2014): 2618–31.

250 seven-minute workouts: See 7-min.com.

250 brain is much less likely to go into panic mode: Jack M. Gorman et al., "Ventilatory Physiology of Patients with Panic Disorder," *Archives of General Psychiatry* 45, no. 1 (1988): 31.

251 a transient hypofrontality: Arne Dietrich, "Transient Hypofrontality as a Mechanism for the Psychological Effects of Exercise," *Psychiatry Research* 145, no. 1 (2006): 79–83.

251 activates the endocannabinoid system: P. B. Sparling et al., "Exercise Activates the Endocannabinoid System," *Neuroreport* 14 (2003): 2209–11; A. Dietrich and W. F. McDaniel, "Cannabinoids and Exercise," *British Journal of Sports Medicine* 38 (2004): 50–57; David A. Raichlen et al., "Exercise-Induced Endocannabinoid Signaling Is Modulated by Intensity," *European Journal of Applied Physiology* 113, no. 4 (2013): 869–75.

251   **rewarding effects both during and after exercise:** David A. Raichlen et al., "Wired to Run: Exercise-Induced Endocannabinoid Signaling in Humans and Cursorial Mammals with Implications for the "Runner's High," *Journal of Experimental Biology* 215, no. 8 (2012): 1331–36.

251   **In lab rats, even a single session:** Giovane Galdino et al., "Acute Resistance Exercise Induces Antinociception by Activation of the Endocannabinoid System in Rats," *Anesthesia and Analgesia* (2014).

251   **Myofascial manipulation:** John M. McPartland, "Expression of the Endocannabinoid System in Fibroblasts and Myofascial Tissues," *Journal of Bodywork and Movement Therapies* 12, no. 2 (2008): 169–82.

252   **positive effects of exercise on memory:** Matthew N. Hill et al., "Endogenous Cannabinoid Signaling Is Required for Voluntary Exercise-Induced Enhancement of Progenitor Cell Proliferation in the Hippocampus," *Hippocampus* 20, no. 4 (2010): 513–23.

252   **exercise-induced memory formation improves:** Talita H. Ferreira-Vieira et al., "A Role for the Endocannabinoid System In Exercise-Induced Spatial Memory Enhancement in Mice," *Hippocampus* 24, no. 1 (2014): 79–88.

252   **Mice allowed to run obsessively:** Timothy J. Schoenfeld et al., "Physical Exercise Prevents Stress-Induced Activation of Granule Neurons and Enhances Local Inhibitory Mechanisms in the Dentate Gyrus," *Journal of Neuroscience* 33, no. 18 (2013): 7770–77.

252   **helps to lower high blood pressure:** Rod K. Dishman et al., "Neurobiology of Exercise," *Obesity* 14, no. 3 (2006): 345–56.

252   **Motor skills training and exercise:** Ibid.

253   **Inactivity physically shrinks your brain:** Ratey with Hagerman, *Spark*.

253   **massively increases neurogenesis:** Andrea K. Olson et al., "Environmental Enrichment and Voluntary Exercise Massively Increase Neurogenesis in the Adult Hippocampus Via Dissociable Pathways," *Hippocampus* 16, no. 3 (2006): 250–60.

253   **"apt to zap . . . the nervous system":** Nicholas A. Mischel et al., "Physical (in) Activity-Dependent Structural Plasticity in Bulbospinal Catecholaminergic Neurons of Rat Rostral Ventrolateral Medulla," *Journal of Comparative Neurology* 522, no. 3 (2014): 499–513.

253   **BDNF helps to promote serotonin neuron growth:** Keri Martinowich and Bai Lu, "Interaction Between BDNF and Serotonin: Role in Mood Disorders," *Neuropsychopharmacology* 33, no. 1 (2007): 73–83.

253   **exercise creates a cascade of neurotransmitters:** Ratey with Hagerman, *Spark*.

253   **One author likens going for a run:** Ibid.

253   **Exercise has anti-inflammatory properties:** Anne Marie W. Petersen and Bente Klarlund Pedersen, "The Anti-inflammatory Effect of Exercise," *Journal of Applied Physiology* 98, no. 4 (2005): 1154–62.

253   **cytokines from skeletal:** Called myokines.

253   **proinflammatory cytokines:** Called adipokines.

253   **Decrease inflammation and you lower your risk:** Michael Gleeson et al., "The Anti-inflammatory Effects of Exercise: Mechanisms and Implications for the Prevention and Treatment of Disease," *Nature Reviews Immunology* 11, no. 9 (2011): 607–15.

254   **those with higher inflammatory markers:** C. D. Rethorst et al., "Pro-inflammatory Cytokines as Predictors of Antidepressant Effects of Exercise in Major Depressive Disorder," *Molecular Psychiatry* 18 (2013): 1119.

254   **Mice fed a high-fat diet:** Pontus Boström et al., "A PGC1-[Agr]-Dependent Myokine That Drives Brown-Fat-like Development of White Fat and Thermogenesis," *Nature* 481, no. 7382 (2012): 463–68.

255   **it feels easier if their "voices" tell them:** Anthony W. Blanchfield et al., "Talking Yourself Out of Exhaustion: The Effects of Self-Talk on Endurance Performance," *Medicine and Science in Sports and Exercise* 46, no. 5 (2014): 998–1007.

255   **Use your smartphone:** Abby C. King et al., "Promoting Physical Activity Through Handheld Computer Technology," *American Journal of Preventive Medicine* 34, no. 2 (2008): 138–42.

255   **"I say that inner beauty":** Osmel Sousa, *New York Times* quote of the day, November 7, 2003.

255   **girls learn . . . they will be judged on their looks:** Joan Jacobs Brumberg, *The Body Project: An Intimate History of American Girls* (New York: Random House, 1998); Joan Jacobs Brumberg, *Fasting Girls: The Emergence of Anorexia Nervosa as a Modern Disease* (Cambridge, MA: Harvard University Press 1998).

255   "For women ... eyes of others": Germaine Greer, *The Female Eunuch* (London: MacGibbon and Kee, 1970), 28.

256   Plucked eyebrows, collagen-enhanced lips: Mitchel P. Goldman and Arnost Fronek, "Anatomy and Pathophysiology of Varicose Veins," *Journal of Dermatologic Surgery and Oncology* 15, no. 2 (1989): 138–46; Grant L. Peters et al., "The Effect of Crossing Legs on Blood Pressure: A Randomized Single-Blind Cross-Over Study," *Blood Pressure Monitoring* 4, no. 2 (1999): 97–102.

256   Women need at least 17 percent body: Rose E. Frisch, "Fatness, Menarche, and Female Fertility," *Perspectives in Biology and Medicine* 28, no. 4 (1985) 611-33.

256   Mannequins have become thinner: Minna Rintala and Pertti Mustajoki, "Could Mannequins Menstruate?" *British Medical Journal* 305, no. 6868 (1992): 1575.

256   as have Playboy centerfolds: Martin Voracek and Maryanne L. Fisher, "Shapely Centerfolds? Temporal Change in Body Measures: Trend Analysis," *British Medical Journal* 325, no. 7378 (2002): 1447.

256   Barbie, the doll many of us: Kevin I. Norton et al., "Ken and Barbie at Life Size," *Sex Roles* 34, no. 3-4 (1996): 287–94.

256   Our consumer culture: Williams, *Breasts*.

256   More than half of women surveyed in *Glamour* magazine: Laura Fraser, "Body Love, Body Hate" *Glamour* 201, October 1998.

257   Women who don't feel good: Jacobs, *The Body Project*.

257   Girls who look at fashion magazines: Eric Stice et al., "Exposure to Media-Portrayed Thin-Ideal Images Adversely Affects Vulnerable Girls: A Longitudinal Experiment," *Journal of Social and Clinical Psychology* 20, no. 3 (2001): 270–88.

257   literature linking the "thin-ideal": M. P. Levine and L. Smolak, "Media a Context for the Development of Disordered Eating," in *The Developmental Psychopathology of Eating Disorders*, L. Smolak, M. P. Levine, and R. Striegel-Moore, eds., (Mahwah, NJ: Erlbaum, 1996), 183–204; R. H. Striegel-Moore et al., "Toward an Understanding of Risk Factors for Bulimia," *American Psychologist* 41 (1986): 246–63; J. K. Thompson et al., *Exacting Beauty: Theory, Assessment, and Treatment of Body Image Disturbance* (Washington, DC: American Psychological Association, 1999).

257   "seduction of inadequacy": Lupita Nyong'o, *Essence* speech, February 27, 2014, http://www .essence.com/2014/02/27/lupita-nyongo-delivers-moving-black-women-hollywood-acceptance -speech/.

258   men are hardwired to respond to a woman's: S. M. Platek and D. Singh, "Optimal Waist-to-Hip Ratios in Women Activate Neural Reward Centers in Men," *PLoS One* 5, no. 2 (2010): e9042.

258   waist-hip ratio: Maryanne L. Fisher and Martin Voracek, "The Shape of Beauty: Determinants of Female Physical Attractiveness," *Journal of Cosmetic Dermatology* 5, no. 2 (2006): 190–94.

<u>258</u>   perception of attractiveness: Many researchers have arrived at the number 0.7 as the ideal, and universally most attractive, ratio.

258   "reliable and honest indicator": Devendra Singh, "Body Shape and Women's Attractiveness: The Critical Role of Waist-to-Hip Ratio," *Human Nature* 4, no. 3 (1993): 297–21.

259   more variability of women's breasts: Williams, *Breasts*.

259   one breast is usually one-fifth of a cup size: Z. Hussain et al., "Estimation of Breast Volume and Its Variation During the Menstrual Cycle Using MRI and Stereology," (2014).

259   Many men are aroused by darker areolas: Barnaby J. Dixson et al., "Eye Tracking of Men's Preferences for Female Breast Size and Areola Pigmentation," *Archives of Sexual Behavior* 40, no. 1 (2011a): 51–58.

260   the mammary gland needs: Williams, *Breasts*.

260   Breast implants will often make it: S. Bondurant et al., "Safety of Silicone Breast Implants: Report of the Committee on the Safety of Silicone Breast Implants (Washington, DC: Institute Of Medicine, 1999).

260   More than 80 percent of women surveyed: Roy Levin and Cindy Meston, "Nipple/Breast Stimulation and Sexual Arousal in Young Men and Women," *Journal of Sexual Medicine* 3, no. 3 (2006): 450–54.

260   Women with ruptured implants: Williams, *Breasts*; S. Brown et al., "An Association of Silicone-Gel Breast Implant Rupture and Fibromyalgia," *Current Rheumatology Reports* 4, no. 4 (2002): 293–98.

260   "doorknob effect": Neal Handel et al., "A Long-Term Study of Outcomes, Complications, and Patient Satisfaction with Breast Implants," *Plastic and Reconstructive Surgery* 117, no. 3 (2006): 757-67.

260   rare cancer can grow: FDA, 2013, http://www.fda.gov/medicaldevices/productsandmedicalprocedures/implantsandprosthetics/breastimplants/ucm239995.htm.

260 implants can make it harder for mammograms: Harry Hayes Jr. et al., "Mammography and Breast Implants," *Plastic and Reconstructive Surgery* 82, no. 1 (1988): 1–6.

261 In the women studied who didn't wear bras: Shaunacy Ferro, "Brassiere Support Is a Lie, Say French Scientists," *Popular Science*, April 11, 2013.

261 Wearing a bra 24/7: Sydney Singer and Soma Grismaijer, *Dressed to Kill: The Link Between Breast Cancer and Bras* (New York: Avery Publishing Group, 1995); Sydney Singer and Soma Grismaijer, *Get It Off! Understanding the Causes of Breast Pain, Cysts, and Cancer* (ISCD Press, 2000).

261 Premenopausal women who don't wear bras: C-C. Hsieh and D. Trichopoulos, "Breast Size, Handedness and Breast Cancer Risk," *European Journal of Cancer and Clinical Oncology* 27, no. 2 (1991): 131–35.

261 Sleeping without a bra: A. Q. Zhang et al., "Risk Factors of Breast Cancer in Women in Guangdong and the Countermeasures," *Journal of Southern Medical University* 29, no. 7 (2009): 1451–53.

261 bisphenol-A (BPA), an artificial estrogen: A. G. Recchia et al., "Xenoestrogens and the Induction of Proliferative Effects in Breast Cancer Cells Via Direct Activation of Estrogen Receptor A," *Food Additives and Contaminants* 21, no. 2 (2004): 134–44.

261 BPA basically turns on and off the genes: Sandra Viviana Fernandez and Jose Russo, "Estrogen and Xenoestrogens in Breast Cancer," *Toxicologic Pathology* 38, no. 1 (2010): 110–22.

261 When young rats are fed BPA: Leo F. Doherty et al., "In Utero Exposure to Diethylstilbestrol (DES) or Bisphenol-A (BPA) Increases EZH2 Expression in the Mammary Gland: An Epigenetic Mechanism Linking Endocrine Disruptors to Breast Cancer," *Hormones and Cancer* 1, no. 3 (2010): 146–55.

262 When developing mice are exposed to atrazine: Jennifer L. Rayner et al., "Adverse Effects of Prenatal Exposure to Atrazine During a Critical Period of Mammary Gland Growth," *Toxicological Sciences* 87, no.1 (2005): 255–66.

262 at least two hundred chemicals: Ruthann A. Rudel et al., "Chemicals Causing Mammary Gland Tumors in Animals Signal New Directions for Epidemiology, Chemicals Testing, and Risk Assessment for Breast Cancer Prevention," *Cancer* 109, no. S12 (2007): 2635–66.

262 when our government tests chemicals... they leave out looking at breasts: Williams, *Breasts*.

263 laser surgery lawsuits: H. Ray Jalian et al., "Increased Risk of Litigation Associated with Laser Surgery by Nonphysician Operators," *JAMA Dermatology* 150, no. 4 (2014): 407–11.

263 Shaving and waxing: Claire Dendle et al., "Severe Complications of a 'Brazilian' Bikini Wax," *Clinical Infectious Diseases* 45, no. 3 (2007): e29–e31; Allyssa L. Harris and Heidi Collins Fantasia, "Community-Associated MRSA Infections in Women," *Journal for Nurse Practitioners* 6, no. 6 (2010): 435–41.

264 vulnerability to the viruses molluscum contagiosum: François Desruelles et al., "Pubic Hair Removal: A Risk Factor for 'Minor' STI Such as Molluscum Contagiosum?" *Sexually Transmitted Infections* 89, no. 3 (2013): 216.

264 herpes: Charlotte Castronovo et al., "Viral Infections of the Pubis," *International Journal of STD & AIDS* 23, no. 1 (2012): 48–50.

264 contaminated wax or strips of cloth: Dendle et al., "Severe Complications of a 'Brazilian' Bikini Wax," e29–e31.

264 How someone smells affects us: Karl Grammer et al., "Human Pheromones and Sexual Attraction," *European Journal of Obstetrics & Gynecology and Reproductive Biology* 118, no. 2 (2005): 135–42.

264 demand for plastic surgery (called vulvoplasty) in this area: Lih Mei Liao and Sarah M. Creighton, "Requests for Cosmetic Genitoplasty: How Should Healthcare Providers Respond?" *British Medical Journal* 334, no. 7603 (2007): 1090–92.

264 alter your inner labia: V. Braun and C. Kitzinger, "The Perfectible Vagina: Size Matters," *Culture Health Sexuality* 3 (2001): 263–77; R. Bramwell et al., "Expectations and Experience of Labial Reduction: A Qualitative Study," *BJOG* 114, no. 12 (2007): 1493–99.

Chapter Twelve: You. Need. Downtime.

268 people prefer to give themselves an electric shock: Timothy D. Wilson et al., "Just Think: The Challenges of the Disengaged Mind," *Science* 345, no. 6192 (2014): 75–77.

269 When we are fully present in nature: Richard Louv, *The Nature Principle: Human Restoration and the End of Nature-Deficit Disorder* (New York: Algonquin Books, 2012).

269 A nature walk can lead to: Rodney H. Matsuoka, "Student Performance and High School Landscapes: Examining the Links." *Landscape and Urban Planning* 97, no. 4 (2010): 273–82.

269 restoring attention and decreasing mental fatigue: S. Kaplan, "The Restorative Benefits of Nature: Toward an Integrative Framework," *Journal of Environmental Psychology* 15 (1995): 169–82;

S. Kaplan, "Meditation, Restoration, and the Management of Mental Fatigue," *Environment and Behavior* 33 (2001): 480–506.

269 **Directed-attention fatigue:** Rachel Kaplan and Stephen Kaplan, *The Experience of Nature: A Psychological Perspective* (Cambridge, Eng.: Cambridge University Press, 1989).

269 **When kids with ADHD played outside:** A. F. Taylor et al., "Coping with ADD: The Surprising Connection to Green Play Settings," *Environment and Behavior* 33 (2001): 54–77.

270 **significantly better concentration:** Andrea Faber Taylor and Frances E. Kuo, "Children with Attention Deficits Concentrate Better After Walk in the Park," *Journal of Attention Disorders* 12, no. 5 (2009): 402–9.

270 **outdoor immersion program:** Kaplan and Kaplan, *The Experience of Nature*.

270 **reduction in anxiety:** Alan Ewert, "Reduction of Trait Anxiety Through Participation in Outward Bound," *Leisure Sciences* 10, no. 2 (1988): 107–17.

270 **helplessness:** Richard S. Newman, "Alleviating Learned Helplessness in a Wilderness Setting: An Application of Attribution Theory to Outward Bound," in Leslie J. Fyans and American Educational Research Association, *Achievement Motivation* (U.S.: Springer, 1980), 312–45.

270 **improved cognitive reasoning:** Ruth Ann Atchley et al., "Creativity in the Wild: Improving Creative Reasoning Through Immersion in Natural Settings," *PloS One* 7, no. 12 (2012): e51474.

270 **Being outside in nature:** Melanie Rudd et al., "Awe Expands People's Perception of Time, Alters Decision Making, and Enhances Well-Being," *Psychological Science* 23, no. 10 (2012): 1130–36.

270 **three-quarters of us are deficient:** Jordan Lite, "Vitamin D Deficiency Soars in the U.S.," *Scientific American*, March 23, 2009.

270 **twenty minutes of sunshine:** That's if you're light skinned; if you're dark skinned, you may need ten times this amount.

270 **Low vitamin D levels:** Michael Berk et al., "Vitamin D Deficiency May Play a Role in Depression," *Medical Hypotheses* 69, no. 6 (2007): 1316–19; Robert H. Howland, "Vitamin D and Depression," *J Psychosoc Nurs Ment Health Serv* 49, no. 2 (2011): 15–18.

270 **giving patients adequate doses of vitamin D:** F. M. Gloth III et al., "Vitamin D Vs. Broad Spectrum Phototherapy in the Treatment of Seasonal Affective Disorder," *Journal of Nutrition, Health & Aging* 3, no. 1 (1999): 5; R. Jorde et al., "Effects of Vitamin D Supplementation on Symptoms of Depression in Overweight and Obese Subjects: Randomized Double Blind Trial," *Journal of Internal Medicine* 264, no. 6 (2008): 599–609; Jason Hawrelak and Stephen P. Myers, "Vitamin D for Depression," *Journal of Complementary Medicine* 8, no. 2 (2009): 62

270 **One study of people in an ER:** G. A. Plotnikoff and J. M. Quigley, "Prevalence of Severe Hypovitaminosis D in Patients with Persistent, Nonspecific Musculoskeletal Pain," *Mayo Clinic Proceedings* 78 (2003): 1463–70.

271 **fashionable sunglasses:** Most opthalmologists recommend wearing sunglasses at all times to protect against UV exposure, especially if you have light-colored eyes.

271 **the sunlight needs to hit your retinas:** S. N. Young, "How to Increase Serotonin in the Human Brain Without Drugs," *Journal of Psychiatry and Neuroscience* 32 (2007): 394–99; Mahmut Alpayci et al., "Sunglasses May Play a Role in Depression," *Journal of Mood Disorders* 2, no. 2 (2012).

272 **Phototherapy lamps:** lighttherapyproducts.com.

272 **Depression is aggravated in lab animals:** Hiroyuki Mizoguchi et al., "Lowering Barometric Pressure Aggravates Depression-like Behavior in Rats," *Behavioral Brain Research* 218, no. 1 (2011): 190–93.

272 **A survey of thousands of suicides:** Laura Hiltunen et al., "Atmospheric Pressure and Suicide Attempts in Helsinki, Finland," *International Journal of Biometeorology* 56, no. 6 (2012): 1045–53.

272 **temperature and humidity:** See Michael Persinger, *The Weather Matrix and Human Behavior* (New York: Praeger, 1980).

273 **Studies using negative ion generators:** N. Goel et al., "Controlled Trial of Bright Light and Negative Air Ions for Chronic Depression," *Psychological Medicine* 35, no. 7 (July 2005): 945–55; N. Goel and G. R. Etwaroo, "Bright Light, Negative Air Ions and Auditory Stimuli Produce Rapid Mood Changes in a Student Population: A Placebo-Controlled Study," *Psychological Medicine* 36, no. 9 (September 2006): 1253–63.

273 **lower stress and inflammatory markers:** H. Nakane et al., "Effect of Negative Air Ions on Computer Operation, Anxiety and Salivary Chromogranin A-Like Immunoreactivity," *International Journal of Psychophysiology* 46, no. 1 (October 2002): 85–89.

273 **increase alertness and mental energy:** Pierce J. Howard, *The Owner's Manual for the Brain: Everyday Applications from Mind-Brain Research* (Austin, TX: Bard Press, 2000).

273 **ability to cope with stress and recover:** Roger S. Ulrich et al., "Stress Recovery During Exposure to Natural and Urban Environments," *Journal of Environmental Psychology* 11, no. 3 (1991): 201–30.

273 **Green exercise boosts resilience:** Q. Li et al., "Forest Bathing Enhances Human Natural Killer Activity and Expression of Anti-Cancer Proteins," *International Journal of Immunopathology and Pharmacology* 20, no. 2 Suppl. (2007): 3.

273 **city folks also have greater anterior cingulate activity:** F. Lederbogen et al., "City Living and Urban Upbringing Affect Neural Social Stress Processing in Humans," *Nature* 474 (June 2011): 498.

273 **anterior cingulate . . . implicated in depressive symptoms:** C. G. Davey et al., "Regionally Specific Alterations in Functional Connectivity of the Anterior Cingulate Cortex in Major Depressive Disorder," *Psychological Medicine* 42, no. 10 (2012): 2071–81.

273 **more positive outlook on life:** Kaplan and Kaplan, *The Experience of Nature.*

273 **genuinely happy people recover from illness:** Louv, *The Nature Principle.*

273 **22 percent of people felt more depressed:** *Ecotherapy: The Green Agenda for Mental Health. Executive Summary,* Mind, 2007. http://www.mind.org.uk/media/211252/Ecotherapy_The_green_agenda_for_mental_health_Executive_summary.pdf.

273 **The medical mile:** Louv, *The Nature Principle,* 85.

274 **Patients who have a view of a tree:** Roger S. Ulrich, "View Through a Window May Influence Recovery from Surgery," *Science* 224, no. 4647 (1984): 420–21.

274 **Canadian studies report that children:** James Raffan, "Nature Nurtures: Investigating the Potential of School Grounds," http://www.evergreen.ca/docs/res/Nature-Nurtures.pdf.

274 **people in indoor workspaces with a window:** Peter H. Kahn Jr. et al., "A Plasma Display Window?—The Shifting Baseline Problem in a Technologically Mediated Natural World," *Journal of Environmental Psychology* 28, no. 2 (2008): 192–99.

274 **The research of Frances Kuo shows that:** Frances E. Kuo and William C. Sullivan, "Environment and Crime in the Inner City Does Vegetation Reduce Crime?" *Environment and Behavior* 33, no. 3 (2001a): 343–67.

274 **Chicago public-housing projects:** Frances E. Kuo and William C. Sullivan, "Aggression and Violence in the Inner City Effects of Environment Via Mental Fatigue," *Environment and Behavior* 33, no. 4 (2001): 543–71.

274 **Couples in which both partners use cannabis:** Phillip H. Smith et al., "Couples' Marijuana Use Is Inversely Related to Their Intimate Partner Violence Over the First 9 Years of Marriage," *Psychology of Addictive Behaviors* 28, no. 3 (2014): 734.

274 **makes us more caring and generous:** Netta Weinstein et al., "Can Nature Make Us More Caring? Effects of Immersion in Nature on Intrinsic Aspirations and Generosity," *Personality and Social Psychology Bulletin* 35, no. 10 (2009): 1315–29.

275 **hunter-gatherers . . . egalitarian and communal:** Elizabeth A. Cashdan, "Egalitarianism Among Hunters and Gatherers," *American Anthropologist* 82, no. 1 (1980): 116–20.

275 **Antibacterial soaps and overprescribed antibiotics create "superbugs":** H. Okada et al., "The 'Hygiene Hypothesis' for Autoimmune and Allergic Diseases: An Update," *Clinical & Experimental Immunology* 160, no. 1 (2010): 1–9; Graham A. W. Rook, "Hygiene Hypothesis and Autoimmune Diseases," *Clinical Reviews in Allergy & Immunology* 42, no. 1 (2012): 5–15.

275 **Babies born by a Caesarean section:** Michael Pollan, "Some of My Best Friends Are Germs," *New York Times Magazine,* May 15, 2013; Josef Neu and Jona Rushing, "Cesarean Versus Vaginal Delivery: Long-Term Infant Outcomes and the Hygiene Hypothesis," *Clinics in Perinatology* 38, no. 2 (2011): 321.

276 **children born by C-section are more likely:** J. Blustein et al., "Association of Cesarean Delivery with Child Adiposity from Age 6 Weeks to 15 Years," *International Journal of Obesity* 37, no. 7 (2013): 900–6.

276 **combine high-calorie foods with antibiotics in mice:** L. Cox et al., "Altering the Intestinal Microbiota During a Critical Developmental Window Has Lasting Metabolic Consequences," *Cell* 158, no. 4 (2014): 705–21.

276 **triclosan and triclocarban . . . disrupting thyroid function:** K. M. Crofton et al., "Short-Term in Vivo Exposure to the Water Contaminant Triclosan: Evidence for Disruption of Thyroxine," *Environmental Toxicology and Pharmacology* 24 (2007): 194–97.

276 **amplifying hormone levels:** R. H. Gee et al., "Oestrogenic and Androgenic Activity of Triclosan in Breast Cancer Cells," *Journal of Applied Toxicology* 28 (2008): 78–91.

276 **promoting drug-resistant infections:** M. Braoudaki and A. C. Hilton, "Low Level of Cross-Resistance Between Triclosan and Antibiotics in Escherichia Coli K-12 and E. Coli O55 Compared to E. Coli O157," *FEMS Microbiology Letters* 235 (2004): 305–9.

276 **antibacterial chemicals are found in our urine:** A. M. Calafat et al., "Urinary Concentrations of Triclosan in the U.S. Population: 2003–2004," *Environmental Health Perspectives* 116, no. 3 (2008): 303–7.

276   **our breast milk:** M. Allmyr et al., "Triclosan in Plasma and Milk from Swedish Nursing Mothers and Their Exposure Via Personal Care Products," *Science of the Total Environment* 372, no. 1 (2006): 87–93.

276   **Mice given live *M. vaccae*:** Christopher A. Lowry et al., "Identification of an Immune-Responsive Mesolimbocortical Serotonergic System: Potential Role in Regulation of Emotional Behavior," *Neuroscience* 146, no. 2 (2007): 756–72.

276   **regulating the stress response:** T. G. Dinan and J. F. Cryan, "Regulation of the Stress Response by the Gut Microbiota: Implications for Psychoneuroendocrinology," *Psychoneuroendocrinology* 37 (2012): 1369–78.

276   **administering *Lactobacillus helveticus*:** M. Messaoudi et al., "Assessment of Psychotropic-like Properties of a Probiotic Formulation (Lactobacillus Helveticus R0052 and Bifidobacterium Longum R0175) in Rats and Human Subjects," *British Journal of Nutrition* 105 (2011): 755–64.

276   **certain bacteria are essential for normal social development:** L. Desbonnet et al., "Microbiota is Essential for Social Development in the Mouse," *Molecular Psychiatry* 19, no. 2 (2014): 146.

276   **autistic-like behavior improves:** Elaine Y. Hsiao et al., "Microbiota Modulate Behavioral and Physiological Abnormalities Associated with Neurodevelopmental Disorders," *Cell* 155, no. 7 (2013): 1451–63.

277   **"Minimize unnecessary antibiotics... in the dirt and with animals":** Pollan, "Some of My Best Friends Are Germs."

277   **higher levels of hormones in their urine:** Thomas Heberer, "Tracking Persistent Pharmaceutical Residues from Municipal Sewage to Drinking Water," *Journal of Hydrology* 266, no. 3 (2002): 175–89.

277   **Hormones in the drinking water:** David Margel and Neil E. Fleshner, "Oral Contraceptive Use Is Associated with Prostate Cancer: An Ecological Study," *British Medical Journal Open* 1, no. 2 (2011).

277   **women's risk of breast cancer:** Mark Clemons and Paúl Goss, "Estrogen and the Risk of Breast Cancer," *New England Journal of Medicine* 344, no. 4 (2001): 276–85.

277   **When plastics are heated in a microwave:** Mariah Blake, "The Scary New Evidence on BPA-Free Plastics and the Big Tobacco–Style Campaign to Bury It," *Mother Jones,* March/April 2014.

277   **chronic exposure brings on puberty:** Kembra L. Howdeshell et al., "Environmental Toxins: Exposure to Bisphenol A Advances Puberty," *Nature* 401, no. 6755 (1999): 763–64.

278   **asthma, heart and liver ailments, ADHD, and cancer:** Blake, "The Scary New Evidence on BPA-Free Plastics."

278   **switch off genes that suppress tumor growth:** Ana M. Soto and Carlos Sonnenschein, "Environmental Causes of Cancer: Endocrine Disruptors as Carcinogens," *Nature Reviews Endocrinology* 6, no. 7 (2010): 363–70.

278   **"A poison kills you":** Blake, "The Scary New Evidence on BPA-Free Plastics."

278   **No industry-funded studies have reported significant effects:** Saal Vom et al., "An Extensive New Literature Concerning Low-Dose Effects of Bisphenol A Shows the Need for a New Risk Assessment," *Environmental Health Perspectives* 113, no. 8 (2005): 926.

278   **it's been replaced by other chemicals:** Chun Z. Yang et al., "Most Plastic Products Release Estrogenic Chemicals: A Potential Health Problem That Can Be Solved," *Environmental Health Perspectives* 119, no. 7 (2011): 989.

278   **The billion-dollar plastics industry:** Blake, "The Scary New Evidence on BPA-Free Plastics."

278   **Phthalates... correlated with cancers and birth defects:** Evanthia Diamanti-Kandarakis et al., "Endocrine-Disrupting Chemicals: An Endocrine Society Scientific Statement," *Endocrine Reviews* 30, no. 4 (2009): 293–42.

278   **decreased sperm quality:** Elisabeth Carlsen et al., "Evidence for Decreasing Quality of Semen During Past 50 Years," *British Medical Journal* 305, no. 6854 (1992): 609.

278   **abnormal testes development:** N. E. Skakkebaek et al., "Association Between Testicular Dysgenesis Syndrome (TDS) and Testicular Neoplasia: Evidence from 20 Adult Patients with Signs of Maldevelopment of the Testis," *APMIS* 111, no. 1 (2003): 1–9.

278   **interfere with testosterone production:** Juliane-Susanne Schmidt et al., "Effects of Di (2-Ethylhexyl) Phthalate (DEHP) on Female Fertility and Adipogenesis in C3H/N Mice," *Environmental Health Perspectives* 120, no. 8 (2012): 1123.

278   **lower fertility:** Germaine M. Buck Louis et al., "Urinary Bisphenol A, Phthalates, and Couple Fecundity: The Longitudinal Investigation of Fertility and the Environment (LIFE) Study," *Fertility And Sterility* (2014).

278   **reproductive toxins:** Vanessa R. Kay et al., "Reproductive and Developmental Effects of Phthalate Diesters in Females," *Critical Reviews in Toxicology* 43, no. 3 (2013): 200–19.

278   **brings on puberty earlier:** Jonathan R. Roy et al., "Estrogen-like Endocrine Disrupting Chemicals Affecting Puberty in Humans—a Review," *Medical Science Monitor: International Medical Journal of Experimental and Clinical Research* 15, no. 6 (2009): RA137–45; Jefferson P. Lomenick et al., "Phthalate Exposure and Precocious Puberty in Females," *Journal of Pediatrics* 156, no. 2 (2010): 221–25.

278   **linked with breast cancer:** P. D. Darbre, "Environmental Oestrogens, Cosmetics and Breast Cancer," *Best Practice & Research Clinical Endocrinology & Metabolism* 20, no. 1 (2006): 121–43; Sandra Viviana Fernandez and Jose Russo, "Estrogen and Xenoestrogens in Breast Cancer," *Toxicologic Pathology* 38, no. 1 (2010): 110–22.

278   **diabetes, and obesity:** Richard W. Stahlhut et al., "Concentrations of Urinary Phthalate Metabolites Are Associated with Increased Waist Circumference and Insulin Resistance in Adult U.S. Males," *Environmental Health Perspectives* (2007): 876–82; P. Monica Lind et al., "Circulating Levels of Phthalate Metabolites Are Associated with Prevalent Diabetes in the Elderly," *Diabetes Care* 35, no. 7 (2012): 1519–24; Tamarra James-Todd et al., "Urinary Phthalate Metabolite Concentrations and Diabetes Among Women in the National Health and Nutrition Examination Survey (NHANES) 2001–2008," *Environmental Health Perspectives* 120, no. 9 (2012): 1307.

279   **indigenous cultures, nature is where the spirit is:** Ralph Metzner, "The Split Between Spirit and Nature in European Consciousness," *Trumpeter* 10, no. 1 (1993), http://trumpeter.athabascau.ca/index.php/trumpet/article/viewArticle/407/658.

279   **cannabis-based medicines... resilience to stress:** R. J. Bluett et al., "Central Anandamide Deficiency Predicts Stress-Induced Anxiety: Behavioral Reversal Through Endocannabinoid Augmentation," *Translational Psychiatry* 4, no. 7 (2014): e408.

279–280 **Hemp and cannabis... fiber, fuel, and food:** Holland, *The Pot Book.*

280   **go out and find beauty in the world:** O. R. W. Pergams and P. A. Zaradic, "Is Love of Nature in the U.S. Becoming Love of Electronic Media? 16-Year Downtrend in National Park Visits Explained by Watching Movies, Playing Video Games, Internet Use, and Oil Prices," *Journal of Environmental Management* 80 (2006): 387–93.

280   **actually disrupt our endocrine system and cause cancer:** Soto and Sonnenschein, "Environmental Causes of Cancer," 363–70.

280   **We eat artificial sweeteners:** Qing Yang, "Gain Weight by 'Going Diet?' Artificial Sweeteners and the Neurobiology of Sugar Cravings: Neuroscience 2010," *The Yale Journal of Biology and Medicine* 83, no. 2 (2010): 101.

280   **Men ogle plastic breasts:** Donald L. Hilton Jr, "Pornography Addiction–A Supranormal Stimulus Considered in the Context of Neuroplasticity," *Socioaffective Neuroscience & Psychology* 3 (2013).

280   **Chemicals in plastics:** Steven F. Hotze, *Hormones, Health, and Happiness* (Houston: Forrest Publishing, 2005); Laura E. Corio, *The Change Before the Change* (New York: Bantam, 2000); Tyrone N. Hayes et al., "Atrazine Induces Complete Feminization and Chemical Castration in Male African Clawed Frogs (Xenopus Laevis)," *Proceedings of the National Academy of Sciences* 107, no. 10 (2010): 4612–17; Vanessa R. Kay, Christina Chambers, and Warren G. Foster, "Reproductive and Developmental Effects of Phthalate Diesters in Females," *Critical Reviews in Toxicology* 43, no. 3 (2013): 200–219.

281   **Exposure to others' traumas:** P. Vasterman et al. "The Role of The Media and Media Hypes in the Aftermath of Disasters," *Epidemiological Review* 27 (2005): 107–14; K. M. Wright et al., "The Shared Experience of Catastrophe: An Expanded Classification of the Disaster Community," *American Journal of Orthopsychiatry* 60, no. 1 (1990): 35–42; Alison E. Holman et al., "Media's Role in Broadcasting Acute Stress Following the Boston Marathon Bombings," *Proceedings of the National Academy of Sciences* 111, no. 1 (2014): 93–98.

281   **America now has more Internet-connected devices:** NPD Group, Connected Intelligence, *Connected Home Report*, press release quoted in *USA Today*, January 2, 2013.

281   **"continuous partial attention":** Linda Stone, "Continuous Partial Attention–Not the Same as Multi-Tasking," *Businessweek* 24 (2008).

281   **drains our ability to focus:** Louv, *The Nature Principle.*

281   **When a research subject hears his phone ring:** Martin Lindstrom, "You Love Your iPhone. Literally," *New York Times*, September 30, 2011.

281   **A new term, *nomophobia*:** Manjeet Singh Bhatia, "Cell Phone Dependency—a New Diagnostic Entity," *Delhi Psychiatry Journal* 11, no. 2 (2008): 123–24.

282   **it is impossible to get enough of something:** Maté, *When the Body Says No.*

282   **When we're tense or fearful:** Walton T. Roth et al., "Voluntary Breath Holding in Panic and Generalized Anxiety Disorders," *Psychosomatic Medicine* 60, no. 6 (1998): 671–79; Patricia Hill Bailey, "The Dyspnea-Anxiety-Dyspnea Cycle—COPD Patients' Stories of Breathlessness: 'It's Scary/When You Can't Breathe,'" *Qualitative Health Research* 14, no. 6 (2004): 760–78.

285 **Meditation can decrease stress:** Maria B. Ospina et al., "Meditation Practices for Health," Agency for Healthcare Research and Quality, publication no. 07-E010, 2007.

285 **improve resilience:** Perla Kaliman et al., "Rapid Changes in Histone Deacetylases and Inflammatory Gene Expression in Expert Meditators," *Psychoneuroendocrinology* 40 (2014): 96–107.

285 **tamp down inflammation:** T. W. Pace et al., "Effect of Compassion Meditation on Neuroendocrine, Innate Immune and Behavioral Responses to Psychosocial Stress," *Psychoneuroendocrinology* 34 (2009): 87–98; C. Reardon et al., "Lymphocyte-Derived Ach Regulates Local Innate but Not Adaptive Immunity," *PNAS* 110 (2013): 1410–15.

285 **benefiting genes that control energy metabolism:** M. K. Bhasin et al., "Relaxation Response Induces Temporal Transcriptome Changes in Energy Metabolism, Insulin Secretion and Inflammatory Pathways," *PLoS One* 8, no. 5 (2013): e62817.

285 **Meditation practices are associated with neuroplastic changes:** Lisa A. Kilpatrick et al., "Impact of Mindfulness-Based Stress Reduction Training on Intrinsic Brain Connectivity," *Neuroimage* 56, no. 1 (2011): 290–98.

285 **strengthening these connections improves self-regulation:** Britta K. Hölzel et al., "How Does Mindfulness Meditation Work? Proposing Mechanisms of Action from a Conceptual and Neural Perspective," *Perspectives on Psychological Science* 6, no. 6 (2011a): 537–59.

285 **longer people have an established meditation practice:** Eileen Luders, "The Unique Brain Anatomy of Meditation Practitioners: Alterations in Cortical Gyrification," *Frontiers in Human Neuroscience* 6 (2012).

285 **Meditation can help you be more resilient to stress:** Richard J. Davidson and Sharon Begley, *The Emotional Life of Your Brain: How Its Unique Patterns Affect the Way You Think, Feel, and Live— and How You Can Change Them* (New York: Penguin, 2012).

285 **"top-down" control:** Dennis S. Charney, "Psychobiological Mechanisms of Resilience and Vulnerability. Implications for Successful Adaptation to Extreme Stress," *FOCUS: The Journal of Lifelong Learning in Psychiatry* 2, no. 3 (2004): 368–91.

285 **stronger connections between the PFC and the hippocampus:** Negar Fani et al., "White Matter Integrity in Highly Traumatized Adults with and without Post-traumatic Stress Disorder," *Neuropsychopharmacology* 37, no. 12 (2012): 2740–46.

286 **Advanced meditators are better at inhibiting:** Christopher A. Brown and Anthony K. P. Jones, "Meditation Experience Predicts Less Negative Appraisal of Pain: Electrophysiological Evidence for the Involvement of Anticipatory Neural Responses," *Pain* 150, no. 3 (2010): 428–38.

286 **Even after just eight weeks of mindfulness training:** Britta K. Hölzel et al., "Mindfulness Practice Leads to Increases in Regional Brain Gray Matter Density," *Psychiatry Research: Neuroimaging* 191, no. 1 (2011): 36–43.

286 **People who meditate are not only more:** Teresa M. Edenfield and Sy Atezaz Saeed, "An Update on Mindfulness Meditation as a Self-Help Treatment for Anxiety and Depression," *Psychology Research and Behavior Management* 5 (2011): 131–41; R. J. Davidson et al., "Alterations in Brain and Immune Function Produced by Mindfulness Meditation," *Psychosomatic Medicine* 65, no. 4 (2003): 564–70; P. Grossman et al., "Mindfulness-Based Stress Reduction and Health Benefits. A Meta-analysis," *Journal of Psychosomatic Research* 57, no. 1 (2004): 35–43; Peter Sedlmeier et al., "The Psychological Effects of Meditation: A Meta-analysis," *Psychological Bulletin* 138, no. 6 (2012): 1139–71.

286 **Meditation:** Check out mindspace.com for an app that can help you learn to meditate.

286 **job is to be there:** Staying "on task" will make you feel great. Instead, most of us tend to think up how to torture ourselves when we've nothing better to do. While we make the bed and wash dishes, we court drama and replay scenes where we were wronged or excluded instead of allowing ourselves those few moments of the pleasure of a well-made bed and hydrotherapy.

287 **Having a sense of awe:** Rudd et al., "Awe Expands People's Perception of Time," *Psychological Science* 23, no. 20 (2012): 1130–36.

Conclusion: Staying Sane in an Insane World

289 **Too many of us are out of sync:** John Bowlby, "Maternal Care and Mental Health," *Journal of Consulting Psychology* 16, no. 3 (1952): 232; Maté, *When the Body Says No.*

289 **compulsive consumers:** Americans pour seven million dollars into the U.S. retail industry every minute, purchasing an average of 1,440 McDonald's burgers, 5,695 Starbucks' drinks, and eighty-four thousand dollars' worth of Amazon items.

294 **Women are made to be in tune:** Winnifred Berg Cutler et al., "Lunar and Menstrual Phase Locking," *American Journal of Obstetrics & Gynecology* 137, no. 7 (1980): 834–39; W. B. Cutler, "The Moon and Menses," *American Journal of Obstetrics & Gynecology* 160, no. 2 (1989): 522–23.

Appendix: Naming Names: A Guide to Selected Drugs

321 **this time by:** Rosemary Bassoon et al., "Efficacy and safety of viagiain estrogedized women with sexual Dysfunction Associated with Female Sexual Aromsal Disorder," *International Journal of Gynecolosy* and obstetries supp 1.5 (2002).

333 **manufacturing of the drug oxycodone:** Katherin Eban, "OxyContin: Purdue Pharma's Painful Medicine" *Fortune* 164, no. 8 (2011): 76.

333 **Emergency room visits:** R. E. Cai et al., "Emergency Department Visits Involving Nonmedical Use of Selected Prescription Drugs in the United States, 2004–2008," *Journal of Pain and Palliative Care Pharmacotherapy* 24, no. 3 (2010): 293–97.

334 **until our bodies finally say no:** Gabor Mate, *When the Body Says No* (Hoboken: Wiley, 2011).

334 **women with a history of childhood sexual abuse:** James Morrison, "Childhood Sexual Histories of Women," *American Journal of Psychiatry* 146, no. 2 (1989): 239–41; Page Ouimette et al., "Physical and Sexual Abuse Among Women and Men with Substance Use Disorder,." *Alcoholism Treatment Quarterly* 18, no. 3 (2000): 7–17.

335 **prescriptions for stimulants:** What Is prescription Drug Abuse? NIDA, August 7, 2012, nida .nih.gov/researchreports/prescription/prescription?.html.

337 **Cocaethylene is even more likely:** W. L. Hearn, et al., "Cocaethylene Is More Potent Than Cocaine in Mediating Lethality," *Pharmacology Biochemistry and Behavior* 39, no. 2 (1991): 531–33.

337 **visits reporting Ecstasy use:** SAMHSA, 2012, oas.samsa.gov/2kll/DAWN027/ecstasy.htm.

338 **Nineteen substances were so obscure:** Frank Owen and Lera Gavin, "Molly Is the New Club Drug, But What's in It?" *Playboy*, Oct. 20, 2013.

338 **no guarantee of purity:** See ecstasydata.org for examples of pill and powder testing.

338 **medically supervised settings:** Michael C. Mithoefer et al.,"The Safety and Efficacy of 3-, 4-Methylenedioxymethamphetamine-Assisted Psychotherapy in Subjects with Chronic, Treatment-Resistant Posttraumatic Stress Disorder: The First Randomized Controlled Pilot Study," *Journal of Psychopharmacology* 25, no. 4 (2011): 439–52.

338 **recreational setting:** For more information on MDMA please see the nonprofit book *Ecstasy: The Complete Guide*, edited by Julie Holland, M.D. (Rochester, VT: Park Street Press) 2001.

339 **Eighty-two percent:** Rasmussen Report "82% Say US Not Winning the War on Drugs" August 18, 2013.

339 **believe cannabis should be legal:** Pew Research, "Majority Now Supports Legalizing Marijuana" April 4, 2013.

340 **lower their use of opiates significantly:** D. I. Abrams et al.,"Cannabinoid–Opioid Interaction in Chronic Pain," *Clinical Pharmacology & Therapeutics* 90, no. 6 (2011): 844–51.

340 **makers of Oxycontin and Vicodin:** Lee Fang et al., "The Anti-Pot Lobby's Big Bankroll: The Opponents of Marijuana-Law Reform Insist That Legalization Is Dangerous—But the Biggest Threat Is to Their Own Bottom Line," *Nation* 299, nos. 3–4 (2014): 12–18.

340 **and go on to become addicted:** James C. Anthony, Lynn A. Warner, and Ronald C. Kessler, "Comparative Epidemiology of Dependence on Tobacco, Alcohol, Controlled Substances, and Inhalants: Basic Findings from the National Comorbidity Survey," *Experimental and Clinical Psychopharmacology* 2, no. 3 (1994): 244.

341 **Sucking releases endorphins:** Ester Fride et al., "Critical Role of the Endogenous Cannabinoid System in Mouse Pup Suckling and Growth," *European Journal of Pharmacology* 419, no. 2 (2001): 207–14.

341 **Acupuncture involving ear stimulation:** Mehdi Tahiri et al., "Alternative Smoking Cessation Aids: A Meta-Analysis of Randomized Controlled Trials," *The American Journal of Medicine* 125, no. 6 (2012): 576–84.

366 **The hippy gynoid shape:** Corio, *The Change Before the Change.*

366 **Cortisol counteracts insulin:** Claudia Gragnoli, "Depression and Type 2 Diabetes: Cortisol Pathway Implication and Investigational Needs," *Journal of Cellular Physiology* 227, no. 6 (2012): 2318–22.

366 **stops the production of a transporter:** Soonho Kwon and Kathie L. Hermayer, "Glucocorticoid-Induced Hyperglycemia," *American Journal of the Medical Sciences* 345, no. 4 (2013): 274–77; Paul E. Marik and Rinaldo Bellomo, "Stress Hyperglycemia: An Essential Survival Response," *Critical Care* 17, no. 2 (2013): 305; Nyika D. Kruyt et al., "Stress-Induced Hyperglycemia in Healthy Bungee Jumpers Without Diabetes Due to Decreased Pancreatic B-Cell Function and Increased Insulin Resistance," *Diabetes Technology & Therapeutics* 14, no. 4 (2012): 311–14.

367 **Estrogen increases the expression:** C. L. Bethea et al., "Ovarian Steroids and Serotonin Neural Function," *Molecular Neurobiology* 18, no. 2 (1998): 87–123.

367 **directly increases serotonin activity:** I. Hindberg and O. Naesh, "Serotonin Concentrations

in Plasma and Variations During the Menstrual Cycle," *Clinical Chemistry* 38, no. 10 (1992): 2087–89.

367 **while estrogen creates high levels:** Corio, *The Change Before the Change.*

367 **High progesterone also inhibits:** Ibid.

367 **Leg spasms occur in 40 percent:** Corio, *The Change Before the Change.*

368 **Two androgens:** Corio, *The Change Before the Change.*

368 **Tibolone, a medicine that raises:** Susan R. Davis, "The Effects of Tibolone on Mood and Libido," *Menopause* 9, no. 3 (2002): 162–70.

369 **In women with higher SHBG:** Barbara A. Gower and Lara Nyman, "Associations Among Oral Estrogen Use, Free Testosterone Concentration, and Lean Body Mass Among Postmenopausal Women," *Journal of Clinical Endocrinology & Metabolism* 85, no. 12 (2000): 4476–80.

369 **biodentical products are delivered:** Gail A. Greendale etal., "Symptom Relief and Side Effects of Postmenopausal Hormones," *Obstetrics o' Gynecology* 92, no.6 (1998); 982–88.

371 **Perhaps the new or full moon can serve:** Northrup, *The Wisdom of Menopause.*

377 **If you stress lab rats:** C. Pugh, et al "Role of Interleukin-1 Beta in Impairment of Contextual Fear Conditioning Caused by Social Isolation," *Behavioural Brain Research* 106, no. 1 (1999): 109–18.

377 **If you block the IL1-beta:** R. M. Barrientos et al., "Brain-Derived Neurotrophic Factor Mrna Downregulation Produced by Social Isolation Is Blocked by Intrahippocampal Interleukin-1 Receptor Antagonist," *Neuroscience* 121, no. 4 (2003): 847–53.

378 **When the junk food is removed:** Johnson et al., "Dopamine D2 Receptors in Addiction-like Reward Dysfunction," 635–41.

379 **Rats show they prefer saccharine-sweetened water:** Magalie Lenoir et al., "Intense Sweetness Surpasses Cocaine Reward." *PloS One* 2, no. 8 (2007): e698.

381 **half the fat of coconut oil is lauric acid:** Shari Lieberman et al., "A Review of Monolaurin and Lauric Acid: Natural Virucidal and Bactericidal Agents," *Alternative & Complementary Therapies* 12, no. 6 (2006): 310–14.

383 **Anxious patients are more deficient:** Joanne J. Liu et al., "Omega-3 Polyunsaturated Fatty Acid (PUFA) Status in Major Depressive Disorder with Comorbid Anxiety Disorders," *Journal of Clinical Psychiatry* 74, no. 7 (2013): 732–38.

383 **those with more severe social anxiety disorders:** Pnina Green et al., "Red Cell Membrane Omega-3 Fatty Acids Are Decreased in Nondepressed Patients with Social Anxiety Disorder," *European Neuropsychopharmacology* 16, no. 2 (2006): 107–13.

383 **supplementation decreases anxiety-like behaviors in rodents:** Venugopal Reddy Venna et al., "PUFA Induce Antidepressant-like Effects in Parallel to Structural and Molecular Changes in the Hippocampus," *Psychoneuroendocrinology* 34, no. 2 (2009): 199–211.

383 **nonhuman primates:** Nina Vinot et al., "Omega-3 Fatty Acids from Fish Oil Lower Anxiety, Improve Cognitive Functions and Reduce Spontaneous Locomotor Activity in a Non-Human Primate," *PLoS One* 6, no. 6 (2011): e20491.

383 **medical students:** Janice K. Kiecolt-Glaser et al., "Omega-3 Supplementation Lowers Inflammation and Anxiety in Medical Students: A Randomized Controlled Trial," *Brain, Behavior, and Immunity* 25, no. 8 (2011): 1725–34.

383 **they need to be high in EPA:** Liu et al., "Omega-3 Polyunsaturated Fatty Acid (PUFA) Status in Major Depressive Disorder," *The Journal of Clinical Psychiatry* 174, no. 7, (2013): 732–38.

384 **Chronic treatment with the bacteria:** M. E. O'Brien et al., "SRL172 (Killed Mycobacterium Vaccae) in Addition to Standard Chemotherapy Improves Quality of Life Without Affecting Survival, in Patients with Advanced Non-Small-Cell Lung Cancer: Phase III Results," *Annals of Oncology* 15, no. 6 (2004): 906–14.

384 **reducing levels of cytokines:** R. Hernandez-Pando and G. A. Rook, "The Role of TNF-Alpha in T-Cell-Mediated Inflammation Depends on the Th1/Th2 Cytokine Balance," *Immunology* 82, no. 4 (1994): 591.

384 **Treatment with bifidobacteria:** J. Rao et al., "Regulation of Cerebral Glucose Metabolism," *Minerva Endocrinologica* 31, no. 2 (2006): 149.

385 **Endocannabinoids:** Chu Chen and Nicolas G. Bazan, "Lipid Signaling: Sleep, Synaptic Plasticity, and Neuroprotection," *Prostaglandins & Other Lipid Mediators* 77, no. 1 (2005): 65–76; Eric Murillo-Rodriguez et al., "Anandamide Enhances Extracellular Levels of Adenosine and Induces Sleep: An in Vivo Microdialysis Study," *SLEEP* 26, no. 8 (2003): 943–47.

386 **In depressive disorders, insomnia is:** Maurice M. Ohayon and Thomas Roth, "Place of Chronic Insomnia in the Course of Depressive and Anxiety Disorders," *Journal of Psychiatric Research* (2003).

390 **SSRIs are often used:** M. P. Kafka, "Successful Antidepressant Treatment of Nonparaphilic Sexual Addictions and Paraphilias in Men," *Journal of Clinical Psychiatry* 52 (1991): 60–65.

390 **If you are on SSRIs and have the genotype:** Jeffrey R. Bishop et al., "The Association of Serotonin Transporter Genotypes and Selective Serotonin Reuptake Inhibitor (SSRI)–Associated Sexual Side Effects: Possible Relationship to Oral Contraceptives," *Human Psychopharmacology: Clinical and Experimental* 24, no. 3 (2009): 207–15.

390 **Double-SERT people are more likely:** G. L. Hanna et al., "Serotonin Transporter and Serotonin Transporter Promoter Affects Onset of Paroxetine Treatment Seasonal Variation in Blood Serotonin in Families With Obsessive-Compulsive Disorder," *Neuropsychopharmacology* 18 (1998): 102–11.

390 **better responders to SSRIs than double-S people:** Nada Bozina et al., "Association Study of Paroxetine Therapeutic Response with SERT Gene Polymorphisms in Patients with Major Depressive Disorder," *World Journal of Biological Psychiatry* 9, no. 3 (2008): 190–97.

390 **In experiments, THC led to delayed time:** T. L. Crenshaw and J. P. Goldberg, *Sexual Pharmacology: Drugs That Affect Sexual Function* (New York: Norton, 1996).

390 **In the female rat, levels of brain endocannabinoids:** Heather B. Bradshaw et al., "Sex and Hormonal Cycle Differences in Rat Brain Levels of Pain-Related Cannabimimetic Lipid Mediators," *American Journal of Physiology-Regulatory, Integrative and Comparative Physiology* 291, no. 2 (2006): R349–R358.

390 **Female rats receiving an endocannabinoid antagonist:** Hassan H.López et al., "Cannabinoid Receptor Antagonism Increases Female Sexual Motivation," *Pharmacology Biochemistry and Behavior* 92, no. 1 (2009): 17–24.

390 **if you stimulate pleasure centers chemically:** James Olds and Peter Milner, "Positive Reinforcement Produced by Electrical Stimulation of Septal Area and Other Regions of Rat Brain," *Journal of Comparative and Physiological Psychology* 47, no. 6 (1954): 419; Robeht G. Heath, "Depth Recording and Stimulation Studies in Patients," *Surgical Control of Behavior* (1971): 21–37.

390 **The dopamine and endorphin release:** Doidge, *The Brain That Changes Itself.*

391 **To insure against "poachers":** Ryan and Jethá, *Sex at Dawn.*

391 **Even babies in the womb:** Israel Meizner, "Sonographic Observation of in Utero Fetal 'Masturbation,'" *Journal of Ultrasound in Medicine* 6, no. 2 (1987): 111; Harry Bakwin, "Erotic Feelings in Infants and Young Children," *Archives of Pediatrics & Adolescent Medicine* 126, no. 1 (1973): 52.

391 **Sexual pleasure from exercise:** Debby Herbenick and J. Dennis Fortenberry, "Exercise-Induced Orgasm and Pleasure Among Women," *Sexual and Relationship Therapy* 26, no. 4 (2011): 373–88.

392 **fascinating research on just how the uterus contracts:** G. Kunz et al., "Uterine Peristalsis During the Follicular Phase of the Menstrual Cycle: Effects of Estrogen, Antioestrogen and Oxytocin," *Human Reproduction Update* 4, no. 5 (1998): 647–54.

392 **all mediated by oxytocin:** H. Newton, "The Role of the Oxytocin Reflexes in Three Interpersonal Reproductive Acts: Coitus, Birth and Breastfeeding," *Clinical Psychoneuroendocrinology in Reproduction* 22 (1978): 411–18.

392 **prosocial, trusting behaviors:** P. Kirsch et al., "Oxytocin Modulates Neural Circuitry for Social Cognition and Fear in Humans," *Journal of Neuroscience* 25, (2005): 11489–93.

394 **hippocampal neuroplasticity:** Zhen Zhang et al.,"Blockade of 2-Arachidonoylglycerol Hydrolysis Produces Antidepressant-Like Effects and Enhances Adult Hippocampal Neurogenesis And Synaptic Plasticity," *Hippocampus,* August 27, 2014.

Index

Abilify, 4, 16, 316, 317–18
acetylcholine, 125–26
acid cider vinegar, 176, 382n
Acomplia (rimonabant), 325–26
acupuncture
  for opiate addiction, 335
  for sleep, 212
  for smoking cessation, 341
Adderall, 310–11, 325, 335–36
addiction, 60–61
  ADHD medications, 335–36
  dopamine and, 60, 166
  food, 168–69
  internet porn, 224–26
  opiate painkillers, 333–35
ADHD, 201–2, 269–70, 310
  abuse of ADHD medications, 335–36
  stimulants for, 310–12
adipokines, 397n
adrenal glands, 148
adrenaline, 21, 343
advertising, by pharmaceutical industry,
    4, 5, 14–16
aerobic exercise (cardio), 42, 246–48. *See also*
    exercise
aggression, 20, 22
  maternal, 96, 101
aging. *See also* menopause; perimenopause
  graceful, 141–44
  inflammation and, 158–59
  stress and, 158–59
  telomeres, methods for lengthening, 158–59
agonist, 343
air, 272–73
alcohol, 340
  cocaine and, creating cocaethylene, 336–37
  sex and, 222–23
  sleep and, 212
alexithymia, 21
algae, 181
alkanizing, 176, 381n
alloparenting, 228
almond milk, 179
alpha male, 50–51
Alzheimer's disease

estrogen and, 126
hormone replacement therapies and, 136
Ambien (zolpidem), 33, 209–10, 210–11, 326–28
amino acids, 42
amphetamines
  for appetite suppression, 325–26
  for attention-deficit disorder, 310–12
amygdala, 20, 64, 124, 150, 273, 285, 286, 343
Anafranil, 308–9
anal sex, 242–43
anandamide, 161, 162, 343
anaplastic large cell lymphoma, 260
androgens, 128, 129, 343
android shape, 366n
andropause, 128
anger
  libido and sexual responsiveness decreased
      by, 217
  suppression of, and depression, 29
anovulatory cycles, 119
antagonist, 343
anterior cingulate cortex, 64, 149, 273, 343
anterior fornix errogenous zone (AFE), 242
anthocyanins, 181
antiandrogen, 343
antibacterial soaps, 275, 276
antibiotics, 275, 276
antidepressants, 290–91, 301–9
  advertising of, 4, 5, 15
  bupropion, 220, 306–8
  effects of, 26–30
  hippocampal neurogenesis effect of, 309
  MAOIs, 308–9
  overprescription of, 5, 14–18
  sex and, 26, 66–67, 216, 219–21, 302–3, 390n
  SNRIs, 43–44, 219, 305–6, 347
  SSRIs (*See* serotonin reuptake inhibitors
      (SSRIs))
  tetracyclics (Remeron), 16, 308, 332
  tricyclics, 308–9
antihistamines, and sexual dysfunction, 216–17
antioxidants, 181
antipsychotics, 4, 14–18, 316–19
anxiety
  adaptive advantage conferred by, 25

anxiety (*Cont.*)
　increased risk in women, 23–25
　magnesium for, 125
　perimenopause and, 124–25
　pregnancy, medication use during, 98–99
　probiotics and, 184–85
　sleep and, 196, 387n
apigenin, 140
Aplenzin, 220
Apomorphine, 323
appetite suppressant medications, 324–26
apples, 178
aromatherapy, 212
arousal addiction, 392n
artichokes, 183
artificial nighttime light, and sleep disruption, 203
artificial sweeteners, 167, 179–80, 183
asparagus, 183
aspartame, 180
A-spot, 242
assertiveness, 30
Ativan, 210, 312, 313, 314, 329
atrazine, 262
attachment and bonding, 59–60
　chemistry of, 75–78
　parenthood and, 103–4
attention restoration, and nature, 269–70
attraction, 59–68
　brain-derived neurotrophic factor (BDNF)
　　and, 64–65
　chemistry of, 59–63
　dopamine and, 60, 65
　lust, distinguished, 67–68
　oxytocin and, 63–64
　serotonin and SSRIs impact on, 65–67
autism
　older sperm and risk of, 128
　SSRIs and, 98–99
autoimmune diseases, 148
　bacteria and, 275–76
　inflammation and, 151–52
　leaky gut syndrome and, 186
　mood disorders and, 373n
awareness, 5–6
Axiron, 323

baby blues, 105–6
bacteria
　balance of good and bad, 184
　beneficial role of, 275–77
　gut, 182–85, 206, 275–76
　sleep and, 205–6
Bacteroides fragilis, 276
bananas, 41
barometric pressure, 272
Basson, R., 321
BDNF. *See* brain-derived neurotrophic factor
　(BDNF)
beans, 183
beets, 181
Belviq, 326

Benadryl, 210, 332–33
benzodiazepines
　for anxiety, 312–15
　for sleep, 210, 329–30
Berman, Dr., 240, 320–21
beta carotenoids, 181
Better Homes and Gardens, 15
Bifidobacterium longum, 276, 385n
binge eating, 187, 192–93, 197
bioidentical hormones, 135, 370n
biological clock, 97–100
biome, 182
bipolar disorder, 99
　mood stabilizers as treatment for, 315–19
birth, 100–101
　Caesarean sections, 275–76
birth control pills. *See* oral contraceptives
　(the Pill)
bisphenol-A (BPA), 262, 277–78, 344
　estrogenic activity of, effects of, 277–78
black cod (sablefish), 181
black cohosh, 139
black tea, 181
blueberries, 181
blue blocking sunglasses, 208
body, 245–65
　acceptance of, 264–65, 292–93
　bra use, dangers of, 261–62
　breast augmentation, 258–60
　cultural messages regarding ideal, 255–57
　exercise, benefits of (*See* exercise)
　inactivity, effects of, 245–46
　male response to curvaceousness, 257–58
　pubic hair, 262–64
body autonomy, 111
body dimorphism, 85–86
bonding. *See* attachment and bonding
bonobos, 85, 86, 215
Botox, 141
BPA. *See* bisphenol-A (BPA)
brain, 19–23
　aging and, 125–26
　conflict response and, 21–22
　depression and, 149
　development of, 19–20
　emotion processing and, 22–23
　intuition and, 20–21
　women's versus men's, 19–23
brain-derived neurotrophic factor (BDNF)
　antidepressants and, 309, 344
　estrogen as increasing BDNF in brain's
　　learning and memory centers, 126
　exercise and, 248, 252, 253, 309
　falling in love and, 64–65
brain stem, 184
bran, 183
bra use, 261–62
bread, 181, 185
breast augmentation, 258–60
breast cancer
　bra use and, 261

chemicals and, 261–62
hormone replacement therapies and, 136–37
nighttime light exposure and, 203
rationality and anti-emotionality as risk
  factors for death from, 153
breast milk, 101–2
breath/breathing, 267, 282–84
Breathe Right strips, 207
Bremalanotide, 323
brown fat cells, 254
brussel sprouts, 139
buprenorphine, 335
bupropion, 220, 306–8
Buspirone (Buspar), 321

cad versus dad dilemma, 50–51, 54, 76
Caesarean section, 275–76
caffeine, 42, 206–7, 212
calcium
  for insomnia, 210
  for premenstrual syndrome (PMS), 42
cancer
  breast, 136–37, 153
  rationality and anti-emotionality as risk factor
    for death from, 153
candida, 185–86
cannabidiol (CBD), 140
cannabinoids, 344. See also endocannabinoid
    system
  in breast milk, 102
  stress resilience and, 161–63
cannabis, 181, 279–80, 339–40
  for insulin resistance, 172–73
  for menstrual cramps, 163
  for nausea in pregnancy, 163
  for perimenopausal symptoms, 139, 140–41
  sex and, 222–23
  stress, resilience and, 161–63
carbohydrates, 168, 175, 178
  complex, 172
  insulin and, 171–73
  light exposure and, 204
  stress triggering cravings for, 189–90
cardio (aerobic exercise), 42, 246–48
cardiovascular disease
  exercise and, 246
  hormone replacement therapies and, 135,
    136, 137
  low-carb diets and, 175
casein, 179
catechins, 181
caudate nucleus, 60
CB1, 252, 344
CB2, 141, 344
CB2 agonists, 141
Celexa, 18, 303
cerebellum, 23
cervical tapping, 242
chamomile, 210
chasteberry (vitex), 140
child rearing, 106–9

chimps, 85, 86
chocolate, 41, 181
cholesterol, 140, 175, 176, 177, 178, 381n
choline, 178, 383n
chromium picolinate, 172
chronotherapy, 208–9
Cialis, 320
cigarettes, 212, 340–42
cinnamon, 172
circadian rhythms, 202–3, 205, 208–9
coital alignment technique, 238–39
climacteric psychosis. See perimenopause
clitoral body, 227
clitoris, 226–28, 237, 238–39, 392n
Clomid, 98
cocaethylene, 336–37
cocaine, 60, 333, 336–37
coconut milk, 179
coconut oil, 176, 381n
cognitive performance
  estrogen and, 125–26, 367n
  and sleep, 201–2
  testosterone and, 126
companionate love, 76
computer use at night, and sleep, 207–8, 212
Concerta, 312
conflict response, 21–22
consensual nonmonogamy, 90–91
contraceptives
  in early perimenopause, 135
  oral (the Pill), 44–48
Coolidge effect, 87–88
Cooper's ligaments, 261
corn, 186
cortisol, 125, 148, 190, 344
cougar phase, of perimenopause, 126–29
CPAP machine, 207, 344
crying, 27–28
  premenstrual syndrome (PMS) and, 37–38
cuddling, 64, 69, 72, 103
Cymbalta, 43, 306, 332
Cyproheptadine, 321
Cyrus, Miley, 61
cytokines, 149, 150–51, 158, 248, 249, 251, 344

dad versus cad dilemma, 50–51, 54, 76
dairy, 179, 185, 186
damiana, 139
date nights, 113–14
DDT, 262
decongestants, and sexual dysfunction, 216–17
Deep Sleep, 210
Depakote, 315, 316
Depo Provera, 132
depression, 23–30
  adaptive advantage conferred by, 25
  anger suppression and, 29
  bacterial exposure and, 276
  brain areas implicated in, 149
  estrogen levels and, 26
  increased risk in women, 23–25

depression (*Cont.*)
  inflammation and stress creating, 148–52
  insomnia and, 200–201, 387n
  leaky gut syndrome and, 186
  major, 36, 124, 200, 346
  medications for (*See* antidepressants)
  obesity and, 248–49
  postpartum, 104–6
  pregnancy, medication use during, 98–99
  probiotics and, 184–85
  reproductive, 24, 123–24
  sex as natural anti-depressant, 244
  stress and inflammation creating, 148–52
desperate housewife phase, of perimenopause,
  126–29
Dexedrine, 310–11, 325, 335
DHEA, 344
diabetes, 175, 176, 178
  combating, 172–73
  hormone replacement therapies and, 135
  risk factors, 172
  type 1, 172
  type 2, 172–73, 197, 205
*Diagnostic and Statistical Manual of Mental
  Disorders*, 36
diet and nutrition, 165–94, 292
  anti-inflammatory diet, 180–82, 186
  biological basis of gorging, 166–69
  dopamine circuitry and, 166, 168
  eating process, 187–94
  endocannabinoid system and, 169–70, 172–73
  food addiction, 168–69
  genetic component of weight, 173
  ghrelin, role of, 173–74
  gluten-free diet, 186–87
  gut bacteria and, 182–85
  high-protein, low-carb diet, benefits of, 172
  insulin, role of, 171
  leaky gut syndrome, 185–87
  leptin, role of, 170, 173
  low-carb, 175
  mental health and, 167–68
  paleo, 175
  perimenopause and, 139–40
  premenstrual syndrome (PMS) and, 42–43
  probiotics, 183–85
  stress and, 168, 189–90
  what to drink, advice on, 179–80
  what to eat, advice on, 174–79
diet soda, 179, 181
dildos, 242
Dior, Christian, 255–56
directed attention fatigue, 269
direct-to-consumer advertising, 4, 14–16
division of labor, 81–83
divorce
  initiated by women at midlife, 143
  rates of, 78
DLPA, 335
Dodson, Betty, 233, 236, 240
Doidge, Norman, 224, 225

dopamine, 22, 344
  addiction and, 60, 166
  attachment and, 75
  attraction and, 60, 65
  exercise and, 253
  food and, 166, 168–69
  lust and, 67
  novel experiences and, 91–92
  orgasm and, 70, 71, 73
  sex and, 69, 70, 219–20
double L SERT, 391n
Dow Corning, 260
downtime, 267–87, 292
  breath/breathing and, 267, 282–84
  importance of, 267–69
  mindfulness/meditation and (*See*
    mindfulness/meditation)
  nature, restorative properties of (*See* nature)
  screens, unhealthy effects of, 281–82
driving, effects of sleep deprivation on, 197–98
drugs/drug therapy, 3–5, 290–91
  abuse of prescription drugs, 333–36
  advertising and, 4, 5, 14–16
  antidepressants (*See* antidepressants)
  antipsychotics, 4, 15, 316–19
  appetite suppressants, 324–26
  benzodiazepines, 312–15
  mood stabilizers, 315–19
  overuse of, in U.S., 5, 8, 14–18
  during pregnancy, 98–99
  prosexual medicines, 319–24
  research on women, lack of, 33
  sleep aids, 196–97, 209–11, 213, 326–33
  statins, 16
  stimulants, 310–12
dysthymia, 344

eating process, 187–94
  binge eating, 187, 188, 192–93
  intuitive versus emotional, 190–92
  nighttime eating, 192–93
  remaining conscious while eating, 188–89
  sleep and, 197
  slowing down, 189–90
  stress affecting, 168, 189–90
ecopsychology, 279–81
Ecstasy, 337–38
Edluar, 328
EEMT HS, 323
Effexor, 43, 305–6
eggs, 178, 181, 186
Eichel, Edward, 239
Elavil, 308–9, 331
embodiment, 265
emotional connectedness, 76–77, 359n
emotions
  health and emotional stress, 152–54
  positive, and stress, 157–58
empathy, 14, 21, 26–27
Emsam, 309
endocannabinoid, 344

endocannabinoid system, 7, 161–63, 345.
    See also cannabinoids
    deficient functioning of, effects of, 161–62
    exercise as activating, 251–52
    feeding behavior and, 169–70
    insulin resistance and, 172–73
    pregnancy and, 101, 363n
    sex and, 222
    sleep and, 386n
    stress response and, 161–63
endocrine system, 345
endometriosis, 44
endorphins, 187, 345
    attraction and, 61–62
    in breast milk, 102
    orgasm and, 71
    sex and, 69, 70, 222
enzymes, 183
Equal, 183
Estrace, 133
Estratest, 323
Estring, 133
estrogen, 18, 22, 25–26, 125–26
    attachment and, 76
    attraction and, 61, 62
    caffeine metabolism and, 207
    cognitive functioning and, 125–26, 367n
    depression and, 26
    dominance, 120–21, 125, 136
    FAAH/estrogen interaction, 162–63
    hormone replacement therapies and, 134–35
    in late perimenopause, 120–21
    libido and, 131
    lust and, 67
    menstrual cycle and, 35–36, 39
    oral contraceptives and, 45, 46–47
    perimenopause stages and levels of, 120–21,
        122, 124–25, 126, 128–29, 130, 132–33
    pheromone detection and, 52
    serotonin levels and, 25–26, 124, 352n, 367n
    sex and, 69–70
    supplementation, 134–35
    types of, 349n
    xenoestrogens, 121, 132, 277–78
estrus, 48–49
eszopiclone (Lunesta), 210, 328–29
euthymia, 24
evening primrose oil, 139
excitation transfer, 92
executive function, 220, 252, 345
exercise, 291, 292
    anti-inflammatory properties of, 253–54
    benefits of, 246–48
    CDC recommendations for amount of, 246
    endocannabinoid system activated by, 251–52
    forms of, 249–51
    insulin resistance and, 172
    integrating, into daily regime, 250–51
    learning and, 252–53
    memory and, 247–48, 252
    motivational self-talk and, 254–55

neuroplasticity and, 247–48
    perimenopause and, 138–39
    premenstrual syndrome (PMS) and, 42
    resilience to stress and, 252–53
    running, 249–50
    sex and, 138–39, 235, 247
    top-down control and, 252
exorphins, 186–87
extended sexuality, 48

Facebook, 282
fantasies, 230–34, 393n
farro, 172
fat cells, 254
fatigue
    parental, 108–9
    perimenopause and, 125
    during pregnancy, 99
fats, 166–67, 172, 175
    monounsaturated, 175
    saturated, 175
    trans, 175
fatty acid amide hydrolase (FAAH),
        162–63
fear, 20, 64
Female Brain, The (Brizendine), 77
fermented foods, 183, 184
fertility, 48
    melatonin and, 98
    SSRIs and, 98
fertility drugs, 98
fetus, effect of SSRIs on, 98–99
fiber, 183
fibromyalgia, 31
fidelity, 86–88. *See also* monogamy
    testosterone levels and, 86–87
    vasopressin and, 86
Fifty Shades of Grey (James), 230
fight or flight mode, 21
fish, 181–82
Fisher, Helen, 60, 77
5-hydroxytrytophan (5HTP), 42
flame retardants, 102
flaxseed, 181
Flibanserin, 322
flour, 179, 180, 181
fluoxetine (Prozac), 18, 26–27, 220, 303
f.lux, 208
folate, 139
folliculitis, 263
food. *See* diet and nutrition
food cravings, and premenstrual syndrome
        (PMS), 41–42
foreplay, 237–39
Foria, 140
free radicals, 181
free T4 test, 123
Freud, Sigmund, 240
frontal cortex, 72, 345
frontal lobes, 252
fructose, 177

fruit juices, 177
fruits, 174, 177

GABA, 124, 184–85
gabapentin, 210
galanin, 193
galattorphins, 102
gastric bypass surgery, 183
ghrelin, 173–74, 183, 190, 193, 197, 204, 345
gibbons, 85
Glamour, 256–57
glans, 227
GlaxoSmithKline, 15
glucose, 177, 254
glutamate, 151
gluten, 185, 186
gluten-free diet, 186–87
glycemic index, 172
Goldstein, Irwin, 131
Good Housekeeping, 15
gorillas, 85–86
grapeseed oil, 176
Gray, John, 114
green tea, 181
G-spot (Grafenberg spot) orgasm, 241–42, 394n
gut bacteria, 182–85, 206, 275–76
gynoid shape, 122, 366n

Halcion, 210
Haldol, 316
halibut, 181
HDL cholesterol, 178, 381n
headaches, 130
heart attacks, 178
heat, 48–49
hemp, 279–80
hemp seed, 181, 182
hemp seed oil, 182
herbal remedies
    for insomnia, 210, 212
    for perimenopausal symptoms, 133, 139–40
    for vaginal atrophy, 133
heroin, 333
high blood pressure, 178
high-fructose corn syrup, 177
high-protein, low-carb diet, 172
hippocampal neurogenesis, 309
hippocampus, 20, 124, 247–48, 252, 285–86, 345
hops, 139, 210
hormone replacement therapy (HRT), 134–37
    Alzheimer's and, 136
    benefits of, 134–35
    breast cancer risk and, 136–37
    cardiovascular disease and, 135, 136, 137
    diabetes and, 135
    estrogen supplementation, 134–35
    progesterone supplementation, 135
    testosterone supplementation, 134–35
    time to initiate, 136
hormones. *See also* specific hormones
    appetite and, 171–74

circadian rhythms and, 202
in drinking water, 277
drop-off in, in postpartum period, 105
mood variability and, 24–27
neurotransmitters and, link between, 18
variations and cycles in, 2
horniness. *See* libido
hot flashes, 119–20
Hot Monogamy (Love), 112
HRT. *See* hormone replacement therapy (HRT)
hugging, 63–64, 160
hydrocodone, 333
hydrotherapy, 273
hyperphagia. *See* binge eating
hypnosis, 341
hypoglycemia, 171
hypothalamus, 124–25, 345
hypothyroidism, 123
hysterectomies, 32–33
hysteria, 30–31, 236

immune system, 147, 199, 202, 206, 275–76
inactivity
    health problems resulting from, 245–46
    as risk factor for insulin resistance, 172
infancy, bonding during, 103–4
infections, 149–50
    antibacterial soaps and, 276
    chronic stress and increased risk of, 152
    fewer, in breast-fed babies, 101
    inflammation and, 151–52
    mood disorders and, 373n
    pubic hair removal and, 263–64
infidelity, 83–84, 89–90
inflammation, 147–63
    aging and, 158–59
    anti-inflammatory diet, 180–82, 186
    autoimmune disorders and, 151–52
    emotional stress and health, 152–54
    endocannabinoid system as anti-
        inflammatory, 161–63
    exercise and, 253–54
    infections and, 151–52
    isolation and, 160
    leaky gut syndrome and, 186
    obesity and, 148
    oxytocin as anti-inflammatory, 160
    probiotics and, 183–84
    resilience and, 154–56
    sleep deprivation and, 148, 196
    stress-inflammation-depression mechanism,
        7, 148–52
insomnia. *See also* sleep; sleep deprivation
    anxiety disorders and, 196, 387n
    depression and, 196, 200–201, 387n
    incidence of, women versus men, 195
    magnesium for, 125, 210
    natural remedies for, 212–13
    nonprescription aids for, 332–33
    perimenopause and, 119, 124–25
    pregnancy and, 99–100

prescription aids for, 196–97, 209–11, 213, 326–32
    sleep hygiene and, 212–13
    stress and, 196
Instagram, 282
insula, 21, 32
insulin, 171–73, 204
insulin resistance, 172–73, 197
intercourse, 238–39
interferon, 149
Intermezzo, 328
Intrinsa patch, 138, 322
intuition, 14, 20–21
    men's lack of, 28
    premenstrual syndrome (PMS) and, 40
intuitive eating, 190–92
irisin, 254
isolation, 160, 377n

jet lag, 203, 388n
junk food, 166–67, 379n

kale, 181
kefir, 183
Kegelcizer, 236
Kegel exercises, 235–36
kimchi, 183
Kinsey, Alfred, 234
Klonopin, 210, 312, 314–15, 329
knyurenine, 150–51
kombucha, 183
Komisaruk, Barry, 72
Kuo, Frances, 274
kynurenine, 248, 345

labor, 100–101
Lactobacillus helveticu, 276, 385n
lactose, 185
Lamictal, 318–19
laser hair removal, 263
Last Picture Show, The (movie), 127
lazy position, 239
LDL cholesterol, 177, 381n
leaky gut syndrome, 185–87
leaky gut theory, 151
learning, and exercise, 252–53
lemon, 176
lentils, 41
leptin, 170, 173, 190, 197, 204–5, 345, 380n
leptin resistance, 170, 204
Levitra, 320
Lexapro, 18, 43–44, 303–4, 307, 390n
libido
    chemistry of lust, 67–69
    Coolidge effect and, 87–88
    cougar phase, of perimenopause, 126–29
    estrogen levels and, 131
    low, in perimenopause, 129–32
    menstrual cycle and fluctuations in, 48–50
    motherhood and, 109–12
    novel experiences and, 91–92, 231

oral contraceptives and decrease in, 47–48, 132
    ovulation and, 49–50
    postpartum, 110
    testosterone levels and, 62, 131–32
Libigel, 322–23
licorice, 139
lifestyle illnesses, 178
limbic system, 124, 345
lipopolysaccharides (LPS), 184
lithium, 315, 316
Little, Tony, 54
lordosis, 61
Lorexys, 321–22
love, 6, 59–91
    attachment phase, 59–60, 75–78
    attraction phase, 59–68
    lust, chemistry of, 67–69
    marriage and, 77–94
    orgasm and, 71–73
    sex, chemistry of, 69–71
Love, Pat, 112
low-carb diets, 175
L-tryptophan, 42
lubricants, 133
lubrication issues, 133
Lunesta (eszopiclone), 210, 328–29
lupus, 152
Luramist, 323
lust. See libido
Lybrido, 322
Lybridos, 321, 322
lycopene, 181

maca, 133, 139–40
magnesium
    for anxiety, 125
    for insomnia, 125, 210
    for perimenopause symptoms, 125, 130
    for premenstrual syndrome (PMS), 41, 42
    for restless leg syndrome, 125
major depression, 36, 124, 200, 346
major histocompatibility complex (MHC), 53, 78, 346
mangoes, 178
MAOIs, 308–9
Marplan, 309
marriage, 77–94
    balancing needs for intimacy and isolation in, 89
    communication and, 93–94
    consensual nonmonogamy and, 90–91
    Coolidge effect and, 87–88
    division of labor in, 81–83
    infidelity and, 83–84, 89–90
    making love last, 91–94
    mindfulness and, 80
    negativity, impact of, 93
    novelty and, 91–93
    opposite partners, and completion as team in, 78–81

marriage (*Cont.*)
  projection of childhood traumas onto partners,
    80
  repulsion phase, 79–80
  separateness and, 88–89
Maslow hierarchy of human needs, 78
Masters and Johnson, 234, 240
masturbation, 232–33, 234
mate selection, 49–55
  alpha-male attraction during fertile period,
    50–51
  dad versus cad dilemma, 50–51, 54, 76
  different immunities and MHC of mate as
    factor in, 53, 78
  oral contraceptives and, 51, 54–55
  pheromones and, 52–54
  SSRIs effect on, 66–67
Mating in Captivity (Perel), 90
MDMA (methyene-dioxy-meth-amphetamine),
  337–38
meadow voles, 86
medical research, male bias in, 33
medicines. *See* drugs/drug therapy
meditation. *See* mindfulness/meditation
melatonin, 98, 202–6, 207–8, 210, 213, 388n
melons, 178
memory/memories
  emotions and, 20
  exercise and, 247–48, 252
  isolation and, 160, 377n
menarche, 36, 346
Men Are from Mars, Women Are from Venus
  (Gray), 114
menopause, 117. *See also* perimenopause
  aging gracefully and, 141–44
  average age for, 117
menopot, 121–23
menstrual cycle, 35–55
  depression/anxiety risk and, 24–25
  estrogen and, 35–36, 39
  follicular phase, 35
  keeping track of, 37, 38
  luteal phase, 35–36
  mate selection and, 49–55
  orgasm and, 218–19
  ovulation, 48–51
  pain sensitivity and, 32
  during perimenopause, 120–21
  premenstrual syndrome (PMS), 36–44
  progesterone and, 35–36, 40
Metadate, 312
microglia, 199
midwives, 100
migraines, 130, 368n
MILFs, 114–15
milk, 41, 179
millet, 172
mindfulness/meditation, 8, 267, 268, 269,
  285–87, 291
  benefits of, 285–86
  inflammatory marker levels improved by, 159

marriage and, 80
neuroplastic changes fostered by, 285
sleep and, 212
stress resilience and, 285–86
telomerase activity and, 158–59
top-down control and, 80, 285
weight loss from stress reduction through, 190
minerals, 42
Mirtazapine (Remeron), 16, 308, 332
missionary position, 238–39
mittelschmerz (middle pain), 354n
Molly, 337–38
monkeys, 103, 153
monogamy
  benefits of, 94
  maintaining relationship, 91–94
  in nature, 84–86
  serial, 90, 91
monogamy gene (vasopressin receptor gene), 77
monounsaturated fats, 175
moods/moodiness, 1–9, 20, 289–95
  anger, 29, 217
  awareness and, 5–6
  body, awareness and acceptance of (*See* body)
  brain and, 19–23
  crying, 27–28, 37–38
  downtime and (*See* downtime)
  drug therapy and (*See* drugs/drug therapy)
  expression of, 27–30
  female diagnoses and, 30–33
  food and (*See* diet and nutrition)
  hormonal fluctuations and, 18, 24–27
  inflammation and (*See* inflammation)
  marriage and (*See* marriage)
  memories and, 20
  menstrual cycle and (*See* menstrual cycle)
  motherhood and (*See* motherhood)
  neurotransmitters and, 18–19
  perimenopause and (*See* perimenopause)
  sex and (*See* sex)
  sleep and (*See* sleep)
  stress and (*See* stress)
mood stabilizers, 315–19
motherhood, 95–115
  aggression and, 22, 101
  biological clock, 97–100
  bonding with baby, 103–4
  child rearing and, 106–9
  fertility drugs, use of, 98
  increase in age for starting family, 97–98
  libido and, 109–12
  nesting and, 40, 98
  neuroplasticity induced by, 95–96
  nursing and, 101–2, 106
  postpartum period, 25, 104–6, 110
  sex during, 109–15
  "village" alternative for, 107–9
motivational self-talk, and exercise, 254–55
mula bandha, 235
multiple orgasms, 241
multiple sclerosis, 152

Mycobacterium vaccae, 276, 385n
myokines, 397n

naloxone, 167
naps, 198
Nardil, 309
natural foods, 174
natural labor, 100–101
nature, 267–68, 269–75, 287, 293
    air, effects of, 272–73
    attention restoration and, 269–70
    bacteria, beneficial role of, 275–77
    barometric pressure, effects of, 272
    ecopsychology and, 279–81
    learning stillness from, 269–70
    monogamy in, 84–86
    pollution and (*See* pollutants/pollution)
    resilience and, 156
    sunlight, effects of, 270–71
    as therapy, 273–75
    weather, effects of, 272
negative ion exposure, 272–73
negativity, 93
nesting, 40, 98
neurogenesis, and exercise, 252, 253
neuroplasticity, 151, 346
    exercise and, 247–48
    internet porn and, 224, 225
    meditation and, 285
    motherhood and, 95–96
    stress and, 248
neurotransmitters, 18–19, 346. *See also*
        dopamine; norepinephrine; serotonin;
        specific neurotransmitters
    circadian rhythms and, 202
    exercise and, 253
    gut bacteria and, 183
    high-fructose diets and, 177
    hormones and, link between, 18
    inflammation and, 180
    leaky gut syndrome and, 186
    negative feedback loop in eating behavior
        and, 168
    production in gut, 168
New York Times, 16, 211
nicotine, 212, 340–42
nighttime eating, 192–93
nighttime light exposure, and sleep
        disruption, 203
9/11 terrorist attacks, and pharmaceutical
        advertising, 15
nipple stimulation, 237–38
nocturnal orgasms, 240–41
noise, and sleep, 207
nomophobia, 281
norepinephrine, 346
    attachment and, 75
    attraction and, 61
    exercise and, 253
    novel experiences and, 92
    sex and, 70

novel experiences, 91–93, 231
nursing, 101–2, 110
    benefits of, 101–2
    breast augmentation, and lactation
        insufficiency, 260
    downside of, 102
    postpartum depression and, 106
nutrition. *See* diet and nutrition
nuts, 175, 181, 183, 186

oats, 172, 183
Obama, Barack, 223
obesity, 178
    abdominal
        in perimenopause, 121–23, 366n
        telomere length and, 158
    circadian timing and, 205
    depression and, 248–49
    gut bacteria and, 182
    inflammation and, 148
    phytotherapy and, 205
    as risk factor for insulin resistance, 172
olanzapine (Zyprexa), 182
olive oil, 176
omega-3 fatty acids, 42, 172, 181–82, 383n
omnisexual women, 228–30
1L-1beta, 249
onions, 183
open marriages, 90–91
opiate painkillers, abuse of, 333–35
opiod system, 222
oral contraceptives (the Pill), 44–48
    emotional side effects of, 45–46
    mate selection and, 51, 54–55
    pheromone processing and, 54
    for premenstrual syndrome (PMS), 44–45
    sexual drive and desire, decrease in, 47–48,
        132, 216
    weight gain and, 46–47
oral sex, 238
orangutans, 85–86
oregano, 139
orgasms, 71–73, 217–19
    A-spot, 242
    brain blood flow and, 72–73
    chemistry of, 71–72
    clitoral stimulation and, 233
    exercise-induced, 235, 393n
    G-spot, 241–42, 394n
    masturbation and, 232–33, 234
    menstrual cycle and, 218–19
    multiple, 241
    pelvic floor, 240
    penile penetration and, 233–34
    spontaneous, 240–41
    SSRIs and, 67
    timing and, 218
    types of, 239–43
orthorexia, 380n
outdoor immersion programs, 270
overprescription, 5, 8, 14–18

ovulation, 48–51, 354n
oxidative stress, 181
oxycodone, 333
Oxycontin, 333
oxytocin, 22
    attachment and, 76, 77
    attraction and, 63–64
    lust and, 67, 69
    motherhood and, 96
    orgasm and, 70, 71
    parenthood and, 103
    sex and, 64, 69–70
    as stress hormone, 159–60

pain, 31–32
Pain, 32
paleo diet, 175
palm oil, 176
Pamelor, 308–9, 331
pancreas, 172
parasympathetic system, 70, 189, 218, 346
paraurethral glands (Skene's glands), 242
parental impulse, in men
    testosterone and, 76, 86–87
    vasopressin and, 103
Parnate, 309
partible paternity, 108
pasta, 181, 185
Paxil, 6, 15, 18, 43, 304–5, 332, 390n
Paxil CR, 305
PEA. *See* phenylethylamine (PEA)
pears, 178
pelvic floor orgasm, 240
penguins, 84
penis, 227, 392n
peppers, 181
peptide Y, 190
Percocet, 333
Perel, Esther, 90
perimenopause, 7, 36, 117–44
    abdominal obesity in, 121–23, 366n
    aging gracefully and, 141–44
    anxiety and, 124–25
    cannabis for, 139, 140–41
    cognitive functioning and, 125–26, 367n
    cougar/desperate housewife phase of, 126–29
    diet and, 139–40
    estrogen dominance, 120–21, 125
    estrogen levels and, 120–21, 122, 124–25, 126,
        128–29, 130, 132–33
    exercise, benefits of, 138–39
    hormone replacement therapy, 134–37
    insomnia and, 119, 124–25
    low libido in, 129–32
    menopot and, 121–23
    menstrual cycles during, 120–21
    progesterone levels during, 120–21, 122
    supplements and, 139–40
    symptoms of, 119–20, 124–26
    vaginal atrophy and, 132–33
pesticides, 121, 132, 262, 277–78

Pfaus, Jim, 220
Pfizer, 304
phallus, 227
pharmaceutical industry advertising, 4, 5, 14–16
pharmakon, 4
Phentermine, 324–25
Phentolamine, 323–24
phenylethylamine (PEA), 346
    attachment and, 75
    attraction and, 62
    orgasm and, 71
pheromones, 52–54, 63
phthalates, 278
phytoestrogens, 139
phytotherapy, 205, 271–72
pickled products, 176
Pilates, 138, 235
the Pill. *See* oral contraceptives (the Pill)
pine bark extract (pycnogenol), 139
Pitocin, 100
plastics, 277–78, 280–81
    BPA in (*See* bisphenol-A (BPA))
    phthalates in, effects of exposure to, 278
    xenoestrogens in, 121, 132, 277
PMS. *See* premenstrual syndrome (PMS)
Pollan, Michael, 276–77
pollutants/pollution, 261–62, 277–78
    breast cancer risk and, 261–62
    in breast milk, 102
    pesticides, 121, 132, 262, 277–78
    phthalates, 278
    plastics, 121, 132, 261, 262, 277–78, 280–81
    xenoestrogens, 121, 132, 277, 347
polyamorous, 90–91
polybrominated diethyl ethers (PBDEs), 102
polygyny, 86
polymorphism, 346
polyphenols, 181
pomegranates, 181
porn, 224–26, 229, 263
postmenopausal period, 24
postpartum period
    depression, 104–6
    psychosis, 105
    risk of depression/anxiety and, 25
    sex during, 110
post-traumatic stress disorder (PTSD),
    20, 346
Pot Book, The (Holland), 340
prairie voles, 86
prebiotics, 183, 385n
prefrontal cortex (PFC), 184, 220, 252,
    285–86, 346
pregnancy
    birth and, 100–101
    depression/anxiety risk and, 25
    fatigue during, 99
    insomnia during, 99–100
    labor and, 100–101
    medication use prior to and during, 98–99
Premarin, 136, 370n

premenstrual dsyphoric disorder (PMDD), 36
premenstrual syndrome (PMS), 36–44
    diet and, 42–43
    exercise and, 42
    food cravings and, 41–42
    learning from, 38–40
    oral contraceptives and, 44–45
    orgasm and, 218–19
    rejection sensitivity and, 37–38
    serotonin levels and, 36, 39, 41–42
    sex and, 43, 218–19
    symptoms of, 36
    treatment options, 41–44
    vitamins, minerals and nutritional
        supplements for, 42
Prempro, 370n
primates, 84–86, 103, 259
Pristiq, 43
probiotics, 183–85, 277
processed foods, 166–67, 174, 177, 181, 183
Procter & Gamble, 138
progesterone, 25
    deficiency, and breast cancer risk, 136–37
    hormone replacement therapies and, 135
    menstrual cycle and, 35–36, 40
    oral contraceptives and, 45–46
    during perimenopause, 120–21, 122
    for relief of painful intercourse, 133
    serotonin levels and, 367n
progestins, 136
    and headache, 130
    hormone replacement therapies and, 135, 136
    side effects of, 135
prolactin, 206, 390n
    depression and, 105
    parental bonding and, 103
    sex and, 220
Prolixin, 316
prosexual medicines, 319–24
proteins, 172, 174, 175
Provera, 130, 135
proximate separation, 104
Prozac (fluoxetine), 18, 26–27, 220, 303
psychic autonomy, 111–12
psychobiotics, 185
PTSD, 20, 346
pubic hair, 263–64
    laser removal of, 263
    purpose of, 264
    shaving/waxing, health risks associated with,
        263–64
pycnogenol (pine bark extract), 139

quinoa, 172
Qysmia, 325

raloxifene, 135
Ramelteon (Rozerem), 331
rear entry, 239, 242
receptor, 346
red clover, 139

red meats, 181
red wine, 181
Reich, Wilhelm, 232–33
rejection sensitivity, 37–38
relaxation techniques, 212
Remeron (Mirtazapine), 16, 308, 332
REM (rapid eye movement) sleep, 198–99
repressive behavior, and stress, 153–54
reproductive cycle, 18
reproductive depression, 24, 123–24
resilience, 154–56
    cannabinoids and, 161–63
    chronic trauma, effects of, 154–55
    exercise and, 252–53
    meditation and, 285–86
    nature and, 156
    nurturing and, 155–56
    social support and, 160
    stress inoculation and, 154
restless leg syndrome, 125, 367n
Restoril, 329
Restylane, 141
reverse cowgirl, 239
Reynolds, Joshua, 163
rice milk, 179
rimonabant, 170
Risperdal, 17, 316
Ritalin, 312, 335
role playing, 393n
Roth, Geneen, 188
Rouillon, Jean Denis, 261
Rozerem (Ramelteon), 331
Rules, The (Fein and Schneider), 61
running, 249–50

saccharine, 180
salads, 176
salience, 60
salmon, 181
salt, 166–67
saturated fats, 175
sauerkraut, 183
schizophrenia, 128
screens (computers/phones/tv)
    nighttime use, and sleep, 207–8, 212
    unhealthy effects of, 281–82
seasonal affective disorder, 271–72
Seasonale, 44
Seasonique, 44
seeds, 181
seizures, 199
selective estrogen receptor modulators
        (SERMs), 135
selenium, 181
self-esteem, 22, 30
semen, 243–44
senile vagina, 132–33
sensitivity, 14, 40
separateness, 88–89
Serax, 313
serial monogamy, 90, 91

serial orgasms, 241
SERMS. *See* selective estrogen receptor
    modulators (SERMs)
Seroquel, 316, 332
serotonergic, 347
serotonin, 18–19
    attachment and, 75
    attraction/infatuation process and, 65–67
    estrogen levels and, 25–26, 124, 352n, 367n
    exercise and, 253
    as melatonin precursor, 203
    natural methods for boosting, 41–42
    premenstrual syndrome (PMS) and, 36, 39,
        41–42
    progesterone and, 367n
    receptor numbers and sensitivity, gender
        differences in, 352n
    sex and, 219–20
serotonin and norepinephrine reuptake
    inhibitors (SNRIs), 43–44, 219, 305–6, 347
serotonin reuptake inhibitors (SSRIs), 18–19,
    291, 301–5, 347
    attraction/infatuation process, impact on,
        65–67
    complacency and, 28–29
    exercise combined with, 253
    fertility and, 98
    fetus, effect on, 98–99
    mechanism of action, 301–2
    for premenstrual syndrome (PMS), 43–44
    sex and, 26, 66–67, 219–21, 302–3, 390n
    suppression of emotions and, 26–30
    time when pill should be taken, 303–4
    withdrawal issues, 305
serotonin reuptake transporter (SERT), 150, 347,
    352n, 391n
seven-year itch, 83–84
sex, 6, 7–8, 215–44
    alcohol and, 222–23
    anal, 242–43
    antidepressants and, 26, 66–67, 216, 219–21,
        302–3, 390n
    antihistamines and, 216–17
    arousal, requirements for, 216–17
    benefits of, 215–16
    casual, and triggering of attraction and love,
        68–69
    chemistry of, 69–71
    clitoris and, 226–28, 237, 238–39, 392n
    date nights, 113–14
    decongestants and, 216–17
    drug use (illegal) and, 222–23
    dysfunction
        categories of, 390n
        factors causing, 216–17
    egalitarian marriages and, 82–83
    exercise and, 138–39, 235, 247
    fantasies and, 230–34
    gender differentiation and, 83
    getting in the mood for, 234–35
    intercourse, 238–39

Kegel exercises and, 235–36
libido (*See* libido)
MILFs and, 114–15
during motherhood, 109–15
nipple play, 237–38
omnisexual women and, 228–30
oral, 238
oral contraceptives and, 47–48, 216, 221
orgasms (*See* orgasms)
porn and, 224–26, 229
premenstrual syndrome (PMS) and, 43,
    218–19
prosexual medicines, 319–24
spontaneity and, 113–14
SSRIs and, 26, 66–67, 219–21, 302–3, 390n
technique, 237–39
VENIS (very erotic, non-insertive sex), 134
Viagra and, 133–34, 216, 320–21
vibrators and, 236–37
sex holiday, 220–21, 390n
sex hormone binding globulin (SHBG), 46
sexual assaults, 223
sexual drive and desire. *See* libido
Sexy Mamas (Winks and Semans), 48, 113
SHBG, 128–29, 347
shellfish, 186
shift work, 203
short-chain fatty acids, 183–84
sickness behavior, 149–50
Sinequan, 331
Skene's glands (paraurethral glands), 242
sleep, 195–213, 386n. *See also* insomnia; sleep
    deprivation
    bacteria and, 205–6
    caffeine and, 206–7
    chronotherapy and, 208–9
    circadian rhythms and, 202–3, 205, 208–9
    cognitive functioning, 201–2
    computer use at night and, 207–8
    consolidated, 198
    depression and, 196, 200–201, 387n
    feeding and, 197
    hormones of hunger/fullness, relationship to,
        204–5
    ideal amount of, 198
    importance of, 195–96
    melatonin and, 202–6, 207–8, 210, 213
    noise and, 207
    nonprescription aids for, 332–33
    prescription aids for, 196–97, 209–11, 213,
        326–32
    quality of, and longevity, 195
    restorative role of, 199
    seizures prevented by, 199
    stages of, 198–99
sleep apnea, 207
sleep deprivation, 195–98. *See also* insomnia;
    sleep
    effects of, 196, 197–98, 199
    inflammation and, 148, 196
    sensitivity to, women versus men, 195

sleep hygiene, 212–13
sleeping pills, 196–97, 209–11, 213
slow-wave sleep, 198–99, 387n
smell, 51–52
smoking cessation, 340–42
SNRIs. *See* serotonin and norepinephrine
    reuptake inhibitors (SNRIs)
soaps, 121
    antibacterial, 275, 276
social media, 282
social support, 159–60
soda, 179
somatosensory cortex, 72
"Some of My Best Friends Are Germs" (Pollan),
    276–77
Sonata (zaleplon), 329
Sousa, Osmel, 255
soy milk, 179
soy products, 139, 186
speed, 60
spinach, 181
Splenda, 183
spontaneity, 113–14
spontaneous orgasms, 240–41
sprouts, 139
squash, 181
SSRIs. *See* serotonin reuptake inhibitors (SSRIs)
starches, 168, 174
statins, 16, 178
stillness, 269–70
stimulants, 310–12
Stone, Linda, 281
stress, 20–21
    aging and, 158–59
    attitudes toward, effects of, 157–58
    cannabinoids and, 161–63
    eating behavior and, 168, 189–90
    emotional, and health, 152–54
    exercise and, 252–53
    high caloric food binges triggered by,
        189–90
    inflammation-stress-depression mechanism,
        7, 148–52
    isolation and, 160
    neuroplasticity and, 248
    oxytocin and, 159–60
    repressive behavior and, 153–54
    resilience and, 154–56, 160, 161–63, 252–53
    social support and, 159–60
    triggers for stress responses, 153
stress inoculation, 154
strokes, 178
sugar, 166–67, 168, 171–72, 175, 177, 179, 180, 181
sunchokes, 183
sunlight, 270–71
swans, 84
sweaty T-shirt experiment, 52–53
Sweet 'n Low, 183
swingers, 90–91
sympathetic system, 70, 189, 218, 252, 347
Synthroid, 179

tamoxifen, 135
tantric sex, 240
technology-aggravated attention deficit, 269
Tegretol, 315, 316, 318
telomeres, 158–59, 347
tend and befriend behavior, 21–22
testosterone, 6
    age and, 128–29
    attachment and, 75–77
    attraction and, 62–63
    brain development and, 19–20
    cognitive functioning and, 125–26
    cougars, 128–29
    dominance, 128
    empathy/intuition impaired by, 21
    FDA approved products for women, lack of,
        137–38, 319
    fidelity and, 86–87
    hormone replacement therapies and, 134–35
    in late perimenopause, 128–29
    libido and, 62, 131–32
    lust and, 67, 68, 69
    menstrual cycle and fluctuations in, 47–48
    motherhood and, 110
    novel experiences and, 92
    oral contraceptives and, 47–48
    oxytocin versus, and social behavior, 22
    parenting phase, and levels of in men, 76,
        86–87
    by prescription, as off-label use, 319–21
    for relief of painful intercourse, 133
    sex and, 69, 70
    supplementation, 131–32, 134–35
    tips for maintaining proper levels of, 132
tetracyclics (Remeron), 16, 308, 332
theaflavin, 181
thin-ideal body image, 256, 257
Thin Thighs in 30 Days (Stehling and Falcone),
    188
Thorazine, 316
thyme, 139
thyroid, 122–23, 130
thyroid-binding globulin, 122–23
Tibolone, 368n
toe sucking, 240
Tofranil, 308–9
tomatoes, 181
Topamax, 324
top-down control, 291, 347
    exercise and, 252
    isolation and, 160
    mindfulness and, 80, 285
    probiotics and, 184
touched out, 110–11
transcranial direct-current stimulation, 347
trans fats, 175
Trazodone, 210, 330–31
tricyclics
    for depression, 308–9, 331
    for sleep, 331
triglycerides, 175, 177

tryptophan, 41–42, 248
  in breast milk, 101–2
  cytokine break down of, in inflammatory
    mechanism, 150
  gut bacteria and, 184
  oral contraceptives and, 46
TSH test, 123
turkey, 41–42
turmeric, 139
type 1 diabetes, 172
type 2 diabetes, 172–73, 197, 205

urinary incontinence, 119
U-spot, 394n

vaginal atrophy, 132–33
valerian, 210
Valium, 210, 312, 314, 315
Vasomax, 323–24
vasopressin, 86
  monogamy and, 76–77
  paternal behavior and, 103
Vasotem, 323–24
vegetables, 174, 176, 181, 183
VENIS (very erotic, non-insertive sex), 134
verbena, 139
Viagra, 133–34, 216, 320–21
vibrators, 236–37
Vicodin, 333
Victoria, Queen, 163
Viibryd, 390n
"village" alternative, for child rearing, 107–9
vinegar, 176
Vital Aging (Wolff), 143
vitamins
  B6, 42, 46, 139
  B12, 139

C, 181
D, 139, 270–71
E, 181
  gut bacteria and, 183
Vivactil, 308–9
vulvoplasty, 264
Vyvanse, 311–12

waist-hip ratio, 258, 398n
Wallace, Sophia, 227
water, 180
weather, 272
Wedekind, Claus, 52–53
Weil, Andrew, 283
Wellbutrin, 16, 220, 221, 306–7, 342, 391n
Wellbutrin SR, 307
Wellbutrin XL, 307
Westermarck effect, 130
white fat cells, 254
whole-grain foods, 172
Wolff, Sara, 143
wrinkles, 119

Xanax, 210, 312, 314, 315, 329–30
xenoestrogens, 121, 132, 277, 347

Yasmin, 46
Yaz, 46
yeast, 184, 185–86
yoga, 80–81, 138, 190, 235
yogurt, 181, 183, 184

zaleplon (Sonata), 329
Zoloft, 4, 6, 18, 65, 302, 304, 390n
zolpidem (Ambien), 33, 209–10, 210–11, 326–28
Zyban, 220, 306, 342
Zyprexa (olanzapine), 182